Flow Experience

László Harmat • Frans Ørsted Andersen
Fredrik Ullén • Jon Wright • Gaynor Sadlo
Editors

Flow Experience

Empirical Research and Applications

Springer

Editors
László Harmat
Department of Neuroscience
Karolinska Institutet
Stockholm, Sweden

Frans Ørsted Andersen
Department of Education
University of Aarhus
Aarhus, Denmark

Fredrik Ullén
Department of Neuroscience
Karolinska Institutet
Stockholm, Sweden

Jon Wright
School of Health Sciences
University of Brighton
Eastbourne, East Sussex, UK

Gaynor Sadlo
School of Health Sciences
University of Brighton
Eastbourne, East Sussex, UK

First Faculty of Medicine
Charles University
Prague, Czech Republic

ISBN 978-3-319-28632-7 ISBN 978-3-319-28634-1 (eBook)
DOI 10.1007/978-3-319-28634-1

Library of Congress Control Number: 2016937673

Printed on acid-free paper

This Springer imprint is published by Springer Nature
The registered company is Springer International Publishing AG Switzerland

Preface

This book is the work of members of The European Flow Researchers Network (EFRN). The EFRN is the first network of its kind in the world. Together we are aiming to develop a common international understanding of the concept and measurement of flow and to stimulate empirical flow research. We believe that these aims are important, not only for academics and students but ultimately for people everywhere whose well-being could be enhanced through experiencing flow. This book represents an important step forward for the EFRN, as it shares our current knowledge regarding flow theory and research and how we are applying what we have learnt in everyday life to promote people's well-being.

The EFRN is an inclusive, dynamic group of individuals who share a passion for flow and believe that is through cooperation and partnership that we can foster scientific progress. We met for the first time in Trier in late November 2012, and since then have ensured that we meet together every year to develop formal and informal opportunities for exchange, cooperation and research. We hope that you are fascinated and inspired by what you read. If you are and would like to join us, please get in touch.

We would like to thank all of the contributors to this book, who are all colleagues within the Network, for sharing their wealth of expertise in and experience in flow research. The contributors were chosen to help demonstrate the range of empirical research and methodologies used within flow research and the different areas of our lives in which flow can occur. We think that they have done this admirably. We are greatful to Emma Louise for her assistant at the final stages of the editorial work. On behalf of the Network, we would also like to thank Springer for the opportunity to publish our work and for all of the support and guidance they have given us.

Since Csikszentmihalyi first described flow and its phenomonology in the mid-1960s, the construct has developed significantly; however, much of the work in the field has been focused on theoretical and philosophical issues. In this volume, we have aimed to focus upon empirical work within flow research. The book is one step towards relating flow research to the main scientific traditions in psychology and psychophysiology, integrating it into the mainstream work of these fields.

In Part I, Chap. 1 provides an overview of flow research that clarifies what is now understood by optimal experience. A co-constructionist perspective of human experience as an interaction between the biological and cultural environment is presented. The chapter introduces us to the processes of psychological selection, emphasizing the role of flow experiences and the meaning given to activities in developing individuals' skills and competencies. Possible individual and environmental explanations for the differences between people in perceiving opportunities for attaining optimal experiences are discussed including: health conditions, social structure and cultural constraints; work and leisure; and family and school environments. The role of both talent and deliberate effort in creating opportunities for optimal experience is explored. The rationale for long-term research that could shed light on the evolutionary significance and role of flow within the dynamics between the individual and the environment is explained.

In Part II, authors discussed flow in relation to arts and sports performances. Chapter 2 addresses a study aimed at investigating self-regulated practice behaviours and flow dispositions in expert musicians. Associations between self-regulated practice behaviours and flow dispositions were explored. Results showed that flow was predominantly a function of self-regulated behaviours. The chapter ends with implications of the findings for musicians, teachers and researchers. Chapter 3 describes and discusses the experience of flow when professional artists create and learn. The author points out that artistic creation happens in a state of deep concentration, and self-forgetting and flow seem to have a specific purpose within artistic processes: triggering, facilitating and guiding the *flow* of creation.

Sport offers rich opportunities to experience flow by posing both mental and physical challenges. Studies specifically investigating flow in sport were first published in 1992. Chapter 4 reviews the methods commonly used to study flow in sport (i.e., interviews, questionnaires and the experience sampling method) and key research themes (i.e., the experience, occurrence, controllability and correlates of flow in sport). The following chapter (Chap. 5) summarises three studies that explored treadmill running in a laboratory context and measured flow-states via self-report data. The authors highlight the work of Dietrich (2003) who postulates within the frame of Transient Hypofrontality Theory (THT) that flow-states are a result of a down-regulated prefrontal cortex. The results, reported in this chapter, provide indirect evidence for the hypothesis that prolonged exercise might result in a state of transient hypofrontality.

The focus of Part III is the association between flow and achievement. Chapter 6 discusses the complex question of how flow relates to creativity. The empirical literature on creativity and flow is summarised and discussed critically in relation to two influential theoretical frameworks: dual-process theories of creativity and the hypofrontality model of flow. The chapter identifies lacunae in our current understanding and ends with several specific suggestions for future empirical work. A concept that is closely related to creativity is intuition. Chapter 7 continues the discussion of themes introduced in Chap. 6, with an analysis of possible relationships between intuition and flow from a dual-process perspective. A conclusion of the chapter is that flow and intuition are related phenomena: flow could be seen as intuitive action; intuition could be construed as cognition in flow. Finally, Chap. 8 discusses novel empirical work on flow and work engagement, a variable of obvious importance for achievement at work. The authors investigate whether the effects of perceived autonomy support are moderated by flow at work. In line with their hypotheses, the authors demonstrate that for individuals with higher flow at work, the relationships between autonomy, support and work engagement – as well as the satisfaction of certain intrinsic psychological needs – are weaker. Individuals with more flow at work are thus likely to show higher work engagement regardless of autonomy support.

In Part IV, we discuss flow in an educational context. Chapter 9 introduces a new tool for educators: a scale for measuring flow in education, based on a longitudinal study of flow experienced by students. The study underlines the importance and relevance of measuring flow in learning. *The EduFlow model: A Contribution Toward the Study of Optimal Learning Environments*. Chapter 10 presents an ESM study of flow during STEM (science, technology, engineering and math) education in lower secondary school, pointing to ways of solving the STEM crisis (i.e., too few students are interested in STEM subjects). The study contributes with new knowledge about factors necessary for increasing student motivation, engagement, learning and flow during STEM education. Chapter 11 presents studies that explore the connection between positive youth development, leisure and flow experience. Their results shed light on how a psycho-social-ecological approach can enhance positive youth development.

In Part V, we focus on investigating flow experience in everyday life. In order to explore this phenomenon, Chap. 12 begins by outlining a definition of consciousness before proceeding to explore subjective experience and the role of perceived challenges and skills in promoting growth in our ability to perform complex activities and improve our well-being. The Experience Sampling Method is presented as a method of collecting everyday experiences in real-time. The Experience Fluctuation Model is then introduced, which enables researchers to explore subjective perceptions of challenges and skills through analysis of real-time data. The empirical findings that support the model are discussed, providing insights into human experience in a variety of contexts and activities. Future research that could advance our knowledge of the phenomenology of conscious experience is suggested including how individuals move from one experience to another. In the following chapter (Chap. 13), reversal theory is introduced that provides a theoretical explanation for how people change between metamotivational states. It is argued that reversal theory and flow theory are compatible theories that together might enhance our understanding of optimal experiences in everyday life. An argument for the importance of phenomenology in the exploration of flow is presented; phenomenology itself is defined and the method considered. A reversal theory perspective of flow experiences in everyday life is given, which suggests that there are eight motivational states, each of which has a core feeling that a person will seek to optimise. The ways in which people may move between states are explained, including the importance protective frames and by reversals between metamotivational states. A justification is given for including reversal theory in future flow research.

In Part VI, we collected works from the field of social psychology. Chapter 14 presents a social psychological study of the connections between flow and the broader socio-cultural environment, thus pointing to the important role of flow experience, not just as an individual growth element but also as a resource for generating social change. Chapter 15 presents studies of team flow during work. The author introduces important new knowledge of components of team flow and point to ways of enhancing it. Chapter 16 presents studies of flow in human-technology interaction and introduces a new model of perfect interaction and knowledge of a new peculiar type of social flow that could be attained by creative groups.

In Part VII, we introduce research about flow and individual differences. A large amount of flow literature demonstrates that situational variables – e.g. environmental opportunities to engage in tasks, which are neither too challenging nor too simple – are important for flow. However, how much flow a person experiences also depends on certain individual variables. This is potentially of both theoretical and practical interest, since flow is related to many positive and valued outcomes. Chapter 17 summarises data from a large Swedish twin cohort, where associations between flow proneness and five basic modalities of individual differences were investigated, i.e. personality, cognitive abilities, motivation, emotional competence and performance on chronometric tasks. In line with flow theory and earlier literature, it was found that flow proneness is substantially related to personality, intrinsic motivation and emotional competence, but not to cognitive abilities or chronometric task performance. The possible importance of these findings for associations between flow, well-being and health is discussed. Chapter 18 focuses on how flow relates to one important outcome, namely personal identity strength, as conceptualised in eudaimonistic identity theory. The authors hypothesise that engaging in flow promoting activities can facilitate personal growth and self definition and find empirical support for this in a multinational investigation. Chapter 19, finally, takes a clinical perspective and discusses possible applications of flow in psychotherapy and mental health rehabilitation. The authors present results suggesting that finding flow may be an important component of psychotherapeutic intervention, by fostering positive change both inside and outside the therapeutic process, and by promoting the clients' integration and active involvement in society.

In last part (Part VIII) of this volume, authors discuss the physiological correlates of flow experience. In Chap. 20, the authors present new psychological and physiological research paradigms to assess and investigate the flow experience. They compare flow theory and research with concepts of challenge and threat as well as with mental effort. They go on to discuss applications for flow research and provide a critical review of existing studies that have aimed to investigate the psychological and physiological mechanisms of flow experience. Chapter 21 provides a condensed summary of findings obtained in research on the state of flow based on experimental paradigms and introduces studies that provide evidence documenting the specific nature of the state of flow – specifically regarding experiential and physiological processes. Chapter 22 proposes a neurobiological mechanism underlying reduced self-awareness during flow. From the perspective of occupational science, it focuses on capturing the last decade of brain imaging studies that analyze neural systems for self-awareness, that show lower levels of activity during externally oriented task performance.

We hope that our anthology provides a thought-provoking overview of current flow research and that the suggestions for new directions will inspire researchers and practitioners within the field of psychology to continue to conduct experimental flow research that will lead to a better understanding of the psychological and physiological mechanisms underlying this fascinating and universally human experience.

Stockholm, Sweden László Harmat
Aarhus, Denmark Frans Ørsted Andersen
Stockholm, Sweden Fredrik Ullén
Eastbourne, East Sussex, UK Jon Wright
Eastbourne, East Sussex, UK Gaynor Sadlo

Contents

About the Editors

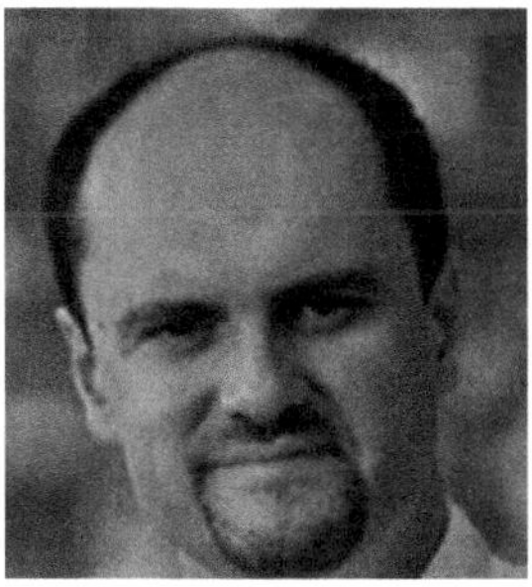

László Harmat, Ph.D. László Harmat was a postdoctoral research fellow at the Department of Neuroscience, Karolinska Institute in Fredrik Ulléns' group from 2011 to 2015. He is currently a researcher at the Department of Psychology, Uppsala University, Sweden. He completed his PhD in 2010 at Semmelweis University, Institute of Behavioral Sciences, Budapest, Hungary, and he was a lecturer in psychology at the same institution for several years. His main research interest involves exploring the physiological correlates of the flow experience and the therapeutic effects of music. He also investigates the neurophysiological underpinnings of expertise and skill learning. He is a graduated music teacher and has been leading a chamber choir in Stockholm, Sweden, since 2012.

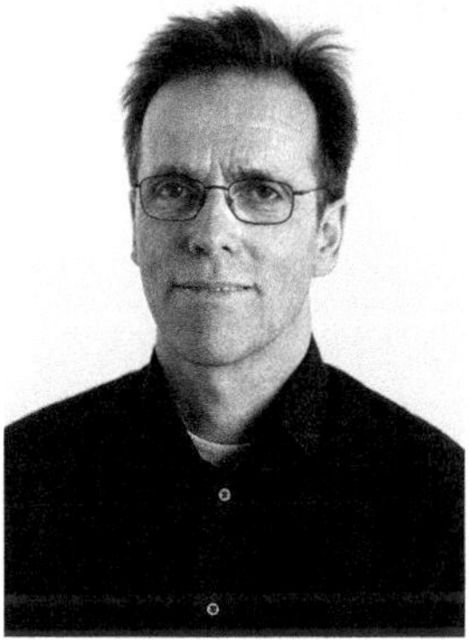

Frans Ørsted Andersen has been Associate Professor at the Department of Education, Aarhus University, Denmark, since 2010. He is involved in school research at many levels and has conducted research within areas like motivation, engagement, cooperation, attention, learning and attention at both primary and secondary school levels, using flow as a concept and a theory to understand optimal learning environments. Teaching and learning in the STEM area (Science Technology Engineering and Math) is another area researched by Frans Ørsted Andersen. He also works with comparative Nordic educational research and has looked especially at the qualities of Finnish education. He has published several books and articles on flow, mainly in Danish and Norwegian, the latest book title being *Flow i hverdagen. Navigation mellem kaos, stress og kedsomhed* [Flow in everyday life. Navigation between chaos, stress and boredom] (2013).

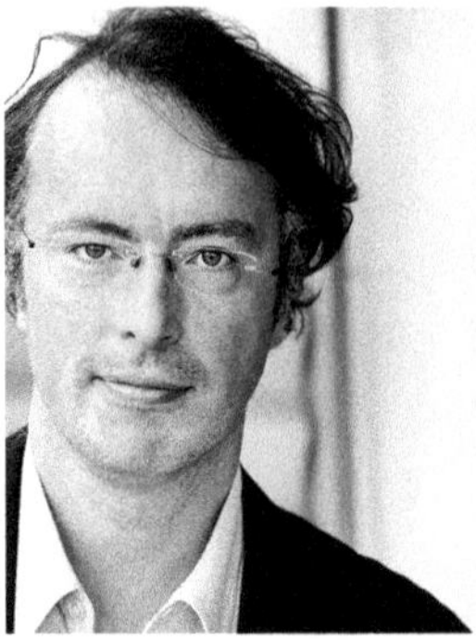

Fredrik Ullén is Professor of Cognitive Neuroscience at the Department of Neuroscience, Karolinska Institutet, since 2010. An overall aim of his research is to analyse the neuropsychology of expert performance, i.e. the various brain mechanisms that allow us to perform at a very high level within a specific domain, after many years of training. One specific research interest is the flow experience, its underlying mechanisms and its importance for motivation and creativity in expertise. The research of Ullén is mainly focused on musicians as a model group. Methodologically, his team combines neuroimaging and behaviour genetic analyses with experimental psychology and physiology. In addition to his career as a scientist, Professor Ullén is active as a professional pianist and is represented as a soloist on around 20 CD records. He is a lifetime fellow of the Swedish Royal Academy of Music since 2007.

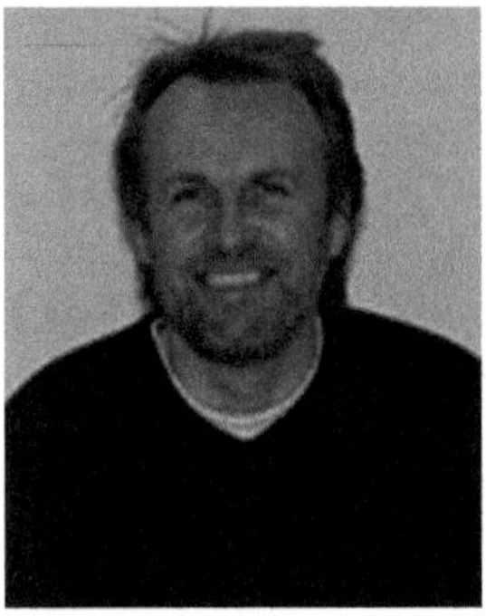

Jon Wright, Ph.D. Jon Wright is Principal Lecturer in the School of Health Sciences at the University of Brighton. He completed his PhD in 2008 exploring the process of optimal experiences utilising a phenomenological approach. Within his research Jon provides an occupational science perspective, a science that underpins his professional background as an occupational therapist. His research has integrated Reversal Theory to help our conceptualisation of flow. Jon's research continues to explore the flow concept, and with a team of Network Partners he is aiming to establish a shared conceptualisation of flow, developing guidelines regarding the utility of different measurements and indicators of flow.

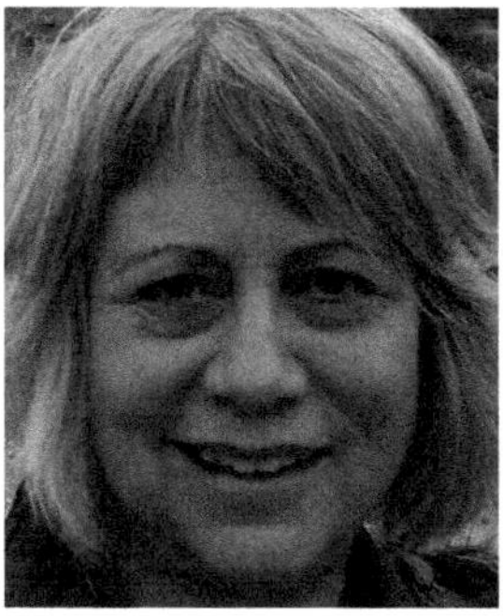

Gaynor Sadlo, Ph.D., PgDTCDHE DipOccThy FCOT NTF Gaynor Sadlo recently retired as Professor of Occupational Science at the University of Brighton, England, following 47 years in occupational therapy practice, teaching and research. She has been interested in flow concepts for about 25 years, promoting undergraduate and postgraduate flow research (with colleague Dr Jon Wright) as crucial to the understanding of the therapeutic properties of 'occupation'; in particular, reduced self-awareness is seen as a crucial aspect of the beneficial effects of deep engagement. Flow within pedagogy is another major interest, and her pioneering research and practice in problem-based learning as a philosophy of optimal educational experience gained the award of National Teaching Fellow in 2007. She is a Fellow of the College of Occupational Therapists. She is currently also a visiting professor at the First Faculty of Medicine, Charles University, Prague, Czech Republic.

The original version of this book was revised. An erratum to this book can be found at http://dx.doi.org/10.1007/978-3-319-28634-1_23

Part I
Flow Experience: General Introduction

Chapter 1
Flow and Psychological Selection

Antonella Delle Fave and Marta Bassi

Abstract Flow or optimal experience is generally defined as a complex and positive state characterized by deep involvement and absorption, supporting personal growth, well-being and optimal functioning in daily life. Since its inception in the 1970s, great effort has been devoted to understand its phenomenological characteristics, antecedents and consequences, as well as its biological, cultural and psychological aspects. This chapter will provide an overview of the related findings, highlighting both the shared understanding of this experience and critical issues deserving further investigation. A specific interpretive framework will be adopted, that takes into account the active role played by individuals in shaping their life trajectories and personal development, though acknowledging the influences and constraints derived from the biological and cultural inheritance and environment. This process of psychological selection is based on personal meanings, goals and quality of subjective experience. Within this conceptual framework, flow contributes to the construction of personal identity, as well as to the co-construction of the individual's sociocultural context, through its influence on the long-term selection and replication of specific activities and information.

1.1 Introduction

The increasingly tangled ties that connect research domains and disciplines exploring human features and behavior represent one of the major problems science is facing today. Psychology is especially affected by this problem, in that it is positioned at the crossroads between biological and social sciences. Human mental processes and behaviors emerge from a multiplicity of events and influences coming from both biology and culture. It is therefore very difficult to investigate them as isolated

A. Delle Fave (✉)
Department of Pathophysiology and Transplantation, University of Milano, Milan, Italy
e-mail: antonella.dellefave@unimi.it

M. Bassi
Department of Biomedical and Clinical Sciences "Luigi Sacco", University of Milan, Milan, Italy
e-mail: marta.bassi@unimi.it

L. Harmat et al. (eds.), *Flow Experience*, DOI 10.1007/978-3-319-28634-1_1

phenomena, without taking into account the two broad inheritance systems to which they are inextricably related (Laland et al. 2000; Richerson and Boyd 2005).

The study of human experience is not exempt from this problem. Experience (*see* Chap. 12 *by Bassi and Delle Fave in this volume*) phenomenologically arises from the interaction of the individual with external or internal stimuli. These stimuli contribute to shaping the experience through both the information contents they carry at the cognitive level, and their qualitative impact at the emotional and motivational levels.

The positioning of individual behavior and experience in the point of intersection of the biological and cultural realms was acknowledged and formalized in the second half of last century by two different perspectives. Bio-cultural theories (Durham 1982; Richerson and Boyd 1978; Ruyle 1973) stressed the co-existence of two trans-generational inheritance systems – the biological and the cultural ones – that shaped human behavior and experience (Massimini and Delle Fave 2000). The bio-psycho-social model (Engel 1977) was developed in the domain of medicine with the aim of broadening the western biomedical approach to disease, prominently focused on the biological aspects of health conditions, by centering it on the patient as a person, with a cultural background and a subjective experience of health, disease, and quality of life (Levin and Browner 2005).

Besides their different disciplinary background and theoretical underpinnings, these two perspectives share a common view: Two sets of information influence human behavior. In particular, the capacity for culture provided humans with an extremely adaptive piece of equipment, allowing them to counterbalance biological constraints and weaknesses. Thanks to the ability to plan, formulate abstract theories, build mental representations of reality, and create basic survival artifacts, humans could survive in every kind of ecological niche (Delle Fave et al. 2011). The information derived by these two evolutionary systems is embodied in the subjective experience people associate to life events and daily activities.

However, by virtue of specific features and properties evolved by humans based on these two inheritance systems, the individual is not just a repository of biological and cultural information, and human experience does not consist in mere and passive elaboration of stimuli provided by the environment. Recent acquisitions in biology have highlighted that already very simple organisms with no centralized brain are able to perform active information processing and to produce goal-oriented behavior (e.g. the search for food in their natural environment) in order to restore homeostasis, defined as an attractor state towards which the system tends to proceed (Ginsburg and Jablonka 2010). With the subsequent emergence of more complex organisms, endowed with a central nervous system and a progressively higher potential for information storage and processing, the behavior of living systems was increasingly guided by associative learning, exemplified by classical and operant conditioning, that implied the ability to select among different possible behaviors according to the contingent situation, based on the systematic memorization of previous experiences and in view of specific adaptive goals (Carillo et al. 1997).

The early emergence in the history of animal evolution of individual agency and end-directed behaviors based on predictions derived from the memory of previous experience was already described by William James (1890, volume I). A further step towards individual autonomy and agentic role was made possible by the specific human capacity for culture, that includes language development, artifacts' building and the production of symbolic information embedded in social customs, norms and values (Jablonka and Lamb 2014).

The crucial role of the individual as an active character in the interaction with the biological and cultural information has become an incontrovertible reality in light of the recent discoveries in the domain of epigenetics. The previously denied assumption, originally formulated by Lamarck, that genetic changes could be derived from behaviors and habits developed from the organism's active and adaptive interaction with the environment, was proved in prokaryotes and eukaryotes (Lachmann and Jablonka 1996). Some of the molecular and biochemical mechanisms underlying this process were clarified for mammalians, and their influence on behavior and psychological functioning of humans were recently evidenced (Zhang and Meaney 2010).

Epigenetic processes imply that through the interaction with the environment individuals may acquire features and assets that can become stable components of the organism's structure, and can be at least partially transmissible to the next generation. From this perspective, epigenetic mechanisms substantially enhance the plasticity and flexibility of individual behavior and functioning (Masterpasqua 2009).

These findings led scientists to represent the interaction between organisms and their environment in terms of a co-construction process; the role of individuals in this interactive process becomes progressively more relevant and active with the increase in species' complexity level. From this perspective, Lamarckian-like processes of inheritance are considered as "emergent phenomena" that are increasingly evident in more evolved species, due to the complex molecular mechanisms that allow for the integration of new material into the genome (Koonin and Wolf 2009). The individual experience and behavior represent the core elements of this co-construction process, and they substantially contribute to shaping both the individual development trajectory and the environmental features. This is especially true of the human species, whose impact on the ecosystem has been massive and to a certain extent even destructive (Diamond 2005; Mesoudi et al. 2006).

This view is also consistent with the conceptualization of living beings as Complex Adaptive Systems (CAS, Couture 2007; Holland 1998). CAS represent examples of dissipative structures (Nicolis and Prigogine 1989), in that the preservation and increase of their complexity require a ceaseless consumption of energy, partly transformed into activities and ordered structures, and partly dissipated due to collateral phenomena. A CAS is an integrated collection of highly differentiated components that dynamically and adaptively interact among each other and with the environment (Fromm 2004). Each of these specialized components contributes to the accomplishment of specific system functions, and it is connected with all the other components in a co-ordinated pattern that allows for the adaptive interaction of the system with the environment (Tononi and Edelman 1998). The higher the system adaptability, the higher is its resilience in presence of perturbations.

Miller (1970) summarized the features of complex systems by highlighting their statistical improbability and predictability: these systems derive from a teleonomic developmental process (Monod 1971), defined as the intrinsic project that shapes their structures, functions, and stable features, as well as their behavioral repertoire in the interaction with the environment. However, without a steady supply of energy from the environment, any complex system tends towards homogeneity, loss of specialization, and entropy, that in living entities can be assimilated to decay and death.

From a co-constructionist and teleonomic perspective, the process of individual development under physiological and adaptive conditions consists in a progressive increase of the system's complexity, by virtue of the ceaseless exchange of information with the environment that leads to more or less stable modifications at both the individual and environmental levels.

1.2 Psychological Selection

Within the evolutionary and co-constructionist perspective outlined in the previous section, the structure of individual behavior and experience throughout the life span emerges from the interaction with the biological and cultural environment. This interaction leads to a ceaseless and bidirectional exchange of information that promotes transformation at both the individual and the environmental levels (Pribram 1996). As concerns individuals, the acquisition of new information is transformed into stable neural connections at the biological level; and into personal skills, beliefs, meanings and purposes at the psychological level. However, the system configuration undergoes continuous changes, by virtue of the progressive integration of new information (Delle Fave 2007).

From the lifelong perspective, the moment-by-moment interaction of the individual with the environment results in the process of daily psychological selection (Csikszentmihalyi and Massimini 1985). This process unfolds from the selective use of attention, as a limited resource that compels individuals to focus on a restricted number of environmental or internal stimuli per time unit (Lavie 2005). Therefore, at each moment the individual effectively perceives only a small part of the available information, subsequently processing and organizing it for future use and transmission. In the long term, this constraint (or asset) leads to a selection trend that affects the biological, social/cultural and psychological features of the person (Delle Fave et al. 2011). To exemplify, at the biological level an individual can invest time and energy in prevention programs and fitness exercises, or on the opposite disregard physical health. At the social/cultural level, a person may decide to become a lawyer, a music teacher or a lab technician; to actively support a political party or union; to devote time to volunteering activities. In one word, each individual throughout his/her life differentially reproduces and transmit a subset of the information available in the environment, through the selective investment of limited attention resources on activities, political ideologies, moral and religious beliefs.

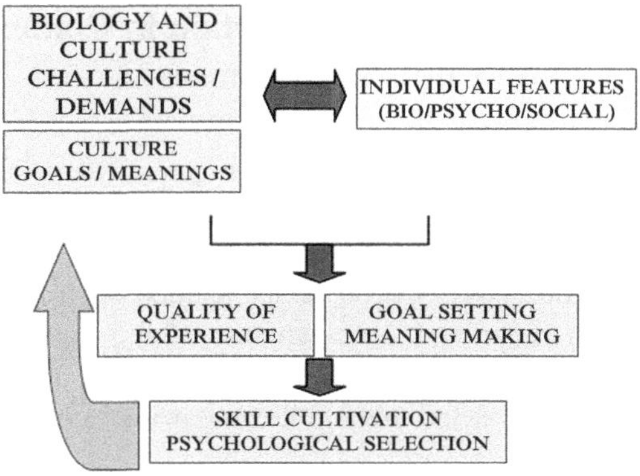

Fig. 1.1 Individual and bio-cultural environment: a dynamic interaction

Although psychological selection can be partially controlled and constrained by cultural features and rules (for example, social stratification based on social status or gender may restrict individual's access to specific information and domains of resource investment), in most societies each person is provided with a relatively wide range of behavioral and developmental alternatives. Overall, it is possible to affirm that individuals actively interact with the bio-cultural milieu, co-constructing it through their differential acquisition, elaboration and replication of environmental information (Delle Fave and Bassi 2014).

Several cross-cultural studies (summarized in Delle Fave et al. 2011) showed that two core elements play a key role in guiding psychological selection. The first one is the association of flow with at least some of activities available to the individual in the daily environment (Massimini et al. 1988). The second component is the perception of long-term meanings and purposes in daily opportunities for action (Delle Fave 2009). Meaning-making represents the way in which people organize their own experience in time around their values and beliefs through goal setting, definition of priorities and action strategies. Through the attribution of meaning to specific life activities and domains, individuals pursue goals deemed relevant, as well as consistent with social values and others' needs (Hicks and King 2009; Steger et al. 2008). Meaning-making is a dynamic process by definition, since individual values and priorities are not necessarily fixed entities: They are related to specific developmental tasks and stages, to the exposure and acquisition of new information, to the organization criteria individuals adopt to integrate the new information into their previous *Weltanschauung* (Delle Fave et al. 2013).

Thus, activities that are perceived as opportunities for engagement and flow, as well as aligned with relevant and meaningful goals, are more likely to be preferentially replicated and cultivated in the long term. Their selective cultivation provides the individual with increasingly complex competences and skills, fostering personal growth and development (Massimini and Delle Fave 2000). The dynamic interplay and ceaseless exchange of information between individuals and environment is summarized in Fig. 1.1.

1.3 Psychological Selection in Context: Biological and Cultural Influences

People differ in their tendency to perceive opportunities for optimal experiences in daily activities. Some people feel challenged by things that other people do not simply take into account as opportunities for action. This can be related to several individual and environmental factors, such as psychological traits and features, health conditions, characteristics of the ecosystem, social and cultural rules and habits, and the dynamic interplay among them. Some of these aspects will be explored in detail in the following paragraphs.

1.3.1 Health Conditions

Health conditions influence the opportunities for and the contents of optimal experiences, both in daily life and in the long term. Cross-cultural studies conducted among people with disabilities and chronic diseases have detected the impact of physical constraints on the access to activities and socialization contexts. After the onset of a chronic disease or disablement, individuals may be forced to identify new patterns of functioning in daily life, new goals and meanings, new life priorities. In some cases they have to dismiss previously gratifying activities and interests, and to look for different opportunities for optimal experiences, more suited to their actual capabilities and resources.

However, the pattern of daily experience fluctuation (*as described in* Chap. 12. *by Delle Fave and Bassi in this volume*) and the features and frequency of optimal experience reported by the participants in these studies are not influenced by physical conditions per se. On the contrary, research studies have emphasized the importance of optimal experience in supporting individual's physical and social functioning especially in conditions of chronic disease and disability. Across different cultural contexts, people with congenital disabilities such as blindness, ostheogenesis imperfecta or cerebral palsy reported optimal experiences and the pursuit of complex long-term goals that enabled them to effectively socialize and participate in active life (Cortinovis et al. 2011; Delle Fave 2010; Delle Fave and Massimini 2004).

As concerns diseases and disabilities acquired during adult life, a peculiar process was identified: the *transformation of optimal experience* (Delle Fave et al. 2011). Physical impairments can make activities previously associated with optimal experiences unavailable to the individual, who is thus forced to find other sources of intrinsic motivation, and engagement. Several studies showed that most persons with disabilities successfully manage to identify new opportunities for optimal experience, sometimes in areas very different from their previous interests (Delle Fave and Massimini 2005). Behavioral flexibility emerges as a crucial feature for adaptation to the environment, enabling the individual to pursue developmental goals despite biological constraints. This flexibility becomes evident soon after the disease onset. A recent study conducted with experience sampling method among people hospitalized in a rehabilitation unit after orthopaedic surgery or stroke highlighted that participants prominently associated rehabilitation activities with optimal experience, clearly distinguishing it from personal care and leisure – the most frequent daily activities – in which they reported low challenging experiences of apathy and boredom instead (Sartori et al. 2014). This was true of both patients with severe impairment, and thus in a condition of complete dependence, and patients who were more autonomous. These findings suggest that the association of flow with rehabilitation tasks can help promote patients' awareness of their active role in recovery and in the cultivation of residual abilities, independent of their level of autonomy. It can also facilitate engagement in autonomous practice at home, where individuals are responsible for their own recovery and development of vicarious abilities, thus influencing well-being in the long run through the pursuit of health and autonomy-related goals.

These findings also challenge the assumptions of adaptation theory (Brickman and Campbell 1971), which states that within few weeks after a trauma individuals tend to psychologically adapt to the new condition: they report an increase in positive emotions and their average mood returns to the levels reported before trauma. Research findings, on the contrary, highlighted that individuals can actively search for new interests, meanings and life goals after the onset of a chronic disease, even identifying benefits in the illness condition (Sodergren and Hyland 2000; Tennen and Affleck 2002). Optimal experience plays a crucial role in this process, supporting resource investment, skill development, and personal growth (Bassi et al. 2014a; Delle Fave et al. 2015).

In line with this empirical evidence, an increasing amount of studies conducted within the perspective of positive psychology showed that the subjective perception of functioning in daily activities and situations affects the quality of life of people with chronic and degenerative disease besides and beyond physical conditions. These studies (synthetically summarized in Delle Fave 2013) highlight the pivotal role of psychological resources, strengths and potentials in promoting individuals' effective coping and adjustment to disease, and in contributing to well-being and flourishing.

These issues were addressed also within the domain of mental health. Mental disorders negatively impact on individual agency and perceived resourcefulness, thus undermining the evaluation and exploitation of opportunities for flow in daily life. Attention to psychological resources and promotion of positive experiences such as flow represent useful assets for psychotherapists, as reported in several studies (Bassi et al. 2012; Delle Fave and Massimini 1992; Lanfranchi et al. 2011) and by Riva, Bassi and Freire (*see* Chap. 19 *in this volume*).

1.3.2 Cultural and Social Features

Psychological selection seems to be a universally shared mechanism for the reproduction of environmental information, as well as for the creation of new information that can be shared with other individuals and ultimately integrated in the cultural pool. Similarly, human behavior arises from motivations, emotions, and cognitive functions such as memory, learning strategies and abstract reasoning which are common psychic features of human beings. Every member of our species can accurately describe his/her feelings, thoughts, quality of experience in coping with daily activities and interactions. Similarly, every human being, as a complex adaptive system with an intrinsic tendency towards higher levels of complexity, pursues the acquisition of progressively increasing knowledge, competences and social integration across the life span.

This view, although conceptualized in different ways, is shared by non-western philosophical and cultural traditions (Morandi and Delle Fave 2013). Nevertheless, the meaning of complexity can astonishingly differ among cultural contexts. In western societies it is prominently related to the concept of self-actualization; it means to fulfil one's own desires, at the same time meeting culturally determined ethical and social expectations. However in other contexts, such as within Hinduism and Buddhism, it means attaining supreme detachment from desires and earthly goals.

Similarly, the importance attributed to personal feelings and expectations, individual autonomy and freedom of choice depends upon the cultural system in which people are raised and live; it is a product of the hierarchy of values that individuals develop during their life, according to ideal models acquired through the learning process. In particular, the emphasis on self-actualization and personal achievements specifically characterizes western cultures, in comparison with other societies. Western culture emphasizes personal initiative and resources in dealing with the environment, and the imperative of asserting one's own power and freedom in interpersonal relationships. In contrast, non-western collectivistic societies foster the adoption of indirect and collective control strategies, which entail the sharing of responsibility among individuals participating in the same task, and the preservation of harmony even in case of failure or negative outcomes (Delle Fave 2014). The so-called harmony control (Morling and Fiske 1999) leads individuals to recognize the agency residing in contextual, social, or spiritual forces rather than in their own person. By adopting this control strategy individuals attempt to merge with these forces instead of opposing them, thus accepting their own roles and their environment, without direct attempt to modify or change them.

The focus on the individual as the central unit of society led, for example, to the strong personalization of the artistic and scientific works in European history. Information about the identity and life history of the authors of philosophical theories, frescoes, poems and mathematical models is systematically documented and continuously implemented by new details discovered in archives. On the contrary, in several Asian societies the names of painters, sculptors, architects and scientists have never been recorded, although these individuals substantially contributed to the enrichment of human cultural heritage with their masterpieces and discoveries. The distinction between individualistic and collectivistic societies (Hofstede 1980; Hofstede et al. 2010) and between independent and interdependent self construals (Markus and Kitayama 1991) provide a solid framework in support of this evidence.

The relevance attached to the role of the individual by the cultural norms and values dominating in a society has deep consequences on psychological selection as well, promoting the development of specific patterns of individual resource investment, goal setting and pursuit, meaning attribution and identification of opportunities for flow. In particular, the social structure and cultural constraints contribute to defining the range and variety of potential flow activities available to the person in the different life domains. The daily exposure of individuals to more or less challenging and complex environments influences the quality of experience associated with daily activities.

In the work domain, the enrolment in repetitive, low-challenge and merely executive tasks strongly limits the availability of occasions for optimal experiences (Delle Fave and Bassi 2014). In these conditions, optimal experiences can and must be found outside the work context, in leisure, family or social relations. Nevertheless, finding flow at work is particularly relevant from the perspective of psychological selection, since work activities occupy a conspicuous amount of daily time and life years; the possibility to identify in one's own job both an opportunity for flow and a source of goals and meaning represents a good prerequisite for global well-being promotion.

In modernized contexts, research recurrently highlighted some peculiar features of the flow experience associated with work activities, such as below average scores of affect and intrinsic reward, however counterbalanced by the perception of the short- and long-term relevance of the activity. This experiential profile was reported by a variety of professionals, prominently including office employees and factory workers. This phenomenon – not surprising, given the compulsory nature of work – was labeled the work paradox (Csikszentmihalyi and Lefevre 1989).

More recent studies conducted among teachers and physicians, however, showed a different picture, indicating the coexistence of autonomous and extrinsic regulation in the flow experience at work, and the need to more carefully consider this issue taking into account the typology of job under examination (Bassi and Delle Fave 2012a; Delle Fave and Massimini 2003). Results contradicting the flow paradox also emerged from a large study involving over 700 participants belonging to different western and non-western cultures (Delle Fave and Bassi 2016). The comparison of the experiential features of flow during traditional and modern job tasks highlighted that the former were characterized by higher values of affect (excitement, enjoyment, and relaxation), and a more autonomous pattern of behavioral regulation (wish to do the activity and effortless concentration). Traditional activities differ according to local ecosystem, customs and history, but they all share features of complexity and challenge that call into play the worker's dexterity, at the same time leading to tangible outcomes that represent either direct means of subsistence for the workers and their families, or useful and often long-lasting artifacts that convey a cultural meaning. In modern jobs, the standardization of behavior and of its products inevitably leads to restrictions in individual initiative and creativity, basic prerequisites for flow onset.

As concerns free time, it can provide occasions for pleasant relaxation and enjoyment through the performance of simple tasks; it can generate experiences of apathy due to the lack of perceived challenges, leading the individual to search for thrill in dangerous or antisocial activities. It can offer flow opportunities in challenging activities that are however not meaningful in the long-term perspective of personal development. Finally, it can be used to practice so-called serious leisure activities (Stebbins 2007), that individuals can cultivate throughout their life as tools to expand their knowledge, increase their competences, and broaden their circle of relationships (Delle Fave and Bassi 2003). An exemplary case is represented by engagement in volunteering activities (Sartori and Delle Fave 2014).

The typology and variety of leisure activities offered to individuals partially depends on the cultural context and on the pattern of modernization vs. adherence to traditional lifestyle that characterizes a community. For example, in a study conducted among Rom gypsies living in the outskirts of an Italian city (Delle Fave et al. 2003a), the most frequent flow occasions reported by participants during free time were traditional Rom activities such as playing music, singing, dancing, and playing cards. They were cited as opportunities for flow across generations, even though younger participants could easily access modern leisure opportunities in the nearby town. In contrast, a generational gap was detected among the members of an extended family living in an Alpine valley in Northern Italy, who had been exposed to deep changes related to modernization and urbanization (Delle Fave and Massimini 1988). Elderly and middle aged participants primarily quoted traditional outdoor recreation, such as walking in nature, alpine skiing, dancing. By contrast, younger participants reported watching TV, ice-skating, reading, riding the bike, going to the disco. Some individuals – predominantly belonging to the middle generation – showed the adoption of an integration strategy, finding flow in both traditional and modernized occupations, such as playing the accordion and riding a motorbike (Delle Fave et al. 2011).

The influence of the cultural context in promoting or hindering access to optimal experiences has been also studied among immigrants. In particular, the adoption of the acculturation pattern of integration versus marginalization (Matsunaga et al. 2010; Tadmor et al. 2009), substantially impacts on opportunities for flow, as highlighted in a study with four groups of foreign citizens living in Italy (Delle Fave and Bassi 2009). In particular, irregular immigrant status, shorter length of residence in the host country and lower educational levels negatively affected individual chances to access complex and meaningful opportunities for flow. These participants relied on unstructured leisure tasks to find positive though low-challenge experiences, in the face of the hardship and stress reported in the other contexts of daily life. In contrast, participants showing a more functional acculturation patterns reported flow in a larger variety of daily activities. It is however worth noticing that in many cases the relevance of these tasks was not directly related to their intrinsic complexity, but to their connection with the person's long-term goals (for example, family reunion or financial support of children's education; Delle Fave et al. 2011).

Similarly, data gathered among people with physical disabilities highlighted that the environmental chances of social integration offered to them are often not matched with their own potentials, skills and resources (Cortinovis et al. 2011). While there is a growing effort to remove architectural barriers and to guarantee the accessibility of private and public places to all citizens, overcoming limitations related to sensory or mobility impairments, less visible communication barriers are still present, including opportunities for jobs not suited to the person's education level, or social isolation, that can undermine both the quality of subjective experience and the social integration process of these people (Delle Fave and Massimini 2005).

Finally, especially in the early developmental stages the proximal environments of family and school have a strong influence on psychological selection and on the discovery and cultivation of optimal activities. The pattern of family interactions can facilitate or hamper the natural tendency of children to selectively engage in and replicate intrinsically rewarding activities. Children may derive positive examples and support in effectively face daily challenges from parents who are committed to self-determined goals (Rathunde 2001; Ryan and Deci 2000) and who perceive high levels of parental self-efficacy (Steca et al. 2011). A notion-centered school environment can lead children to the development of a passive and compulsory learning strategy; alternatively, a learning environment enabling students to find meaningful relations between study contents and personal experience and goals can help them discover the rewarding features of knowledge, and the potential of learning tasks as opportunities for optimal experience (Bassi and Delle Fave 2012b; Shernoff and Csikszentmihalyi 2009; Shernoff et al. 2003).

1.3.3 Psychological Characteristics

Specific talents and innate predispositions may influence the orientations of psychological selection and the perceived opportunities for optimal experience. Studies with talented teenagers (Csikszentmihalyi et al. 1993) have highlighted the relationship between talents in specific domains, such as music or mathematics, and the selective engagement in these domains as opportunities for optimal experiences and skill cultivation.

Talent can drive people, especially during childhood and adolescence, towards the spontaneous discovery of flow opportunities, as often happens with the practice of sports and arts. In these domains, activities originally practiced because of intrinsic enjoyment and reward for the attainment of positive results can become so meaningful and pervasive that they can turn into regular hobbies or occupations. In sports, this is the case of professional athletes, or amateurs who engage in risky sports requiring constant training (Delle Fave et al. 2003b; Jackson and Csikszentmihalyi 1999). In the artistic realm, music represents *par excellence* a domain that can provide remarkable opportunities for flow to talented amateurs and professionals, thanks to the virtually endless possibilities to enhance complexity and to develop innovations in both execution and composition tasks (Bakker 2005; Csikszentmihalyi 1988; MacDonald et al. 2006; Simoens and Tervaniemi 2013).

However, talent is not enough. Without commitment and deliberated effort, complex challenges cannot be faced in any activity domain. This issue emerged very clearly in findings collected among dancers (Massimini et al. 1988) and music students and professional musicians (Delle Fave et al. 2011; Massimini and Delle Fave

1995). This demanding aspect related to practice is well known among artists, who experience it in their own daily life. One of the music students involved in the research work who was raised in a family of musicians, reported a proverb he was taught since childhood: “Talent without discipline is like a car without gasoline”. The opportunities for flow in practicing music or dance can be seized only through massive and persistent investment of mental and physical resources in the activity over prolonged time, facing moments of tiredness, boredom and disengagement especially during the repetitive practice connected with technical skill refinement. Perseverance and long-term commitment however pave the way towards the transformation of music from an occasional and pleasant pastime into a relevant and meaningful component of psychological selection.

Hence, in order to make proper use of flow activities in the long run by successfully including them as components of psychological selection, the intrinsic reward and effortless attention spontaneously arising during their practice must be integrated with intentional and constant resource investment (Oettingen and Gollwitzer 2001). Implementable psychological resources such as self-efficacy (Bandura 1997), an optimistic attributional style (Peterson 1991) and an integrated behavior regulation (Deci and Ryan 2000) represent crucial resources along this pathway.

Personality traits may also play a relevant role in the identification of flow opportunities in daily activities. Csikszentmihalyi (1975/2000) hypothesized a different proneness to flow, defining it as autotelic personality. People showing this trait were assumed to be more curious, creative and intrinsically motivated in daily life than others (Nakamura and Csikszentmihalyi 2009). Moving from the hypothesis that a higher frequency of flow experiences in daily life was a manifestation of autotelic personality, Asakawa (2010) found that autotelic students reported higher levels of well-being and commitment in daily activities, compared with non-autotelic ones. A study by Eisenberger et al. (2005) showed that the combination of high skills and high challenges resulted in an enhanced experience at work for achievement-oriented employees, but not for employees low in need for achievement. Abuhamdeh and Csikszentmihalyi (2009) examined the role of autotelic personality in promoting flow and positive performance in the context of chess competition, classifying autotelic and non-autotelic individuals according to their level of intrinsic motivation in high challenges/high skills situations. Moneta (2012) measured the intrinsic motivation orientation, detecting its positive correlation with optimal experience. In a recent study conducted with Italian adolescents (Bassi et al. 2014b), among the Big Five factors openness to experience emerged as the prominent trait that predicts the occurrence of flow in daily life.

1.4 Final Remarks: The Consequences of Flow

The theoretical approach and empirical findings discussed in this chapter call for a broader view and understanding of flow that too often is investigated as an isolated psychological event within specific domains of daily life. Investigating optimal experience through this lens leads researchers to neglect its relationship with life as a whole, and in particular the crucial issue of the consequences of flow. As a state of consciousness, flow may arise in different contexts and activities, that might be constructive and meaningful for the developmental trajectory of the person, but also harmful and destructive, through its association with illegal activities and drug intake (Delle Fave 2009, 2013). Therefore, its investigation should also take into account the connections of the associated activities with lifelong trajectories, since the short-term benefits of flow as a positive state of absorption promoting the system's complexity and flexibility may be obscured by its long-term disadvantages, as happens with addiction to videogames (Sherry 2004) and risky sports (Partington et al. 2009).

Moreover, flow is often roughly equated to other peculiarly positive states, such as mindfulness, meditation, and peak experiences, again implying its de-contextualization and its evolutionary meaning for the species' adaptation to the demands of the environment (Delle Fave et al. 2011).

Adopting a narrow, strictly analytical perspective does not help evaluate flow in its own essence – a state of consciousness emerging among other daily experiences, that arises in specific conditions depending on contextual and individual features, and that can promote development in the long term when associated with relevant meanings and goals that support adaptation. The studies summarized in this chapter suggest there is a need for a more integrated and articulated perspective, that could shed new light on the evolutionary significance and role of flow within the dynamics of individual/environment interplay and mutual construction. However, in order to promote this approach a more comprehensive and less discipline-bound view of optimal experience is required, that can place flow among the adaptive strategies available to humans, taking into account the universal tendency of living systems towards both inner integration, and information exchange with the external world.

References

Abuhamdeh, S., & Csikszentmihalyi, M. (2009). Intrinsic and extrinsic motivational orientations in the competitive context: An examination of person – situation interactions. *Journal of Personality, 77*, 1615–1635.

Asakawa, K. (2010). Flow experience, culture, and well-being: How do autotelic Japanese college student feel, behave, and think in their daily lives? *Journal of Happiness Studies, 11*, 205–223.

Bakker, A. B. (2005). Flow among music teachers and their students: The crossover of peak experiences. *Journal of Vocational Behavior, 66*, 26–44.

Bandura, A. (1997). *Self-efficacy: The exercise of control*. New York: Freeman.

Bassi, M., & Delle Fave, A. (2012a). Optimal experience among teachers: New insights into the work paradox. *The Journal of Psychology: Interdisciplinary and Applied, 146*, 533–557.

Bassi, M., & Delle Fave, A. (2012b). Optimal experience and self-determination at school: Joining perspectives. *Motivation and Emotion, 36*, 425–438.

Bassi, M., Ferrario, N., Ba, G., Delle Fave, A., & Viganò, C. (2012). Quality of experience during psychosocial rehabilitation: A real-time investigation with experience sampling method. *Psychiatric Rehabilitation Journal, 35*, 447–453.

Bassi, M., Falautano, M., Cilia, S., Goretti, B., Grobberio, M., Pattini, M., Pietrolongo, E., Viterbo, R. G., Amato, M. P., Benine, M., Lugaresi, A., Martinelli, V., Montanari, E., Patti, F., Trojano, M., & Delle Fave, A. (2014a). The coexistence of well- and ill-being in persons with multiple sclerosis, their caregivers and health professionals. *Journal of the Neurological Sciences, 337*, 67–73.

Bassi, M., Steca, P., Monzani, D., Greco, A., & Delle Fave, A. (2014b). Personality and optimal experience in adolescence: Implications for well-being and development. *Journal of Happiness Studies, 15*, 829–843.

Brickman, P., & Campbell, D. T. (1971). Hedonic relativism and planning the good society. In M. Appley (Ed.), *Adaptation-level theory* (pp. 287–305). New York: Academic.

Carillo, M. C., Thompson, L. T., Gabrieli, J. T. E., & Disterhoft, J. F. (1997). Variation of the intertrial interval in human classical conditioning. *Psychobiology, 25*, 152–157.

Cortinovis, I., Luraschi, E., Intini, S., Sessa, M., & Delle Fave, A. (2011). The daily experience of people with achondroplasia. *Applied Psychology: Health and Well-Being, 3*, 207–227.

Couture, M. (2007). *Complexity and chaos – state-of-the-art; overview of theoretical concepts*. Quebec: Defence R&D Canada TM Valcartier.

Csikszentmihalyi, M. (1975/2000). *Beyond boredom and anxiety*. San Francisco: Jossey Bass.

Csikszentmihalyi, M. (1988). Motivation and creativity: Toward a synthesis of structural and energistic approaches to cognition. *New Ideas in Psychology, 6*, 159–176.

Csikszentmihalyi, M., & LeFevre, J. (1989). Optimal experience in work and leisure. *Journal of Personality and Social Psychology, 56*, 815–822.

Csikszentmihalyi, M., Rathunde, K., & Whalen, S. (1993). *Talented teenagers*. New York: Cambridge University Press.

Csikszentmihalyi, M., & Massimini, F. (1985). On the psychological selection of bio-cultural information. *New Ideas in Psychology, 3*, 115–138.

Deci, E. L., & Ryan, R. M. (2000). The "what" and "why" of goal pursuits: Human needs and the self-determination of behavior. *Psychological Inquiry, 11*, 227–268.

Delle Fave, A. (2007). Theoretical foundations of the ESM. In J. Hektner, J. Schmidt, & M. Csikszentmihalyi (Eds.), *Experience sampling method. Measuring the quality of everyday life* (pp. 15–28). New York: Sage.

Delle Fave, A. (2009). Optimal experience and meaning: Which relationship? *Psychological Topics, Special Issue on Positive Psychology, 18*, 285–302.

Delle Fave, A. (2010). Development through disability: The unfolding and sharing of psychological resources. In G. W. Burns (Ed.), *Happiness, healing and enhancement: Your casebook collection for applying positive psychology in therapy* (pp. 88–99). Hoboken: Wiley.

Delle Fave, A. (2013). The psychological roots of health promotion. In A. Morandi & A. N. N. Nambi (Eds.), *An integrated view of health and well-being. Bridging Indian and western knowledge* (pp. 141–162). Dordrecht: Springer.

Delle Fave, A. (2014). Harmony. In A. Michalos (Ed.), *Encyclopedia of quality of life and well-being research*. Dordrecht: Springer.

Delle Fave, A., & Bassi, M. (2003). Italian adolescents and leisure: The role of engagement and optimal experience. In S. Verma & R. Larson (Eds.), *Examining adolescent leisure time across cultures: Developmental opportunities and risks. New directions in child and adolescent development* (pp. 79–93). San Francisco: Jossey-Bass.

Delle Fave, A., & Bassi, M. (2009). Sharing optimal experiences and promoting good community life in a multicultural society. *Journal of Positive Psychology, 4*, 280–289.

Delle Fave, A., & Bassi, M. (2014). Work and the dynamics of development: An integrated model. In C. Biron, R. J. J. Burke, & C.L. Cooper (Eds.), *Creating healthy workplaces* (pp. 37–49). Farnham: Gower Publishing Ltd.

Delle Fave, A., & Bassi, M. (2016). Work, cultures, and the culture of work. In C. J. Fullagar & A. Delle Fave (Eds.), *Flow at work: Measurement and implications*. London: Taylor & Francis.

Delle Fave, A., & Massimini, F. (1988). Modernization and the changing contexts of flow in work and leisure. In M. Csikszentmihalyi & I. Csikszentmihalyi (Eds.), *Optimal experience. Psychological studies of flow in consciousness* (pp. 193–213). New York: Cambridge University Press.

Delle Fave, A., & Massimini, F. (2003). Optimal experience in work and leisure among teachers and physicians: Individual and bio-cultural implications. *Leisure Studies, 22*, 323–342.
Delle Fave, A., & Massimini, F. (1992). The ESM and the measurement of clinical change: A case of anxiety disorder. In M. W. deVries (Ed.), *The experience of psychopathology: Investigating mental disorders in their natural settings* (pp. 280-289). New York: Cambridge University Press.
Delle Fave, A., & Massimini, F. (2004). Bringing subjectivity into focus: Optimal experiences, life themes, and person-centered rehabilitation. In P. A. Linley & S. Joseph (Eds.), *Positive psychology in practice* (pp. 581–597). New York: Wiley.
Delle Fave, A., & Massimini, F. (2005). The relevance of subjective wellbeing to social policies: Optimal experience and tailored intervention. In F. Huppert, N. Baylis, & B. Keverne (Eds.), *The science of wellbeing* (pp. 379–404). Oxford: Oxford University Press.
Delle Fave, A., Bassi, M., & Massimini, F. (2003a). Coping with boundaries: The quality of daily experience of Rom nomads in Europe. *Psychology and Developing Societies, 15*, 87–102.
Delle Fave, A., Bassi, M., & Massimini, F. (2003b). Quality of experience and risk perception in high-altitude rock climbing. *Journal of Applied Sport Psychology, 15*, 82–99.
Delle Fave, A., Massimini, F., & Bassi, M. (2011). *Psychological selection and optimal experience across cultures: Social empowerment through personal growth*. Dordrecht: Springer.
Delle Fave, A., Brdar, I., Wissing, M., & Vella-Brodrick, D. (2013). Sources and motives for personal meaning in adulthood. *The Journal of Positive Psychology, 6*, 517–529.
Delle Fave, A., Fianco, A., & Sartori, R. D. G. (2015). Psychological and relational resources in the experience of disability and caregiving. In S. Joseph (Ed.), *Positive psychology in practice* (2nd ed., pp. 615–633). London: Wiley.
Diamond, J. (2005). *Collapse. How societies choose to fail or succeed*. New York: Viking Books.
Durham, W. H. (1982). Interactions of genetic and cultural evolution: Models and examples. *Human Ecology, 10*, 289–323.
Eisenberger, R., Jones, J. R., Stinglhamber, F., Shanock, L., & Randall, A. T. (2005). Flow experiences at work: For high need achievers alone? *Journal of Organizational Behavior, 26*, 755–775.
Engel, G. L. (1977). The need for a new medical model: A challenge for biomedicine. *Science, 196*, 129–136.
Fromm, J. (2004). *The emergence of complexity*. Kassel: Kassel University Press GmbH.
Ginsburg, S., & Jablonka, E. (2010). Experiencing. A Jamesian approach. *Journal of Consciousness Studies, 17*, 102–124.
Hicks, J. A., & King, L. A. (2009). Meaning in life as a subjective judgment and a lived experience. *Social and Personality Psychology Compass, 3*(4), 638–653.
Hofstede, G. (1980). *Culture's consequences: International differences in work-related values*. London: Sage.
Hofstede, G., Hofstede, G. J., & Minkov, M. (2010). *Cultures and organizations – software of the mind: Intercultural cooperation and its importance for survival*. New York: McGrawHill.
Holland, J. H. (1998). *Emergence: From chaos to order*. Oxford: Oxford University Press.
Jablonka, E., & Lamb, M. J. (2014). *Evolution in four dimensions* (2nd ed.). Cambridge, MA: MIT Press.
Jackson, S.A., & Csikszentmihalyi, M. (1999). *Flow in sports. The keys to optimal experiences and performances*. Champaign, IL: Human Kinetics.
James, W. (1890). *The principles of psychology*. New York: Holt.
Koonin, E. V., & Wolf, Y. I. (2009). Is evolution Darwinian or/and Lamarckian? *Biology Direct, 4*, 42. doi:10.1186/1745-6150-4-42.
Lachmann, M., & Jablonka, E. (1996). The inheritance of phenotypes: An adaptation to fluctuating environments. *Journal of Theoretical Biology, 181*, 1–9.
Laland, K. N., Odling-Smee, J., & Feldman, M. W. (2000). Niche construction, biological evolution, and cultural change. *Behavioral and Brain Sciences, 23*, 131–146.
Lanfranchi, F., Frecchiami, A., & Delle Fave, A. (2011). Interventi riabilitativi ed esperienza ottimale nel contesto montano [Rehabilitation intervention and optimal experience in mountain context]. *Psichiatria di Comunità, 10*, 95–102.

Lavie, N. (2005). Distracted and confused? Selective attention under load. *Trends in Cognitive Sciences, 9*, 75–82.
Levin, B., & Browner, C. (2005). The social production of health: Critical contributions from evolutionary, biological, ad cultural anthropology. *Social Science & Medicine, 61*, 745–750.
Macdonald, R., Byrne, C., & Carlton, L. (2006). Creativity and flow in musical composition: An empirical investigation. *Psychology of Music, 34*, 292–306.
Markus, R., & Kitayama, S. (1991). Culture and the self: Implications for cognition, emotion, and motivation. *Psychological Review, 98*, 224–253.
Massimini, F., & Delle Fave, A. (1995). Qualità dell'esperienza e coltivazione di attività musicali [Quality of experience and cultivation of musical activities]. *Comunicazioni Scientifiche di Psicologia Generale, 14*, 157–180.
Massimini, F., & Delle Fave, A. (2000). Individual development in a bio-cultural perspective. *American Psychologist, 55*, 24–33.
Massimini, F., Csikszentmihalyi, M., & Delle Fave, A. (1988). Flow and biocultural evolution. In M. Csikszentmihalyi & I. Csikszentmihalyi (Eds.), *Optimal experience. Psychological studies of flow in consciousness* (pp. 60–81). New York: Cambridge University Press.
Masterpasqua, F. (2009). Epigenetics and the environmental regulation of the genome and its function. *Review of General Psychology, 13*, 194–201.
Matsunaga, M., Hecte, M. L., Elek, E., & Ndiaye, K. (2010). Ethnic identity development ad acculturation: A longitudinal analysis of Mexican-heritage youth in the Southwest United States. *Journal of Cross-Cultural Psychology, 41*, 410–427.
Mesoudi, A., Withen, A., & Laland, K. N. (2006). Towards a unified science of cultural evolution. *Behavioral and Brain Sciences, 29*, 329–383.
Miller, J. G. (1970). *Living systems*. New York: McGraw-Hill.
Moneta, G. B. (2012). Opportunity for creativity in the job as a moderator of the relation between trait intrinsic motivation and flow in work. *Motivation and Emotion, 36*, 491–503.
Monod, J. (1971). *Chance and necessity: An essay on the natural philosophy of modern biology*. New York: Alfred A. Knopf.
Morandi, A., & Delle Fave, A. (2013). The emergence of health in complex adaptive systems: A common ground for Ayurveda and Western science. In A. Morandi & A. N. N. Nambi (Eds.), *An integrated view of health and well-being. Bridging Indian and western knowledge* (pp. 163–185). Dordrecht: Springer.
Morling, B., & Fiske, S. T. (1999). Defining and measuring harmony control. *Journal of Research in Personality, 33*, 379–414.
Nakamura, J., & Csikszentmihalyi, M. (2009). Flow theory and research. In S. J. Lopez & C. R. Snyder (Eds.), *Handbook of positive psychology* (pp. 195–206). NewYork: Oxford University Press.
Nicolis, G., & Prigogine, I. (1989). *Exploring complexity*. New York: Freeman & Co.
Oettingen, G., & Gollwitzer, P. M. (2001). Goal setting and goal striving. In A. Tesser & N. Schwarz (Eds.), *The Blackwell handbook of social psychology* (pp. 329–347). Oxford: Blackwell.
Partington, S., Partington, E., & Olivier, S. (2009). The dark side of flow: A qualitative study of dependence in big wave surfing. *Sport Psychologist, 23*, 179–185.
Peterson, C. (1991). Meaning and measurement of explanatory style. *Psychological Inquiry, 2*, 1–10.
Pribram, K. H. (1996). Interfacing complexity at the boundary between the natural and social sciences. In E. L. Khalil & K. E. Boulding (Eds.), *Evolution, order and complexity* (pp. 40–60). New York: Routledge.
Rathunde, K. (2001). Family context and the development of undivided interest: A longitudinal study of family support and challenge and adolescents' quality of experience. *Applied Developmental Science, 5*, 158–171.
Richerson, P. J., & Boyd, R. (1978). A dual inheritance model of human evolutionary process: Basic postulates and a simple model I. *Journal of Social and Biological Structures, 1*, 127–154.
Richerson, P. J., & Boyd, R. (2005). *Not by genes alone. How culture transformed human evolution*. Chicago: University of Chicago Press.
Ruyle, E. E. (1973). Genetic and cultural pools: Some suggestions for a unified theory of biocultural evolution. *Human Ecology, 1*, 201–215.

Ryan, R. M., & Deci, E. L. (2000). Self-determination theory and the facilitation of intrinsic motivation, social development, and well-being. *American Psychologist, 55*, 68–78.
Sartori, R. D. G., & Delle Fave, A. (2014). First aid activities and well-being: The experience of professional and volunteer rescuers. *Journal of Social Service Research, 40*, 242–254.
Sartori, R. D. G., Marelli, M., Garavaglia, P., Castelli, L., Busin, S., & Delle Fave, A. (2014). The assessment of patients' quality of experience: Autonomy level and perceived challenges. *Rehabilitation Psychology, 59*, 266–277.
Shernoff, D., & Csikszentmihalyi, M. (2009). Flow in schools. Cultivating engaged learners and optimal learning environments. In R. Gilman, E. Huebner, & M. Furlong (Eds.), *Handbook of positive psychology in schools* (pp. 131–145). New York: Taylor & Francis.
Shernoff, D., Csikszentmihalyi, M., Schneider, B., Shernoff, E. (2003). Student engagement in high school classrooms from the perspective of flow theory. *School Psychology Quarterly, 18*, 158-176.
Sherry, J. L. (2004). Flow and media enjoyment. *Communication Theory, 14*, 328–347.
Simoens, V. L., & Tervaniemi, M. (2013). Musician – instrument relationship as a candidate index for professional well-being in musicians. *Psychology of Aesthetics, Creativity, and the Arts, 7*, 171–180.
Sodergren, S. C., & Hyland, M. E. (2000). What are the positive consequences of illness? *Psychology and Health, 15*, 85–97.
Stebbins, R. A. (2007). *Serious leisure: A perspective for our time*. London: Transaction Publishers.
Steca, P., Bassi, M., Caprara, G. V., & Delle Fave, A. (2011). Parents' self-efficacy beliefs and their children's psychosocial adaptation during adolescence. *Journal of Youth and Adolescence, 40*, 320–331.
Steger, M. F., Kashdan, T. B., Sullivan, B. A., & Lorents, D. (2008). Understanding the search for meaning in life: Personality, cognitive style, and the dynamic between seeking and experiencing meaning. *Journal of Personality, 76*, 199–228.
Tadmor, C. T., Tetlock, P. E., & Peng, K. (2009). Acculturation strategies and integrative complexity. The cognitive implications of biculturalism. *Journal of Cross-Cultural Psychology, 40*, 105–139.
Tennen, H., & Affleck, G. (2002). Benefit-finding and benefit-reminding. In C. R. Snyder & S. J. Lopez (Eds.), *Handbook of positive psychology* (1st ed., pp. 584–597). New York: Oxford University Press.
Tononi, G., & Edelman, G. M. (1998). Consciousness and complexity. *Science, 282*, 1846–1851.
Zhang, T. H., & Meaney, M. J. (2010). Epigenetics and the environmental regulation of the genome and its function. *Annual Review of Psychology, 61*, 439–466.

Part II
Flow in Arts and Sports

Chapter 2
Finding Flow in Music Practice: An Exploratory Study About Self-Regulated Practice Behaviours and Dispositions to Flow in Highly Skilled Musicians

M.V. Araújo and C.F. Hein

Abstract This chapter addresses a study aimed at investigating self-regulated practice behaviours and flow dispositions in expert musicians. A sample of 168 classically trained musicians completed a survey comprising a questionnaire measuring musical self-regulated practice behaviours and the Short Dispositional Flow Scale. Associations of self-regulated practice behaviours and flow dispositions were explored using multivariate regression. Results showed that flow was predominantly a function of self-regulated behaviours Personal Resources and Practice Organization, but not a function of External Resources. Analyses of individual items demonstrated self-regulation seemed to contribute for the experience of flow indicators related to musical skills, tasks, the clarity of goals and feedback, and also concentration and control over the activities. The chapter ends with implications of the findings for musicians, teachers and researchers.

2.1 Introduction

The importance of the 'flow' construct (Csikszentmihalyi 1990) for the domain of musical performance is becoming widely recognised. Defined as a state in which "an individual is completely immersed in an activity without reflective self-consciousness but with a deep sense of control" (Engeser and Shiepe-Tiska 2012,

---

M.V. Araújo (✉)
Communication and Arts Department, University of Aveiro, INET-MD, Campus Universitário de Santiago, 3810-193 Aveiro, Portugal
e-mail: marcosaraujo@ua.pt

C.F. Hein
Department of Social Science, University College London Institute of Education, 20 Bedford Way, WC1H 0DP London, UK
e-mail: chein@ioe.ac.uk

L. Harmat et al. (eds.), *Flow Experience*, DOI 10.1007/978-3-319-28634-1_2

p. 1), flow is often described as an optimal experience, being a highly desirable state to achieve, and one that can improve human performance. In flow, the individual often report one if not all of the following indicators:

> challenge-skill balance (feeling competent enough to meet the high demands of the situation), action-awareness merging (doing things spontaneously and automatically without having to think), clear goals (having a strong sense of what one wants to do), unambiguous feedback (knowing how well one is doing during the performance itself), concentration on the task at hand (being completely focused on the task at hand), sense of control (having a feeling of total control over what one is doing), loss of self-consciousness (not worrying what others think of oneself), transformation of time (having the sense that time passes in a way that is different from normal), and autotelic experience (feeling the experience to be extremely rewarding). (Martin and Jackson 2008, p. 146)

Recently, researchers in the field of music have acknowledged musical performance as an ideal activity for the flow experience (Custodero 2002; Lamont 2012). From a cognitive perspective, music challenges the performer to be completely attentive with mind and body, and music is one of the most demanding tasks for the human central nervous system (Altenmüller and Schneider 2008; Williamon 2004). From a communicative perspective, music challenges the performer to express his/her art via sound and expressive movement according to personal and cultural standards and meanings (Lehmann et al.2007; Davidson 2012). Music performance also challenges the performer perceptually, to organize sound in time, and to explore possible interpretations (meanings) for particular musical sounds (St George et al. 2012). These challenges make musical performance a possible platform for flow experiences.

As a consequence, empirical research about flow in music performance increased significantly. Flow has been investigated in musicians with different levels of expertise and in a variety of contexts such as live performance auditions (Wrigley and Emmerson 2013), wind ensemble rehearsal (Kraus 2003), musical practice activity (Waite and Diaz 2012) and jazz performance (Hart and Di Blasi 2015; Sawyer 2006). Its indicators were related to optimal or successful performances (Bellon 2006; Clark et al. 2014), and flow was also positively related to well-being in music students (Fritz and Avsec 2007), practice time (Marin and Bhattacharya 2013; Waite and Diaz 2012), students' achievement (O'Neill 1999) and emotional intelligence (Marin and Bhattacharya 2013), and negatively related to performance anxiety (Fullagar et al. 2012; Kirchner et al. 2008). Confirming results from domains other than music, no association was shown between flow and demographic variables such as age, genre and level of musical expertise (Marin and Bhattacharya 2013; Sinnamon et al. 2012; Wrigley and Emmerson 2013). Beyond these findings, a particularly important implication of the flow experience for musicians may be that they can experience well-being during the development of their activities, while, at the same time, improving as musicians and deriving enjoyment from within their musical activities.

2.2 Flow in the Context of Music Practice

One activity that may not fit the necessary conditions for the occurrence of flow in music is practice. Practice is an activity that musicians spend much of their time engaged with. For professionals from the Western classical music tradition, practice is usually a solitary and effortful activity, focused on deficiencies and aimed for high levels of proficiency in performance (Chaffin et al. 2002; Lehmann et al. 2007). Because of this, not everyone can always meet the requirements of practice. Where this is the case one might conjecture that flow is not likely to occur.

However, research on music practice demonstrates that individuals with high levels of expertise usually can make practice more efficient (Chaffin et al. 2002). In this context, practice is deliberate and carried out exclusively towards goals and performance improvement. Musicians usually have well-defined tasks, representing musical challenges to overcome. Through intense concentration, skilled musicians rely on their personal strategies when trying to accomplish difficult elements within the task (Chaffin et al. 2002). The practice of professionals is also defined as efficient because it achieves a desired end product in as short a time as possible (Hallam 1997). In this kind of practice, expert musicians also rely heavily on self-regulation (Araújo 2015; Bonneville-Roussy and Bouffard 2014). Self-regulated practice improves performance through the management and planning of practice, and metacognition plays a crucial role, since expert musicians are normally metacognitively engaged with their practice approaches, choosing, modifying and adapting practice strategies (Hallam 1995, 2001). Phases of self-regulation include planning, performance and evaluation of practice outcomes (McPherson and Zimmerman 2011).

In view of all those efficient practice behaviours, one may suppose that efficiency in practice could explain why some musicians are positively engaged with practice, demonstrating some kind of inner drive to continue to enhance and develop it (Bruser 1997; Kurtz 2007; Mach 1991). But would those efficient practice behaviours used by expert performers contribute to making their practice a more enjoyable activity?

Although research on the practice of expert performers usually does not include motivation as dependent variables, many studies have shown associations of flow experience with music practice. Butkovic et al. (2015) found that musical flow proneness was the most significant predictor of total hours of practice throughout the lifetime of a sample of adult musicians. Marin and Bhattacharya (2013) also found that dispositions to flow in student pianists were significantly related to practice time in hours, but not related to the experience of number of years of piano playing. The same result was found in a study with undergraduate music majors (Waite and Diaz 2012). Positive experiences related to practice can also be found in professional musicians' accounts. For instance, Yehudi Menuhin defined music practice as "the search for ever greater joy in movement and expression" (Kurtz 2007, p. 7), and pianists Claudio Arrau and Mark Westcott stated that it is beautiful to practice, and that they love to do it (Chaffin et al. 2002; Mach 1991). In addition, a study conducted by Hallam (1995) found distinct motivations for practice among professional musicians, with some of them presenting intrinsic motivation for practice. If those musicians positively engaged with practice are prone to flow experience, an overall question that needs to be answered is, then, what musicians do in order to have optimal experiences in practice, or what characteristics of their practice might be related to flow?

Few studies have focused on the relationships between musicians' practice behaviours and flow. Although Waite and Diaz (2012) found evidence of flow experience in the practice sessions of twenty undergraduate music majors, their study did not explore associations between specific practice behaviours and flow. Two studies (Bloom and Skutnick-Henley 2005; Kirchner 2011) suggested strategies for the incorporation of flow conditions into music practice. Among several strategies, some of them included the selection of a repertoire within a musician's capacities; focus on the present moment while practicing; a set of clear and specific goals; and avoidance of inner monologue. However, no evidence of the effectiveness of those strategies in the attainment of flow in music practice was provided. In the same research line, Araújo and Andrade (2011) discussed and identified the presence of flow indicators in the musical activities of two professional musicians. When related to practice, the authors found that flow tended to emerge from a combination of continuous sense of challenge and repertoire preference (i.e. the less preferred the repertoire, the more effort was needed). While the set of specific and clear goals were related to a sense of personal accomplishment in practice, both musicians frequently used expressions such as 'a marvellous experience' and 'much happiness' to describe their feelings when they achieved their goals. Conclusively, the authors acknowledged the musicians' self-regulatory processes as "essential components of optimal performance, directing attention and generating the concentration, favouring the flow experience" (Araújo and Andrade 2011, p. 553). Yet, more studies are needed to determine whether these conclusions could be generalized to a more comprehensive sample of expert musicians.

The evidence outlined above suggests that the musicians' experience of flow in practice may be affected by specific practice behaviours, especially self-regulated practice behaviours. In fact, several studies have demonstrated that self-regulation plays a crucial role in the efficiency of practice of musicians from different ages (Araújo 2015; Bonneville-Roussy and Bouffard 2014; McPherson and Zimmerman 2011; Miksza 2011), and the general psychology literature has also found that high levels of self-regulation were related to a sense of psychological stability, personal control and well-being in the general population (Hoyle 2010). People who exert self-regulation typically have well-defined goals and adopt appropriate standards of behaviour (Hoyle 2010). However, little is known about which specific self-regulated practice behaviours are most effective in eliciting flow in the context of music practice. Previous research has not included a more comprehensive set of efficient practice behaviours. Also, a general goal of research on music practice is to find out which specific practice behaviours and strategies are most effective to improve performance (Hallam 1997; Jorgensen 2004; Miksza 2007, 2011), tending to focus on performance achievements rather than optimal experiences. Thus, there is a need for research that incorporates multiple self-regulated practice behaviours, indicators of optimal experiences (i.e. flow) and demographical variables.

The multi-faceted nature of practice results in wide individual differences in musicians' approaches to practice. Specific behaviours such as marking parts, using a metronome, repeating sections, etc. are highly dependent on factors such as the musicians' characteristics (i.e. level of expertise, learning styles, approaches to practice, motivation, personality) and task requirements (i.e. nature of the task, repertoire of the instrument and its characteristics) (Hallam 1997). Because of that, a more general set of self-regulated practice behaviours was considered as a way to investigate relationships with optimal experiences. Thus, the purpose of the research reported here was to examine relationships between self-regulated practice behaviours and dispositions to flow in expert musicians. No studies have explored relationships between a more comprehensive set of self-regulated practice behaviours and dispositions to flow in the music practice of expert musicians. Through this investigation, we expect to offer an opportunity to establish the practice behaviours that might influence flow in musicians, contributing to assisting musicians, teachers and researchers to make practice a meaningful experience.

2.3 Method

2.3.1 Materials

In this study, we explored the relationships between self-regulated practice behaviours and flow dispositions in expert musicians. For this purpose, a cross-sectional survey study was developed using two self-report instruments measuring self-regulated practice behaviours and dispositions to flow.

2.3.2 Self-Regulated Practice Behaviours Questionnaire

The self-regulated practice behaviours questionnaire was used to assess the self-regulation of the expert musicians. Its main section includes 22 items related to three different aspects of self-regulation previously found in an Exploratory Factor Analysis: Practice Organization, Personal Resources and External Resources (Araújo 2015). Self-regulation Through Practice Organization scale includes ten items assessing behaviours related to the organization of practice (e.g. 'I set goals for my practice sessions'; 'I organize the physical environment of my practice sessions'; 'I plan the time of my practice sessions'). Self-Regulation Through Personal Resources includes seven items related to knowledge/regulation of strategies (e.g. 'I am aware of the strategies that I use during practice') and general self-efficacy for goal achievement in practice (e.g. 'I am able to achieve my practice goals satisfactorily'). Lastly, Self-Regulation Through External Resources scale included four items measuring the influence of external aspects in the practice process (e.g. 'I seek information from several sources [books, CDs, videos, internet, biographies, arts, etc.] to support my study'; 'I request help from others [teachers, peers, composers, musicologists and specialists]'). The measure is rated on a 5-point Likert-type scale related to frequency of behaviours (1-never to 5-always) and levels of agreement (1-completely disagree to 5-completely agree). The questionnaire also included a demographical section regarding participants' age, gender, musical instrument, experience in music counting from their first public concert, and daily practice time measured in hours.

2.3.3 Flow Scale

The Dispositional Short Flow Scale (Martin and Jackson 2008) is a brief measure of flow that was validated for the music performance domain. The scale presents nine items each reflecting one of the nine flow indicators, e.g. Challenge-Skill Balance ('I feel I am competent enough to meet the high demands of the situation'), Clear Goals ('I have a strong sense of what I want to do'), Full Concentration ('I am completely focused on the task at hand'), Sense of Control ('I have a feeling of total control'), Autotelic Experience ('The experience is extremely rewarding'). All items were rated on 1 (strongly disagree) to 5 (strongly agree). There are several reasons for the use of this scale in the present study: firstly, this scale achieved good psychometric properties in a sample of musicians (Martin and Jackson 2008); secondly, it seemed to be adequate to the exploration of flow both as a uni- (i.e. global) and multi-dimensional concept; thirdly, according to the scale developers, the "items were selected that appeared to best measure the intended construct" (Martin and Jackson 2008, p. 143), and this can also allow for individual analysis per item, which in turn allows for assessment of individual flow indicators and their relation with music practice behaviours; lastly, being practical and quick to complete, the short version seemed to be a good choice for the undertaking of a study with musicians.

In addition, although there is conceptual and empirical evidence showing that the components of flow are highly correlated, it is premature to conclude that flow can be considered as a one-dimensional concept (Engeser and Shiepe-Tiska 2012), and more research is needed to specify under which conditions components are associated or dissociated. Csikszentmihalyi has conjectured that the action-awareness merging dimension may be the clearest sign of the experience, and some authors concluded, "immersion might, in fact, represent a more central aspect than the other components" (Engeser and Shiepe-Tiska 2012, p. 12). Because of the uncertainty of flow as a one-dimensional concept, this research follows, a priori, the current consideration of flow as an experience with different components, which, in their interplay, represent the experience of flow.

2.3.4 Participants

The participants were volunteers and completed the questionnaire online on a web platform[1] created for this research. For the selection of participants, an invitation for participation in the survey was distributed via email to several music institutions (e.g. universities, colleges, conservatoires) and released in online social networks and digital forums about music research (e.g. *Performance Studies Network*). Those institutions were deemed appropriate because they often include professional musicians and adult students training for professional engagement with music. The invitation included the hyperlinks for access to the web platform for the survey response and information regarding the aims of the research.

From a return rate of 335 questionnaires, only 168 (male = 50.0 %; female = 50.0 %) were used for the present study, as they had more than 10 years of practice experience, satisfying the main criteria to be experts in music (Ericsson et al. 1993). Participants' ages ranged from 18 to 74 years (m = 34.41, SD = 12.39). They were nationals from several countries, but the majority of the respondents were Brazilian (42.8 %), Portuguese (15.7 %) and British (13.9 %). Despite the absence of empirical support for cultural differences affecting both flow and practice behaviours in expert performers (Hallam 1997; Miksza 2011), the present study uses a statistical procedure that is robust to flow and self-regulation reports differing by country.

At the time of this research, the majority of the musicians practiced at least 1–2 h per day and at least 5–6 days a week, confirming that their level of expertise was relatively high. Their main instruments were keyboards (27.4 %), plucked strings (22.6 %), woodwinds (17.3 %), bowed strings (14.9 %), also including singers (9.5 %), brass (4.2 %) and percussion (3.6 %) players.

2.3.5 Procedures

The survey remained open for 5 months, and the participants answered the online questionnaire from October 15th, 2013 to February 28th, 2014. Because the participants were volunteers, they did not need to provide their names or any other data related to their identity. Thus, ethical considerations were only related to assuring the participants of the confidentiality of their responses. The statistical analysis was run with the software IBM SPSS 20 statistics and Stata 13.

We explored the association of self-regulated practice behaviours and flow dispositions using multivariate regression. Following the discussion above, we regressed the same variables on ten different dependent variables. The first model uses factor scores estimated from a Confirmatory Factor Analysis (CFA) using all nine items (named here as Global Flow), the other nine dependent variables are the nine individual items of the Dispositional Short Flow Scale. Using these nine items

[1] http://questionarios.ua.pt/index.php/589964/lang-en

as dependent variables, each on a 5-point Likert scale, we treated these variables as continuous. We made this assumption to be able to compare more easily the corresponding estimates with those of the Flow factor scores, which are on a continuous scale.

We included control variables in the model in order to account for self-regulated behaviours varying systematically by country as well as due to gender, years of experience, musical instrument, whether they have graduated from higher education, whether they have taken part in prize competitions, and hours spent practising per week. Including these control variables also aided inference, as the variance of the error term may not be constant, and instead may be a function of these individual characteristics. We further relaxed this assumption and estimated heteroskedasticity-robust standard errors based on White (1980). We report standardised 'beta' coefficients to ease comparability of our estimates with those from other samples. Thus the reported estimates indicate the change of the dependent variable in standard deviations with a one standard deviation change in the independent variables.

2.4 Results

The results of these regressions can be found in Table 2.1, in which the rows denote the corresponding dependent variables, and the three self-regulated practice behaviours are located in the columns. The first model (in the first row) uses the flow factor scores obtained from a CFA using all items. It therefore can be seen as a summary score of overall flow experience (Global Flow). The estimates suggest that Global Flow is predominantly a function of Practice Organization and Personal Resources, but not a function of External Resources. Analysis of the individual items shows that Challenge-Skill Balance, Clear Goals and Full Concentration appear to follow this pattern. In each of these three cases the estimated correlations are positive for Practice Organization and Personal Resources, whereby the estimated correlation for Personal Resources is twice to three times the size of the corresponding estimate for Practice Organization.

Five of the nine flow indicators appear to only be explained by one of the three self-regulated behaviours. While Unequivocal Feedback and Sense of Control appear to be functions of Personal Resources, Action-Awareness Merging appears to decrease by approximately 0.2 standard deviations (SD) with a standard deviation increase in Practice Organization. On the other hand, Loss of Self-Consciousness and Autotelic Experience appear to be explained by External Resources. The former estimate again is negative and suggests a 0.24 SD decrease. In contrast, a standard deviation increase in External Resources is associated with a 0.3 SD increase in Autotelic Experience. Interestingly, Time Transformation does not seem to vary significantly by any of the three self-regulated behaviours.

Table 2.1 The association of self-regulated practice behaviours and flow experience

Dependent/independent variables	Practice organization	Personal resources	External resources
Global flow	0.11*	0.27***	0.00
	(2.43)	*(2.18)*	*(0.06)*
Challenge-skill balance	0.18*	0.65***	–0.07
	(2.18)	*(5.24)*	*(–0.07)*
Action-awareness merging	–0.20*	–0.07	0.02
	(–2.08)	*(–0.47)*	*(0.15)*
Clear goals	0.30***	0.67***	0.04
	(3.54)	*(6.26)*	*(0.40)*
Unequivocal feedback	0.11	0.28*	0.04
	(1.05)	*(2.07)*	*(0.23)*
Full concentration	0.21*	0.46**	–0.05
	(2.16)	*(2.97)*	*(–0.40)*
Sense of control	0.17	0.33*	–0.05
	(1.49)	*(2.19)*	*(–0.37)*
Loss of self-consciousness	0.14	0.25	–0.24*
	(1.45)	*(1.81)*	*(–2.05)*
Time transformation	0.04	0.08	0.02
	(0.31)	*(0.63)*	*(0.12)*
Autotelic experience	0.114	0.166	0.306*
	(1.04)	*(1.26)*	*(2.14)*

Standardised 'beta' coefficients reported; T-statistics in parentheses based on heteroskedasticity-robust standard errors. Sample size is 168 in all 10 regressions
$*p<0.05$, $**p<0.01$, $***p<0.001$

2.5 Discussion

This study examined relationships between self-regulated practice behaviours and dispositions to flow in the music practice of expert classically trained musicians. Following previous evidence suggesting that efficient practice behaviours may affect flow in musicians, this research is the first empirical evidence of self-regulated practice behaviours affecting dispositions to flow in expert musicians.

Among the three self-regulated behaviours, Self-Regulation Through Personal Resources was a particularly strong predictor of flow dispositions when the estimates are significant. Prior studies have noted that professional musicians usually demonstrate extensive metacognition in their practice processes (Hallam 2001), and, indeed, advanced musicians rely more on self-regulation through personal resources than external ones (Araújo 2015). Thus, this result suggests that self-regulation through personal resources may affect flow in the music practice of expert musicians.

However, the analyses of individual items show that Personal Resources did not predict all the nine flow indicators, but only Challenge-Skill Balance, Clear Goals and Unequivocal Feedback, commonly regarded as conditions to flow in research (Csikszentmihalyi 1990; Fullagar et al. 2012), and Full Concentration and Sense of Control (see Table 2.1). An explanation for this relevant connection between Personal Resources and flow conditions (i.e. balance, goals and feedback) may be that those musicians presenting high capacity for self-regulation through personal resources can make sensible and correct choices of what to do in practice (e.g. musical tasks/challenges, goals, repertoire), contributing to the achievement of a balance between task challenges and their own perceptions of competence. As Hallam (1997) noticed, expert musicians usually "know how to do the right thing at the right time" (p. 181), which may explain the clarity of practice goals. A positive relation between performers' experience and clarity of goals has been found in other studies (Chaffin and Imreh 2001; Chaffin et al. 2002; Chaffin and Lemieux 2004). It is accepted that expert musicians have their own artistic conceptualisations of works to be studied (Chaffin and Lemieux 2004). These characteristics of Self-Regulation Through Personal Resources may, in turn, have enhanced the musicians' concentration in practice, fostering feelings of capacity for being productive and efficient.

Albeit with a lower level of statistical significance, our results show that Self-Regulation Through Practice Organization was also a significant predictor of musicians' dispositions to flow in practice, having a prominent role in the experience of Challenge-Skills Balance, Clear Goals and Full Concentration. These indicators were more related to Personal Resources, which suggests that expert musicians relying on both self-regulated factors (Personal Resources and Practice Organization) may be more prone to achieve those referred to flow indicators. In relation to Challenge-Skills Balance, organized musicians usually set plans and goals for practice (Chaffin et al. 2002; Chaffin and Lemieux 2004; Jorgensen 2004), which may also explain the choice of tasks that are challenging but possible to achieve through practice. Regarding Full Concentration, flow theory suggests that concentration is generally possible because the task has clear goals and immediate feedback (Csikszentmihalyi 1990). This idea was supported by a study conducted by Hallam (2001), in which practice organization was related to concentration in the practice of professional musicians.

On the contrary, the results show Practice Organization negatively related to Action-Awareness Merging, i.e. the more organized the musician, the less prone to the experience of action-awareness merging in practice he/she is. In performing activities, a sense of low attention effort and spontaneity associated with this flow indicator often results in automaticity. According to Jackson et al. (2010), "feelings of automaticity are described by performers, whose well-learnt routines enable them to process subconsciously and pay full attention to their actions" (Jackson et al. 2010, p. 7). Because of that, Action-Awareness Merging may be less likely to occur in practice, and a possible explanation for its negative relation between both variables is that if a musician is executing a task on 'automatic pilot', a clear signal of the experience of this flow indicator in performing activities (Bellon 2006; Clark et al. 2014; Jackson et al. 2010), it is possible that he/she needs no more practice organization, because he/she has probably achieved his/her goals. Perhaps musicians need organization only when seeking to achieve their practice goals, a situation where automaticity may be less likely to occur.

External Resources is the aspect of self-regulation that advanced musicians rely on less (Araújo 2015), and our findings do not suggest that it is a significant predictor of dispositions to flow. However, the analyses of individual items show that Self-Regulation Through External resources was negatively related to Loss of Self-Consciousness and positively related to Autotelic Experience. It is possible that the inclusion of external resources (e.g. teachers, peers, composers, specialists, materials) in the practice process of some expert musicians may have elicited considerations that practice is a rewarding activity in itself, contributing to enjoyment and intrinsic motivation for practice. But further research is needed to confirm if this is the case. On the other hand, a likely explanation for the negative association with Loss of Self-Consciousness is that many studies in music have found problems with the Loss of Self-Consciousness indicator (Marin and Bhattacharya 2013; Sinnamon et al. 2012), which raises uncertainty about the equal importance of this flow indicator for music or about the adequacy of the item in capturing this characteristic of flow.

Finally, time transformation was not related to any aspect of efficient practice. Because Time Transformation is one of the most reported flow dimensions in studies using disposition flow scales in music (Marin and Bhattacharya 2013; Sinnamon et al. 2012), it is possible that other factors might contribute to the experience of this flow indicator in practice.

Self-Regulation is an important element of the expert musicians' practice (Araújo 2015). When related to flow, it seemed to contribute to the experience of flow indicators that were related to musical skills, tasks, the clarity of goals and feedback, and also concentration and control over the activities. Self-Regulation Through Personal Resources and Practice Organization contributed to the achievement of conditions for flow, which, in turn, enhanced the possibility of increased concentration and sense of control in practice. Apparently, expert musicians who also include external elements in their practice processes (e.g. peers, composers, students, materials from distinct sources, etc.) tend to consider practice a more rewarding activity. Overall, it is likely that self-regulated behaviours, which were acquired over more than 10 years of deliberate practice, may have contributed to making the practice of this sample of expert musicians a more rewarding activity. However, the multidimensional nature of the construct and the methods used in this study did not allow the inference of causal relationships between flow and the self-regulated practice behaviours. The methods only weaken the influence of other variables on the flow reports, thereby allowing conclusions in the light of the literature on music practice.

Our findings have important practical implications for musicians, researchers and teachers alike. Although the findings cannot be considered causal, the finding that Self-Regulation Through Personal Resources is a relevant predictor of dispositions to flow in music practice indicates that this aspect of self-regulation may be particularly useful for the achievement of flow in the context of practice. Thus, experimental research could be conducted to test the effect of an intervention of self-regulated strategies in the experience of flow in students. Although relying less on external resources, musicians feeling unmotivated to practice may consider external factors (e.g. teachers, peers, composers, specialists, materials, recordings, etc.) in their practice processes. Teachers could also design specific self-regulatory strategies to help those students who are less motivated to undertake efficient/deliberate practice, contributing to making their practice processes more meaningful and rewarding experiences. This points to a need for more research on aspects of musical practice that are more likely to generate the experience of flow in the practice of students with less experience. This could possibly contribute to a decrease in drop-out in music, allowing students to have meaningful experiences in their music learning processes.

Funding CAPES Foundation, Ministry of Education of Brazil, Brasília – DF 70040-020, Brazil

References

Altenmüller, E., & Schneider, S. (2008). Planning and performance. In S. Hallam, I. Cross, & M. Thaut (Eds.), *The Oxford handbook of music psychology* (pp. 332–343). Oxford: Oxford University Press.

Araújo, M. V. (2015). Measuring self-regulated practice behaviours in highly skilled musicians. *Psychology of Music*. doi:10.1177/0305735614567554.

Araújo, R., & Andrade, M. (2011). Experiência de fluxo e prática instrumental: dois estudos de caso. *Revista DAPesquisa, 8*(1), 01–15.

Bellon, D. (2006). *Application of sport psychology to music performance: A study based on a review of sport psychology literature and selected interviews with professional musicians.* Doctoral dissertation, University of Oregon, Eugene. http://www.oregonpdf.org/index.cfm. Accessed 25 June 2011.

Bloom, A., & Skutnick-Henley, P. (2005). Facilitating flow experiences among musicians. *American Music Teacher, 54*(5), 24–28.

Bonneville-Roussy, A., & Bouffard, T. (2014). When quantity is not enough: Disentangling the roles of practice time, self-regulation and deliberate practice in musical achievement. *Psychology of Music*. doi:10.1177/0305735614534910.

Bruser, M. (1997). *The art of practicing: A guide to making music from the heart.* New York: Three Rivers Press.

Butkovic, A., Ullén, F., & Mosing, M. A. (2015). Personality related traits as predictors of music practice: Underlying environmental and genetic influences. *Personality and Individual Differences, 74*, 133–138. doi:10.1016/j.paid.2014.10.006.

Chaffin, R., & Imreh, G. (2001). A comparison of practice and self-report as sources of information about the goals of expert practice. *Psychology of Music, 29*, 39–69. doi:10.1177/0305735601291004.

Chaffin, R., & Lemieux, A. F. (2004). General perspectives on achieving musical excellence. In A. Williamon (Ed.), *Musical excellence: Strategies and techniques to enhance performance* (pp. 19–39). New York: Oxford University Press.

Chaffin, R., Imreh, G., & Crawford, M. (2002). *Practicing perfection.* Mahwah: Lawrence Erlbaum Associates, Publishers.

Clark, T., Lisboa, T., & Williamon, A. (2014). An investigation into musicians' thoughts and perceptions during performance. *Research Studies in Music Education*. doi:10.1177/1321103X14523531.

Csikszentmihalyi, M. (1990). *Flow: The psychology of optimal experience*. New York: Harper & Row.
Custodero, L. (2002). Seeking challenge, finding skill: Flow experience and music education. *Arts Education Policy Review, 103*(3), 3–9.
Davidson, J. (2012). Bodily movement and facial actions in expressive musical performance by solo and du instrumentalists: Two distinctive case studies. *Psychology of Music, 40*(5), 595–633.
Engeser, S., & Shiepe-Tiska, A. (2012). Historical lines and an overview of current research on flow. In S. Engeser (Ed.), *Advances on flow research* (pp. 1–22). New York: Springer.
Ericsson, K. A., Krampe, R. T., & Tesch-Romer, C. (1993). The role of deliberate practice in the acquisition of expert performance. *Psychological Review, 100*(3), 363–406.
Fritz, B., & Avsec, A. (2007). The experience of flow and subjective well-being of music students. *Horizons of Psychology, 16*(2), 5–17.
Fullagar, C., Knight, P., & Sovern, H. (2012). Challenge/skill balance, flow, and performance anxiety. *Applied Psychology, 62*(2), 236–259.
Hallam, S. (1995). Professional musicians' approaches to the learning and interpretation of music. *Psychology of Music, 23*(2), 111–128.
Hallam, S. (1997). What do we know about practising? Toward a model synthesising the research literature. In H. Jorgensen & A. C. Lehmann (Eds.), *Does practice make perfect? Current theory and research on instrumental music practice* (pp. 179–231). Oslo: Norges Musikkhøgskole.
Hallam, S. (2001). The development of metacognition in musicians: Implications for education. *British Journal of Music Education, 18*(01), 27–39.
Hart, E., & Di Blasi, Z. (2015). Combined flow in musical jam sessions: A pilot qualitative study. *Psychology of Music, 43*(2), 275–290.
Hoyle, R. H. (2010). *Handbook of personality and self-regulation*. West Sussex: Blackwell Publishing Ltd.
Jackson, S., Eklund, B., & Martin, A. (2010). *The FLOW manual: The manual for the flow scales*. www.mindgarden.com. Accessed 2 June 2014.
Jorgensen, H. (2004). Strategies for individual practice. In A. Williamon (Ed.), *Musical excellence: Strategies and techniques to enhance performance* (pp. 85–103). New York: Oxford University Press.
Kirchner, J. M. (2011). Incorporating flow into practice and performance. *Work, 40*, 289–296. doi:10.3233/WOR-2011-1232.
Kirchner, J. M., Bloom, A. J., & Skutnick-Henley, P. (2008). The relationship between performance anxiety and flow. *Medical Problems of Performing Artists, 23*(2), 59–65.
Kraus, B. N. (2003). *Musicians in flow: Optimal experience in the wind ensemble rehearsal*, Doctoral dissertation, Arizona State University, Phoenix.
Kurtz, G. (2007). *Practicing: A musician's return to music*. New York: Random House.
Lamont, A. (2012). Emotion, engagement and meaning in strong experiences of music performance. *Psychology of Music, 40*(5), 574–594.
Lehmann, A. C., Sloboda, J. A., & Woody, R. H. (2007). *Psychology for musicians: Understanding and acquiring the skills*. New York: Oxford University Press.
Mach, E. (1991). *Great contemporary pianists speak for themselves*. New York: Dover.
Marin, M. M., & Bhattacharya, J. (2013). Getting into the musical zone: Trait emotional intelligence and amount of practice predict flow in pianists. *Frontiers in Psychology, 4*, 853–853. doi:10.3389/fpsyg.2013.00853.
Martin, A., & Jackson, S. (2008). Brief approaches to assessing task absorption and enhanced subjective experience: Examining "short" and "core" flow in diverse performance domains. *Motivation and Emotion, 32*(3), 141–157.
McPherson, G. E., & Zimmerman, B. J. (2011). Self-regulation of musical learning: A social cognitive perspective on developing performance skills. In R. Colwell & P. R. Webster (Eds.), *MENC handbook of research on music learning* (Vol. 2, pp. 130–175). New York: Oxford University Press.

Miksza, P. (2007). Effective practice: An investigation of observed practice behaviors, self-reported practice habits, and the performance achievement of high school wind players. *Journal of Research in Music Education, 55*(4), 359–375.

Miksza, P. (2011). A review of research on practicing: Summary and synthesis of the extant research with implications for a new theoretical orientation. *Bulletin of the Council for Research in Music Education, 190*(FALL 2011), 51–92.

O'Neill, S. (1999). Flow theory and the development of musical performance skills. *Bulletin of the Council for Research in Music Education, 141*(1), 129–134.

Sawyer, R. K. (2006). Group creativity: Musical performance and collaboration. *Psychology of Music, 34*(2), 148–165.

Sinnamon, S., Moran, A., & O'Connell, M. (2012). Flow among musicians: Measuring peak experiences of student performers. *Journal of Research in Music Education, 60*(1), 6–25.

StGeorge, J., Holbrook, A., & Cantwell, R. (2012). Learning patterns in music practice: Links between disposition, practice strategies and outcomes. *Music Education Research, 14*(2), 243–263.

Waite, A. K., & Diaz, F. M. (2012). The effect of skill level on instrumentalists' perceptions of flow: An exploratory study. *Missouri Journal of Research in Music Education, 49*, 1–23.

White, H. (1980). A heteroskedasticity-consistent covariance matrix estimator and a direct test for heteroskedacitity. *Econometrica, 48*(4), 807–838.

Williamon, A. (2004). *Musical excellence: Strategies and techniques to enhance performance*. New York: Oxford University Press.

Wrigley, W. J., & Emmerson, S. B. (2013). The experience of the flow state in live music performance. *Psychology of Music, 41*(3), 292–305.

Chapter 3
The Experience of Flow in Artistic Creation

Tatiana Chemi

Abstract In the present chapter I will describe and discuss the experience of flow occurring when professional artists create and learn. The unique findings are part of a larger study that looked at artistic creativity and aimed at describing the ways in which professional and widely recognised artists create, learn and organise their work. The methodological approach was qualitative and based on retrospective narratives of 22 high-achieving professional artists. When asked to describe the ways in which they create, these artists often replied by mentioning a positively felt state of deep concentration and calm. Flow, to them, seems to be at the same time a prerequisite, a constitutive element and an effect of creative processes. Artistic creation happens in a state of deep concentration and self-forgetting and flow seems to have a specific purpose within artistic processes: triggering, facilitating and guiding the *flow* of creation.

3.1 Introduction: Flow in the Arts

The experience of flow in the arts has been variously, but still not thoroughly, documented. Csikszentmihalyi himself has repeatedly contributed to the field by seeing artistic activities as flow-enhancing and by linking the flow experience to creativity (1996). By interviewing a wide variety of professionals and trying to understand the source of their creativity, he repeatedly encountered the experience of deep motivation, described in terms of focused concentration on a given task and autotelic enjoyment. Csikszentmihalyi, whose career began with the study of artistic creativity (Getzels and Csikszentmihalyi 1976; Csikszentmihalyi and Robinson 1990), has indirectly suggested that artistic activities might offer optimal preconditions to the occurrence of flow. Csikszentmihalyi and Robinson (1990) interpret artistic experiences as cognitively challenging and at the same time rewarding – when the artistic jigsaw is approached with solutions and deeper understanding, individuals in his study experienced a deep psycho-emotional gratification. Most of the contributions that specifically focus on the experience of flow in the arts choose music as their artistic modality (Byrne et al. 2006; Custodero 2002; De Manzano et al. 2010;

T. Chemi (✉)
Department of Learning and Philosophy, Aalborg University, Aalborg, Denmark
e-mail: tc@learning.aau.dk

L. Harmat et al. (eds.), *Flow Experience*, DOI 10.1007/978-3-319-28634-1_3

Grape et al. 2003). Perry has looked at writers (1999, 2005), Hefferon and Ollis at professional dancers (2006) and Banfield and Burgess at visual artists (2013).

These studies are often quantitative and focus on a single art form, not systematically taking into consideration commonalities or differences across art forms or genres. In order to fully embrace the complexity of artistic creation and the implications of flow in artistic processes, further focused studies are needed. Especially crucial are distinctions between and within artistic contexts. For instance, the above-mentioned studies range from artistic making to arts appreciation, from educational to artistic settings, from professional to amateur practices, from expressive to educational challenges. However, though contexts, objects of study and artistic experiences vary as much as methodological approaches, the experience of flow in artistic activities seems to be ever-present, consistent to the experience of flow in other human activities, steadily embodied, related to learning through growth and development, and enjoyable.

The present chapter confirms, by means of new empirical data, previous knowledge of and insights into the flow experience in the arts. Its originality lies in the qualitative descriptions and the vivid narratives from the artists who describe flow in their own words. These narratives, by specifying the embodied and emotional experience of flow, allow for original interpretations and novel hypotheses. This chapter intends to address the possibility that the autotelic dimension can be deliberately used in order to facilitate artistic processes and allow for artistic creation to emerge. Moreover, the developmental potential of flow experience is emphasised as an essential part of artistic creation and both its "peaks" and downsides are taken into consideration.

3.2 Looking at Artistic Creativity

In collaboration with my colleagues from the research group ARiEL (Arts in Education and Learning), in 2011–2014 I collected professional artists' narratives on the cognitive, emotional and relational elements of creative processes (Chemi et al. 2015). The overall study focused on the specific qualities of creative and learning processes as interconnected to each other. Even though originally this study was not intentionally focused on understanding flow, it became necessary to include the discussion of the flow experience, because of the consistent findings throughout the interviews and the artists' recurrent references to this experience. Deep concentration is one of the frequent elements that artists describe as necessary to the creation of artworks. How does it feel? What does it look like? What are its effects? Can it be induced and learned? The present chapter looks at flow, described by the artists themselves as embodied and related to motivational aspects of artistic creation. Creativity is here defined as the "interaction among *aptitude*, *process*, *and environment* by which an individual or group produces a *perceptible product* that is both novel and useful as defined within a *social context*" (Plucker et al. 2004) and artistic creativity as the production of a perceptible, novel and useful product that is specific to the domain of the arts.

The methodological approach is qualitative and based on retrospective narratives, collected by means of semi-structured interviews. The 22 interviewed artists (11 females, 11 males, average age 53,5, standard deviation 14.7σ) produced more than 23 interview hours divided in 18 interviews (some collaborating artists were interviewed in pairs). Interviews were recorded, transcribed, where necessary translated and analysed individually and collectively. All the artists contributed to the texts' internal validity by giving us feedback on content and formulations in their own transcribed interview.

Artistic modalities covered were: literature, poetry and scripts; dance and choreography; acting and theatre directing; music (jazz, pop-rock, opera, classic); film-making (motion pictures and documentary); visual arts; digital arts; design; architecture.

The level of creative endeavour looked at is specific to the domain of the arts (Kaufman and Baer 2005) and hinting at the expertise to be found in professional creators -Pro C level of creativity- and high-achieving, widely recognised creators -Big C level of creativity (Simonton 2010). Even though this study did not have an explicit intention of sampling creators in old age, as in Nakamura and Csikszentmihalyi (2003, pp. 188–189), its focus on high achievers necessarily directed the sampling towards experienced and mature artists. The average age was between 40 and 60 (53,5), the youngest being 35 and the oldest being 87 at the time of the interview.

The overall findings of this study show that artists are able and willing to describe how the process of creation feels, in spite of the great difficulty of explaining in a verbal or propositional language the multi-faceted and complex compulsion to create. Even though the interviewed artists describe creativity as a sort of human universal (everyone has it as a potentially expressive force), the full realisation of creative potential in the arts depends on craftsmanship, skills and virtuosity. The specific qualities of artistic creation are characterised by cognitive approaches (wondering, asking questions and being curious, commitment to concentrated artistic practice, experimentation, play and hard work, communication, non-linear enquiry and action), by behavioural choices (starting experiments and connections as well as doing things differently by making detours, staying deliberately in the not-knowing-zone and embracing uncertainty), by relational elements (socio-cultural influences, dialogue with traditions) and by psycho-emotional states.

The latter relates to both positively and negatively perceived states, as well as to the bridging or bypassing of positive/negative states when moving towards acts of creation. It is in this context that the interviewed artists repeatedly describe occurrences of flow experience. In the interviews, flow preconditions and effects were not operationalized nor were Flow Scales taken systematically into consideration. On the contrary, the artists were asked to describe their creative processes by means of life-narratives: "how do you create? In which situations do you experience yourself as the most creative? When do you experience being completely absorbed by artistic work? What inhibits your creativity? How do you generate new material?" Not surprisingly, many described in detail the flow experience and even spontaneously defined it as "flow".

In the interviews, consistently with other flow researches on artists (Csikszentmihalyi 1996; Custodero 2002; Ørsted Andersen and Hanssen 2013; Hefferon and Ollis 2006; Perry 2005), I found clear evidence of the incidence of flow experience in relation to the act of creation. In the present chapter I will discuss the findings that relate specifically to the experience of flow in artistic processes of creation.

3.3 Experiencing Flow

When asked to describe the ways in which they create, the interviewed artists often replied by mentioning a positively felt state of deep concentration and calm. Admittedly, the interviews tended to be positively biased, for the simple reason that the artists were asked to recall retrospectively what they are passionate about: their artistic work. The artists were asked to mention what works optimally for their creativity to unfold and flourish, but also what is disturbing and what inhibits their creativity or communication in artistic communities. Although mentioned in a few places (distrust, lack of communication, frustrations), highly dysfunctional sides of artistic creativity were not systematically looked at in this study.

The interviewed artists describe their favourite creative process as a flow experience. They define this state differently, sometimes explicitly as flow or as the release of endorphins or as a Zen-like learning experience. A 44 year-old female filmmaker says: "you are in do-mode, it's very Zen, in a way, I would describe it, it's a calm level of meditation and very powerful and empowering and when in that moment I feel like I learn the most". A 77 year-old male theatre director describes this state as a radar function that is more similar to mindfulness: "a radar begins to function, a radar which perceives the smallest signs, symptoms, reactions around you". Some performing artists describe a state that is more a relational version of flow, a team flow (musicians from a string quartet), which is perceived as the shared "riding on the same horse" (48 year-old female film director). Team flow is further described in van den Hout's contribution to the present volume, (see Chap. 15 by Hout at al.) The interviewed artists mention flow when they describe their creative processes and they strictly correlate it to creativity, for instance a 47 year-old male designer says: "in reality one experiences flow, when one is in a creative process". According to a 52 year-old male writer, this state is more a movement than a state, a metaphor that seems to be suggested by the "flowing" implicit in the term flow and by Csikszentmihalyi's (1990, 2000) conceptualisation of flow as a dynamic experience. This psychological experience is not inert but rather a vibrant being-in-time or becoming. It is an experience that is delimited to a restricted time-span, even though it can occur often. The psycho-emotional charge of flow makes it a very fulfilling but also an incredibly exhausting experience. As the interviewed quartet members mention, they feel completely absorbed and do not take any breaks. Emotionally fulfilling, focused and deeply concentrated work is not sustainable over long periods, even though individuals can be differently capable of withstanding a lasting performance or concentration. A 42 year-old male writer recurrently defines his creative process in terms of flow experience:

> I enter the flow, where I'm writing and suddenly I must push a lot, and it happens, I write a lot of stuff during maybe an hour or an hour-and-a-half or thereabouts, and there's this flow and creativity that comes at some point during my working day if it's a good working day – but you can't force it. I can't sit down and be in this flow for eight hours. It comes in waves and sometimes it's one wave and sometimes there's a pause and I do something else or just read a manuscript or edit a little or dance about, sometimes I dance with my earphones on, something like that. Something like that and then get on with it.

He goes on to explain the specific compositional technique he uses – automatic writing – and how he approaches it. In order to get started and overcome the possible anxiety of the white page or the blank canvas some artists get their compositional process started by just starting writing or drawing. This process seems to activate unconscious sources of inspiration, giving the artworks a seemingly spontaneous character. It consists in simply writing or drawing without breaks for a continuous period of time, until more shaped ideas and sentences or images are being formulated. The above-mentioned writer describes the sudden transition from random words to structured ideas and the sustained suspension of criticism that this stage of writing needs. Looking back at the process, the writer is almost surprised by the results.

> I just write into a flow and then the ideas come suddenly, things happen and I am writing without thinking, without thinking whether it is good, without being critical. And afterwards, you get that feeling of – bloody hell, where did that come from? Or, oh well – okay. Braw! Or something like that and of course you can, I can get a feeling that I have made something or other or was it me who did it? Or where did that come from?

Several artists mention the surprise in looking at the artwork as it takes shape, as if they have been suspending their conscious presence and suddenly have come back to consciousness. A 47 year-old male designer describes the surprise of going back to the artwork after a process of "letting go" or suspension. The wonder in the presence of a finished work of art or of the tangible emerging of artistic structures and materials is due to the fact that artistic creation might be preconscious, unconscious, partly unconscious or deliberately unconscious. Several other artists mention the feeling of wonder when ideas pop up, for instance a 48 year-old female film director describes the artistic process as an "incredible wonder" and a 35 year-old male digital artist as something that feels like but is not magic: "good ideas can survive anything, and I do not think there is anything magical in the way of the creative process". However, both are aware of the fact that the magical or divine interpretation is nothing but a cultural construction expressing lack of understanding about the source of the creative process: "where the hell did that come from? That is why Bach wrote *Soli Deo Gloria*. [...] I have a different approach to things, but he probably felt the same wonder -where the hell?... it must have come from God. This is not the way I have it, I want to stress this again, but it's really strange", maintains the above female film director. Ideas do not just fall from the sky effortlessly. They must be worked out by means of deep concentration, hard work over time, active experimentation and enjoyment.

What is even more relevant to describing flow is the vibrant statement of purposiveness in the 42 year-old male writer's quote above. This writer makes it clear that the optimal flow in writing does not just happen by itself, but the artist must chase after it, nourish it, create the very conditions for this experience to happen. One more important detail is that the flow experience is in this case not sought after for its own sake, but because in this state artistic creativity unfolds. In his narrative, at the beginning, flow seems to be rather a consequence of the concentration that the writer builds up by means of his automatic writing technique and working rituals. But subsequently, when the writer is caught in the creative waves and their flowing, it appears to be such a gratifying experience that the experience as such seems to be craved for its own sake. Needless to say, in the case of artistic creation the flow experience or state might be instrumental to the main purpose of artistic processes: the creation of artworks. The bodily and psycho-emotional effects of flow may consist of a high level of dopamine, effortless concentration and enjoyment (De Manzano et al. 2013). Because of these positively-felt body changes, flow might be perceived as a state that individuals wish to experience as often as possible and for as long as possible, regardless of its positive spill-over into the creative process. This writer presents us with an incredibly detailed description of his flow experience:

> Well, it feels like a sort of uncontrolled state into which the body falls or floats, where it feels like – what does it feel like? Ah, it's a very emotional state. I mean emotionally, I'm very affected by it. I write, I laugh, I cry and I let go. For me it's about, it feels like letting go of some physical control, both emotional and physical control, where I just float along with it. And it's purely physical, I believe, I have a feeling that my body is different, soft and different, sort of indistinct. Yes, I lose control of myself, physically, mentally and emotionally. I'm not sure if I can, if you can, I don't know if you can talk about it as a control thing. I'm trying to control it some way or other, you know in the creative process. But a lot of the time it's like speed, my heart beats fast and I get warm all over my body and now and again I want to hop up from my chair and go around the house and talk to myself – a bit like that and that's why I don't like being interrupted [...] because I scurry about and make gestures and talk and so [...] I'm filled with something and I let go and am filled with something.

The writer's body is greatly affected: it feels "soft", "warm" or fast ("like speed") and it's both relaxed ("letting go of some physical control") and tense ("I scurry about and make gestures"). He describes this psycho-emotional state as bodily and deeply related to sensory perceptions, but also to the thinking that powers his writing. Embodied cognition explains it through the belief that "thinking is doing, and that cognition is action" (Johnson 2007, p. 92). The materiality implicit in the arts, the involvement of senses, bodies, perception, feelings and emotions is explained in terms of holistic cognitive acknowledgement, because of its embodiment: "Thought can be transformative of our experience precisely because thought is embodied and interfused with feeling" (Johnson 2007, p. 92). The writer's description of flow is an example of embodied meaning and consistent with Hefferon and Ollis (2006) who were looking specifically at dancers' experience of flow. However, the writer seems to suggest between the lines that he consciously induces this state and tries to regulate it in order to create.

3.4 Conceptualising Flow in the Arts

Distinctive elements of the flow experience are conceptualised differently. However, variations among elements are often nuances relating to the same semantic fields. In Csikszentmihalyi's main contribution on creativity (1996, pp. 111–113, but see also 2003), the following are mentioned as elements of flow experience:

- There are clear goals every step of the way
- There is immediate feedback to one's actions
- There is a balance between challenge and skills
  - Action and awareness are merged
- Distractions are excluded from consciousness
  - There is no worry of failure
- Self-consciousness disappears
  - The sense of time becomes distorted
- The activity becomes autotelic.

Perry (2005, p. 26) divides the keys to flow entry into preconditions that arise before the act of creation, clearly related to motivational and psychological aspects, and components that occur during the creative process. Perry's research on writers emphasises the following preconditions for entering a flow state: motivational ("have a reason to write"), cognitive ("think like a writer"), flow-related ("loosen up, focus in, balance among opposites").

I will now discuss the above conceptualisations by looking at the qualitative evidence from the artists' interviews.

3.4.1 Goals Are Clear

Goals are clear looking back at how the interviewed artists describe the modalities of their compositional or interpretive processes, I can infer that they have a clear goal in mind, even when the process is not yet fully defined. A strong sense of purpose and meaningfulness supports the clarity of goals. Moreover, expertise in a given domain gives to artistic discovery a specific focus: the goals that artists meet in the present moment are defined by the challenges of the chosen media and materials. A clear goal might be worked through by means of open heuristics, and this would not change the intelligibility of purpose.

3.4.2 Feedback Is Immediate and Unambiguous

Feedback is immediate and unambiguous artists work with perceptible materials (e.g. colours, clay, bodies, sounds, movements) and media (e.g. radio, film, animation, words). They are always able to see or hear the advancement in their work. They can clearly perceive with senses and bodies the progressive growing of the artwork. No matter if they feel that the process is heading in the right or wrong direction, artists continuously get feedback from their work in the form of a material/medium that is being shaped. They engage in a dynamic dialogue with the artwork and respond to it actively. Moreover, they are keen to choose colleagues or significant others as feedback-givers and to invite them into the compositional process, in stages perceived as appropriate. Artworks in progress are defined as sensitive and fragile, to the extent that feedback given at the wrong time can be unproductive or dangerous.

3.4.3 A Balance Between Skill and Challenge

A balance between skill and challenge in order to dare to be daring and to experiment, artists need to experience the optimal balance between their capacity to face up to their challenges and the actual challenges offered by the material/medium. This is expressed differently in the artists' interviews, for instance, a 48 year-old female film director points out the paradoxical duality of this state, on the one hand encouraging creativity, on the other awkwardness: "I am looking all the time after that [experience], which can be said to be able to express myself within some frames, and I feel a little bit unusual and a little bit uncomfortable, simply because I experience that it directly encourages my creativity". According to a 35 year-old male digital artist, when the artistic process starts generating good ideas "there is a kind of lightness about it, so we're going to be complacent about some things, or not too easy, but all we're going to go easy on some things […] then those things suddenly come and it feels incredibly fruitful". He also stresses the balance between "going easy" and the "not too easy", which we interpret as the attitude he devises in his dialogue with his medium (electronic music). The artistic challenge should be stimulating enough to encourage novelty and originality but not so much that the artist does not experience the process as "fruitful" and enjoyable, losing sight of artistic craftsmanship. A 52 year-old male writer sharply describes this balance, pointing out the gap between artistic creation and everyday life, saying that there is no clear way of being artistically creative, because if there was, then it would be much easier to be creative. A few years earlier, he would have said that the most important precondition for an artist to create is to have no time constraints, but life's challenges had changed his approach:

> It is important that you can just relax in it. It was because I was frustrated over the fact that you have children and you'll never have time to sit and think properly after that. But now

> that I have so many children and never have time to reflect, it has almost been the opposite, so I can have an enormous amount of reflection on how I do [it], but if I go up and just set the timer for an hour and press and say, now I'll just type away this time, and I do not have time to think of editing or anything.

The apparently contradictory needs – quiet, uninterrupted time for the artistic process and the interruptions of everyday life – should be in balance or alternate. This writer, however, admits that the practical-logistical challenge that his daily life brings him has enriched his artistic habits, by means of a new stop-by-the-clock writing routine. Fundamental for him are the pragmatic choices that as an artist he is practically compelled to make, choices that always depart from the recognition of specific needs in the artistic process or the needs of a particular, context-defined compositional challenge.

3.4.4 Total Concentration on the Task at Hand

Total concentration on the task at hand examples of deep concentration during artistic creation are frequent and often detailed in the artists' accounts, as the writer's quotes above demonstrate. A 68 year-old female theatre director describes it in her practice as a shared experience. She focuses on describing her own state, but she extends it to the whole ensemble:

> When for the first time we see something happening on the stage, on the floor. In this moment I don't know where we are, what time it is. Where we are creating, we are really painting a new canvas, a completely white canvas, and we are doing it together, and at this moment it is like a virgin-moment. [...] It's really like stepping out on a white canvas, and of course there, in these moments, I don't think of anything else than that. But most of the time I am absorbed by it, by this... by working, creating, working, creating.

3.4.5 Action-Awareness Merging

Action-awareness merging when action and awareness merge, artists experience that the present is what matters. Living in the present moment is a characteristic that flow shares with mindfulness (Kabat-Zinn 1990, 1994). Both, in different ways, dig into the present moment, flow focusing on a given task or activity, mindfulness focusing on stillness. However, flow achieves it by activating laser-sharp attention to a given task and mindfulness by means of the diffuse awareness about oneself, others and the world around.

Being in the present, for the interviewed artists, is essentially about the task at hand here and now, forgetting about past disappointments or future receptions of their art. A 39 year-old female digital artist feels creative "if you don't ask yourself whether you are tired" and is able to direct all her energies to the task at hand. A 58 year-old female writer maintains a particular differentiation between her study as a working place and her garden as a relaxation place. Rather than the former being related to labour and the latter to leisure, both places seem to be differently related to the task of writing, garden relaxation serving as a break from writing in order to be fresh again for creativity.

Full absorption is not only provided by working or artistic tasks, but also by relaxation tasks. Gardening, unlike physical exercises, enables the writer to let go of her internal narrator, necessary when gathering fresh energy for her work. However, later on in the interview, this female writer specifies a fundamental difference between the two flow occurrences, indicating the studio work as full flow experience, where she forgets time and space, as opposed to garden-flow, where time and space are always present, in spite of full concentration on the task. Common to the two flow occurrences is the feeling of being in the present moment with the given task.

3.4.6 Sense of Control

Sense of control artists are said to take risks (Weisberg 1993) as a 52 year-old male writer suggests, with a metaphor of walking "on thin ice". However, when the creative process "is flowing" the effort involved feels easy, as he says:

> It's always easy. It is never difficult. It can be difficult before, and it can be hard but at the moment it is flowing it is always incredibly easy. I do not think I've ever been in a creative process where I do not feel afterwards that I have cheated. I just think it simply came, so it was amazing that I lost the feeling of time completely and there is a complete lack of feeling that this thing can go wrong. So it is simply when it's there, so it's of course lovely and it is the state I wish to be in. […] That is what keeps one going, I have it when I write, for example, I'm talking out loud, I laugh out loud or I get sad, I literally get touched and thus the entire feeling mechanism is running, but it's not hard, not at the time it is happening.

Control or the feeling of being in control is observable in statements of ease and fun, even in the case of difficult tasks. The above writer displays a whole range of comments on this feeling, from the guilt of perceiving the process as too easy (he feels he has almost "cheated"), to the motivational effect of it ("is what keeps one going"), from the hedonistic drive ("it's of course lovely and it is the state I wish to be in") to the cultural interpretation of artistic creativity as divine ("one can understand that there are some people who think that it just comes from outside or from below or divine inspiration and things like that").

3.4.7 Transformation of Time

Transformation of time the alteration of the sense of time (and often space) is the most recurrent indication of flow. In the interviews this timeless experience is connected to artistic work or parts of it. For instance a 48 year-old female film director does not mention film-making in general as flow enhancing, but specific parts of the film-making process: "I experience it especially when I'm on the shootings or when

I'm in conversations with actors especially about something we have to do. Or when I sit with a writer, so I am fully in it. It is clear that when I miss my family and stuff, it works up here in an area, [...] when I'm shooting, I completely forget time and place". A 58 year-old female writer also seems to suggest that this "highly concentrated work" is enjoyable and effortless. When a long session of work "feels as if it's five minutes" the process has very likely been perceived as comfortable and smooth.

> When I am deep in a novel, the one I am writing now, for example, I will often take one day off during the week, usually Sunday. I take care of business, household chores, the garden. I have discovered that those Sundays last and last. I can't believe how slow the day is...I look up and notice that it's only 11 o'clock in the morning, and I feel that I have already lived through an entire day. When I am at my desk working, however, I am often shocked to look up at the clock and realize that three or four hours have passed and I had no idea. It feels as if it's been five minutes. That's an astonishing effect of highly concentrated work.

The twisted perception of time has a positive influence on the individual artist's feelings about her work, with the consequence of a positively reinforced synergy. Working under flow conditions, because it feels good and effortless, triggers the desire to have more of this state, and getting more of this state might help the artistic process to "flow".

3.4.8 The Loss of Self-Consciousness

The loss of self-consciousness several artists refer to "let-go" strategies. As a 39 year-old female digital artist maintains (and asks herself) "we actually let go of some control or what?" The let-go strategy might in fact aim at getting rid of several constrictions, whether cultural, social or psycho-emotional. Several interviewees emphasise the loss of ego as fundamental for the moment of artistic creation. Artists must forget about their own ego in the moment of idea or material generation, otherwise ideas would not freely emerge. Also in the editing stage of their work, where they need to be their own critic, ego must be set apart. Some artists talk about conscious or unconscious creativity, which perhaps can be interpreted as a form of flow, where the artist is not fully aware of herself consequent to a loss of ego-control and concentration on a given task. For instance a 44 year-old female designer reflects as follows:

> Maybe you could talk about conscious creativity and unconscious creativity. And unconscious creativity is maybe the moments when you just create actually, without thinking about it. I think that it is a thing you are and it's part of you as a person. [...] When I am conscious about creativity as such, that is when I am in a development process together with other people and so that's where I am most creative actually, when we are as a group and somebody has an idea and somebody reacts and then comes up with something.

The conscious/unconscious dilemma does not seem to hint at Freudian interpretations of art (Herbert 2010), but rather at the stepping in and out of a flow experience, where the artist loses track of herself (self-consciousness) in order to create. What seems to be relevant is the creative act in dialogue with others.

3.4.9 Autotelic Experience

In the interviews artists perceive their creative processes as demanding and rewarding at the same time and they positively look at flow as a pre-requisite, a constitutive element and an effect of creative processes. Their capacity for and commitment to concentration, the long-term project of artistic creativity and its relatedness to identity-building make flow a necessity. Artists draw inspiration from a variety of experiences that are sought intentionally, over a long-term exposure. Artistic creation happens in a state of deep concentration and self-forgetting and flow seems to have a specific purpose within artistic processes: to trigger, facilitate, and guide the *flow* of creation. But because professional artists depend professionally and existentially on the act of creation, the triggering of psychological states that bring a sense of control and of ease are fundamental to their processes. Therefore, in spite of its autotelic component, the flow state seems to be deliberately induced in order to facilitate artistic creation. A 52 year-old male writer says: "for me it's much more a matter of a particular state, you can do something to put yourself in it". Another male writer (42 year-old) says that he writes himself into a state of flow and letting-go because he has learned that this is the state where he is more productive and where he most enjoys his work process. Artistic processes are often exhausting or frustrating, but when flow happens, even the most challenging task can be perceived as enjoyable.

3.5 Conclusions

It is important to emphasise how artists look at their creative processes as being dependent on learning and development, on elements of flow experience and on enjoyment. The developmental, engagement-related and hedonic are strictly related in a self-reinforcing relationship, as the flow theory explains. Artists not only generically describe creative processes as flow, but specifically point to their favourite creative states as being flow-like. They describe and experience flow as basically sensory, bodily and dynamic. These experiences, in the arts, can become acts of expression (Dewey 2005) and are dependent on continuous learning and development.

Issues of learning and development have often been brought into discussion in flow conceptualisations. Custodero (2002, p. 3) frames the learning processes activated in the flow experience as a response to challenge-seeking innate behaviours, to which musical experiences give full expression, by means of a "sense of self as an agent of possibility". Jackson and Eklund (2004, p. 5) describes flow even more clearly as an experience leading "to growth and complexity in consciousness", or in other words to development and learning. Individuals who go through flow experiences undergo a transformation by means of enhanced complexity "through the process of differentiation and integration" (Jackson and Eklund 2004, p. 5).

The interviewed artists perceive learning and creativity as interconnected in their artistic work. They tend to develop personal strategies for intentional learning, which are experiential, exploration- and problem-based, mediated, bodily and sensory. In engaging in artistic dialogues with their field they learn their craft by mastering their chosen art form and by simultaneously ensuring opportunities for serendipitous, explorative, self-initiated and on-going creative processes. This means that they depend on the activation of flow states for the optimal unfolding of the creative process and that they possibly deliberately seek out conditions and preconditions for flow to happen.

References

Banfield, J., & Burgess, M. (2013). A phenomenology of artistic doing: Flow as embodied knowing in 2D and 3D professional artists. *Journal of Phenomenological Psychology, 44*, 60–91.

Byrne, C., Carlton, L., & MacDonald, R. (2006). Creativity and flow in musical composition: An empirical investigation. *Psychology of Music, 34*, 262–306.

Chemi, T., Jensen, J. B., & Hersted, L. (2015). *Behind the scenes of artistic creativity: Processes of learning, creating and organising*. New York: Peter Lang.

Csikszentmihalyi, M. (1990). *Flow: The psychology of optimal experience*. New York: HarperCollins.

Csikszentmihalyi, M. (1996). *Creativity. Flow and the psychology of discovery and invention*. London: HarperCollins.

Csikszentmihalyi, M. (2000). *Beyond boredom and anxiety. Experiencing flow in work and play*. San Francisco: Jossey-Bass (1975).

Csikszentmihalyi, M. (2003). *Good business: Leadership, flow, and the making of meaning*. London: Hodder & Stoughton.

Csikszentmihalyi, M., & Robinson, R. E. (1990). *The art of seeing. An interpretation of the aesthetic encounter*. Los Angeles: Paul Getty Museum.

Custodero, L. A. (2002). Seeking challenge, finding skill: Flow experience and music education. *Arts Education Policy Review, 103*(3), 3.

De Manzano, Ö., Theorell, T., Harmat, L., & Ullén, F. (2010). The psychophysiology of flow during piano playing. *Emotion, 10*, 301–311.

De Manzano, Ö., Cervenka, S., Jucaite, A., Hellenäs, O., Farde, L., & Ullén, F. (2013, February 15). Individual differences in the proneness to have flow experiences are linked to dopamine D2-receptor availability in the dorsal striatum. *NeuroImage, 67*, 1–6.

Dewey, J. (2005). *Art as experience*. New York: Perigee Books.

Getzels, J. W., & Csikszentmihalyi, M. (1976). *The creative vision: A longitudinal study of problem finding in art*. New York: Wiley.

Grape, C., Sandgren, M., Hansson, L.-O., Ericson, M., & Theorell, T. (2003). Does singing promote well-being? An empirical study of professional and amateur singers during a singing lesson. *Integrative Physiological and Behavioral Science, 38*, 65–74.

Hefferon, K. M., & Ollis, S. (2006). 'Just Clicks': An interpretive phenomenological analysis of professional Dancers' experience of flow. *Research in Dance Education, 7*(2), 141–159.

Herbert, A. (2010). *The pedagogy of creativity*. London: Routledge.

Jackson, S. A., & Eklund, R. C. (2004). *The flow scales manual*. Morgantown: Fitness Information Technology.

Johnson, M. (2007). *The meaning of the body: Aesthetics of human understanding*. Chicago: Chicago University Press.

Kabat-Zinn, J. (1990). *Full catastrophe living: How to cope with stress, pain and illness using mindfulness meditation*. New York: Hyperion.

Kabat-Zinn, J. (1994). *Wherever you go, there you are: Mindfulness meditation for everyday life*. Westport: Hyperion.

Kaufman, J. C., & Baer, J. (Eds.). (2005). *Creativity across domains: Faces of the muse*. Mahwah: Lawrence Erlbaum Associates.

Nakamura, J., & Csikszentmihalyi, M. (2003). Creativity in later life. In Sawyer et al. (Eds.), *Creativity and development* (pp. 186–217). Oxford: University Press.

Ørsted Andersen, F., & Hanssen, N. (2013). *Flow i Hverdagen: Navigation Mellem Stress, Kaos og Kedsomhed*. København: Dansk Psykologisk Forlag.

Perry, S. K. (1999). *Writing in flow*. Cincinnati: Writer's Digest Books.

Perry, S. K. (2005). Flow and the art of fiction. In J. C. Kaufman & J. Baer (Eds.), *Creativity across domains: Faces of the muse* (pp. 23–40). Mahwah: Lawrence Erlbaum Associates.

Plucker, J. A., Beghetto, R. A., & Dow, G. (2004). Why isn't creativity more important to educational psychologists? *Educational Psychologist, 39*, 83–96.

Simonton, D. K. (2010). Creativity in highly eminent individuals. In J. C. Kaufman & R. J. Sternberg (Eds.), *The Cambridge handbook of creativity* (pp. 174–189). Cambridge: Cambridge University Press.

Weisberg, R. W. (1993). *Creativity: Beyond the myth of genius*. New York: Freeman.

Chapter 4
Flow in Sport

Christian Swann

Abstract Sport offers rich opportunities to experience flow by posing both mental and physical challenges. Studies specifically investigating flow in sport were first published in 1992. Since then a body of empirical research has emerged in this area, which this chapter aims to review in terms of: (i) the methods commonly used to study flow in sport (i.e., interviews, questionnaires, and the Experience Sampling Method); and (ii) key research themes (i.e., the experience, occurrence, controllability and correlates of flow in sport). In turn, current issues within this field are examined, and recommendations are made for future research, including the need to build towards a causal explanation of flow, and potential refinement in understanding how athletes experience these optimal states.

4.1 Introduction

Sports commonly involve highly structured, goal directed and rule-bound activities, competition with oneself and/or others, and require a high level of commitment (Kent 2006). These activities also demand either vigorous physical exertion or the use of relatively complex physical skills, which are often performed in the presence of spectators. Indeed, elements of risk (e.g., injury), exposure to environmental conditions, and interactions with teammates, coaches, opponents and referees can all be present in sporting activities. Importantly, these factors present a variety of both mental and physical challenges, meaning that sporting activities are particularly well suited to the experience of flow states (e.g., Jackson and Csikszentmihalyi 1999).

Flow is highly desirable for athletes due to its association with peak performance (Jackson and Roberts 1992; Landhäußer and Keller 2012). This relationship is particularly relevant to elite athletes for whom the margins between success and failure in competition are often extremely small (Nicholls et al. 2005). Experiencing flow also has a range of psychological benefits, such as enhanced wellbeing (Haworth 1993)

C. Swann (✉)
Early Start Research Institute, University of Wollongong, Wollongong, Australia
e-mail: cswann@uow.edu.au

L. Harmat et al. (eds.), *Flow Experience*, DOI 10.1007/978-3-319-28634-1_4

and self-concept (Jackson et al. 2001). Therefore, understanding and applying the concept of flow within sport is of great interest to athletes, coaches, practitioners (e.g., sport psychologists), and researchers.

Athletes such as rock climbers and basketball players were included in Csikszentmihalyi's (1975) original work, and the first studies of flow to be published in sport journals emerged in 1992 (Jackson 1992; Jackson and Roberts 1992; Kimiecik and Stein 1992). Since then a body of sport-specific flow research has grown, including studies that are considered classics in the field (Jackson 1995, 1996); books (e.g., Jackson and Csikszentmihalyi 1999) and academic book chapters (e.g., Jackson and Kimiecik 2008; Jackson and Eklund 2012); and reviews of this research (e.g., Swann et al. 2012a). Therefore, this field has made important progress since the early 1990s.

Despite these advances in research, however, "there is a degree of uncertainty as to when flow states occur" in sport (Chavez 2008:71). These experiences are often perceived to be elusive, rare, and unpredictable (e.g., Aherne et al. 2011), and the experience of flow has even been regarded as one of the least understood phenomena in sport (Jackson and Csikszentmihalyi 1999). Hence there are a range of unresolved and pressing issues for researchers to address. This chapter aims to review empirical research on flow in sport, in terms of: (i) the methods which have commonly been used; and (ii) empirical findings from studies into key research themes in this area. In doing so, this chapter will examine current issues within this field, and identify recommendations for future research aiming to increase opportunities for individuals to experience flow in sport.

4.2 Methods of Studying Flow in Sport

The nature of flow as a relatively brief, rare, and unpredictable state presents measurement challenges in sport. Indeed, it is suggested that "one of the greatest challenges in flow research is finding ways to assess the experience itself accurately and reliable. No single measurement approach will be able to provide trouble-free assessments of the flow experience" (Jackson and Kimiecik 2008:395). For example, psychophysiological and neuroscientific approaches have been used to study flow in other domains (e.g., de Manzano et al. 2010; Keller et al. 2011; Peifer et al. 2014; Harmat et al. 2015) however little, if any, research using these approaches has been conducted in sport as yet. This is due to issues such as the movement involved in most sporting activities which make such data collection more difficult. As a result, most research in sport has sought to measure flow *after* it has occurred, and three main methods have been employed: (i) interviews; (ii) questionnaires; and (iii) the Experience Sampling Method.

4.2.1 Interviews

The exploration of subjective experience lends itself to qualitative methods, which can provide right insights, detailed descriptions, and important understanding of flow from the athlete's perspective (e.g., Stavrou et al. 2007). In particular, semi-structured interviews have been used to investigate how athletes experience flow, and to understand the factors involved in flow occurrence. For example, Jackson's (1995, 1996) early interview-based studies with elite athletes provided some of the first insights into the experience and occurrence of flow in sport, and are some of the most-cited studies in this field. Subsequently, researchers have attempted to build on this understanding by exploring flow in different sports such as tennis (Young 2000), swimming (Bernier et al. 2009), and golf (Swann et al. 2012b, 2015a, b, 2016). Interviews can therefore be very valuable in exploratory research, especially when studying flow in new sporting contexts.

However, a criticism of interviews is that they rely on memory of events that may have occurred years ago. Due to their retrospective nature, athletes' accounts can be subject to forgetting details (Yarrow et al. 1970) or biased recall of their experiences (e.g., the "rose tinted glasses" effect; Brewer et al. 1991). Small samples appropriate for this type of research and the interpretive biases of researchers may also influence results, especially during analysis of data (Jackson and Kimiecik 2008). In some cases (e.g., Jackson 1995), researchers have provided relatively in-depth definitions of flow during interviews, which could bias the resulting accounts provided by participants (Swann et al. 2012a). Therefore, a challenge for researchers conducting interviews on flow is to introduce a state which athletes may not be immediately familiar with (Jackson 1992) in a way that does not bias their accounts (e.g., see Swann et al. 2015a, b). Researchers should also consider whether 'career-based' or 'event-focused' interviews are most suited to their design (see Swann et al. 2016). Overall, interviews are well suited to the study of subjective states such as flow, and are an important way of refining and developing understanding of flow in sport and in new settings (see Sect. 4.3 in this chapter).

4.2.2 Questionnaires

Questionnaires have also been used extensively to measure flow in sport. This approach is particularly suited to intervention research and that examining relationships between flow and other constructs. Jackson and colleagues developed various scales to assess dispositional flow (or the frequency with which flow is experienced across time) and state flow (the extent to which flow is experienced in a particular event or performance; Jackson and Eklund 2012). The Flow State Scale (FSS) and

Dispositional Flow Scale (DFS), later modified to the FSS-2 and DFS-2 (Jackson and Marsh 1996; Jackson and Eklund 2002), are considered the Long Flow Scales and are most widely used. These 36-item questionnaires have nine subscales, each with four items, to assess Csikszentmihalyi's nine flow dimensions (see Sect. 4.3.1 in this chapter), with respondents indicating their agreement with each statement on a five-point Likert scale. The FSS-2 and DFS-2 have demonstrated good reliability with FSS-2 coefficient alphas ranging between 0.76 and 0.92, and DFS-2 coefficient alphas ranging from 0.78 to 0.90 (Jackson and Eklund 2002; Jackson et al. 2008). Indeed, these scales have been translated into a range of languages including Greek (Stavrou and Zervas 2004), French (Fournier et al. 2007), and Japanese (Kawabata et al. 2007). Short Flow Scales (nine-item versions; Jackson et al. 2008) and Core Flow Scales (ten-item scales; Martin and Jackson 2008) have also been developed to offer brief and practical alternatives to the Long Scales (see Jackson and Eklund 2012).

However, there are also limitations of this approach. Kimiecik and Stein (1992) questioned the appropriateness of using quantitative, objective measures to investigate such a subjective state as flow. For example, over-reliance on questionnaires could reduce these optimal states to numbers and lose the richness of athletes' experiences. Second, FSS-2 questionnaires are distributed after a certain performance to assess any flow state within *that* performance. Given the elusive, unpredictable nature of flow (discussed above), researchers should guard against the assumption that flow will occur in any sport performance. Instead, researchers may need to distribute questionnaires after events that are more likely to be optimally-challenging (e.g., finals), and therefore more likely to facilitate flow than normal performances (Swann et al. 2012a). Third, it could be difficult to be sure that participants in performances measured by the FSS-2 were truly in a state of flow. Currently there is little guidance on how to distinguish between "macro" and "micro" flow experiences (Csikszentmihalyi 1992) using such questionnaires, or at what point participants would qualitatively agree that their experience constituted flow. As a possible revision, it would be helpful if some protocol were established to differentiate flow versus non-flow, or macro-flow from micro-flow. For example, an additional question could ask about the extent to which that athlete would describe the prior performance as flow.

4.2.3 Experience Sampling Method

The Experience Sampling Method (ESM) was developed to obtain data closer to the flow experience – ideally as it is happening (Csikszentmihalyi and Larson 1987). This method requires participants to wear a beeper or watch programmed to signal at random times during a day for a period of one week, during which self-report booklets are used to record characteristics of flow, plus factors such as mood and motivation (Jackson and Kimiecik 2008). Despite notable examples whereby researchers have used the ESM, or a modified version, effectively within sport (e.g., Delle Fave et al. 2003; Schüler and Brunner 2009; Stein et al. 1995), generally, this method has limited use in most sports for practical reasons. For example, the rules of most sports make it difficult, if not impossible, to stop and record one's thoughts and feelings at certain times – especially during competition. The ESM is also intrusive in that the mere act of stopping to reflect on one's experience could actually bring the athlete out of flow in the first place (e.g., Kimiecik and Stein 1992). While the ESM is used less frequently within sport compared to other domains, the endeavour to collect experience-near data on flow is valuable. Researchers should continue to seek alternative ways of collecting data from recent and specific flow states in sport. To achieve this, future studies are encouraged to explore novel, and perhaps mixed-method designs such as that employed by Swann et al. (2016; see Sect. 4.4.1).

4.3 Results: Empirical Research on Flow in Sport

Primary themes for research on flow in sport to date include: (i) understanding the experience of flow from the athlete's perspective; (ii) exploring flow occurrence in terms of influencing factors (i.e., those that facilitate, disrupt and prevent flow); (iii) investigating the potential of controlling and manipulating flow; and (iv) understanding relationships between flow and other constructs (e.g., mindfulness, mental toughness). The following section discusses empirical studies addressing each of these issues.

4.3.1 The Experience of Flow in Sport

Studies exploring the experience of flow in sport have tended to adopt a qualitative approach of interviewing athletes. A number of researchers have adopted a largely deductive approach to analysis whereby the emphasis was on coding data *into* Csikszentmihalyi's framework to understand the relevance of those dimensions across sport (e.g., Jackson 1996) or in specific sports including tennis (Young 2000) and swimming (Bernier et al. 2009). Other researchers have used inductive analysis to let themes/dimensions *emerge* from their data, which have been compared to Csikszentmihalyi's framework afterwards (e.g., Chavez 2008; Swann et al. 2015a). This inductive approach is suggested to encourage more critical descriptions of flow with potential for refined understanding of these experiences within specific sporting contexts (see Swann et al. 2015a for discussion).

Through the research to date, flow in sport is generally understood as nine dimensions: challenge-skill balance, clear goals, unambiguous feedback, concentration on the task at hand, sense of control, action-awareness merging, loss of self-consciousness, time transformation, and autotelic experience (see Jackson and Csikszentmihalyi 1999). In addition, studies have reported concepts that do not easily reconcile with any of the dimensions proposed by Csikszentmihalyi. Jackson's (1996) athletes reported the concepts: *aware of effort*; *remember hearing the crowd*; *feel out of body*; and *as if watching self*. Chavez's (2008) participants reported relaxed, calm aspects of the flow experience, and a heightened perception of the body. Similarly, elite swimmers reported a heightened state of bodily awareness during flow, including a strong heartbeat, a "tingling" sensation in their muscles, and heat in their extremities (Bernier et al. 2009). Elite golfers also reported altered cognitive and kinaesthetic perceptions, as well as awareness of being in flow as it occurred, (Swann et al. 2015a). It is not immediately clear as to which of Csikszentmihalyi's nine dimensions these ideas fit into, and therefore, researchers should not assume that the nine-dimension framework fits perfectly or exhaustively to the experience of flow in sport. It is unclear as to whether these extending dimensions apply across *all* sports, or vary depending on the nature/demands of certain sporting activities. However, it appears that there is scope for further investigation into, and possible refinement of, understanding of the flow experience in sport. In particular, evidence suggests that a further dimension could be developed to represent the bodily/kinaesthetic perceptions reported in these qualitative studies.

4.3.2 The Occurrence of Flow in Sport

To understand how flow occurs in sport, researchers have generally investigated the factors influencing its occurrence using a qualitative approach. In a systematic review of 17 studies in elite sport, Swann et al. (2012a) summarised ten factors which could facilitate, prevent, or disrupt flow: focus, preparation, motivation, arousal, thoughts and emotions, confidence, environmental and situational conditions, feedback, performance, and team play and interaction (see Sect. 15.6. Chap. 15 by van den Hout in this volume). In addition to these 'core' influencing factors, facilitators of flow have also emerged as specific to certain sports. For example, in a study of flow occurrence in jockeys, Jackman et al. (2014) reported *optimal relationship between horse and jockey*, and *positive horse demeanour and performance* to facilitate flow. Therefore, in regard to its occurrence, flow seems to result from the interaction of internal states (e.g., focus, arousal, motivation, confidence, thoughts and emotions), external factors (e.g., environmental and situational conditions, i.e., weather, or course that suited the athlete) and behavioural factors (e.g., preparation) – which is arguably the case across all activities.

Despite the progress made by these studies, flow is still considered to be rare, elusive and unpredictable (see the Introduction of this chapter). Little emphasis has been placed on *how* such factors influence flow. Researchers have arguably reached a point where the core influencing factors are understood (with some task-specific factors expected in new settings). The next step is to understand the mechanisms and processes of flow occurrence, that is, to move towards an explanation of these states. Indeed, most understanding of flow occurrence in sport to date is based on factors *associated* with flow or its inhibition, i.e., causality has not been explored.

New methodological approaches may be needed, such as the connecting analysis (Maxwell 2011) that Swann et al. (2015b) employed to qualitatively explore the interactions between facilitating factors and dimensions of flow in European Tour golfers. To illustrate, that study reported the caddie, effective preparation, and high-quality performance to be most influential on flow occurrence, while confidence and concentration emerged as key constructs underlying the experience. In a separate study, professional golfers reported that flow occurred as a relatively gradual build-up of confidence and momentum in the performance (Swann et al. 2016). The chronological accounts of performance enabled by event-focused interviews hold promise for further exploration of *how* influencing factors combine and interact to produce/inhibit flow, which in turn would be helpful in moving towards an explanation (see Sect. 4.4.1 in this chapter).

4.3.3 The Controllability of Flow in Sport

Investigations into the controllability of flow in sport generally aim to understand if/how flow can be enhanced (e.g., in terms of the frequency and intensity with which it is experienced). Intervention studies have attempted to increase flow using hypnosis (e.g., Pates et al. 2002), imagery (Nicholls et al. 2005), music (Pates et al. 2003), routines (Pain et al. 2011) and mindfulness (Aherne et al. 2011). In some cases, positive results have been reported, for example, in studies where increases in flow were found for all participants after the intervention (Pates et al. 2001, 2002, 2012). Aherne et al. (2011) found that athletes who underwent mindfulness training reported sizeable increases not only in global flow scores but also specifically on the dimensions of "clear goals" and "sense of control" compared to a control group. While advocating the need for further research employing larger samples before firm conclusions can be met, these findings seem to provide initial evidence for the potential of enhancing flow.

However, the results of other interventions are less convincing. For example, increases in flow were reported for only one of three participants in Lindsay et al. (2005) and two of three participants in both Pates et al. (2003) and Pates and Maynard (2000). In some cases findings were small in magnitude which, for example, "makes it unclear whether the changes in flow and performance are due to the imagery intervention" (Nicholls et al. 2005:56). Lindsay et al. (2005) also stated that their findings "do not add conclusive support" to the hypothesis that hypnosis interventions can be used to increase flow and performance (p. 173), and suggest that "there is also the possibility of a Hawthorne effect, meaning changes in performance might merely be a result of being involved in the investigation" (p. 174).

Furthermore, a number of issues are apparent in the interventions reported here. The extent to which these interventions transfer to real-world performance (i.e., their ecological validity) could be questioned as most strategies have focused on skills which athletes could only use *pre*-performance. For example, athletes are unlikely to use hypnosis or be hypnotised during competitive performance; and it is not possible to select or listen to music during competition in many sports. The skills involved should be matched to the influencing factors and dimensions of flow, and the personality characteristics of the individual. Based on the present findings, these could revolve around thorough preparation, task-focus, coping strategies, goal-setting, motivational exercises, confidence building, and arousal manipulation. Furthermore, a number of interventions have assessed flow in the execution of a specific skill, such as golf putting (Pates et al. 2001) or shooting in basketball (Pates et al. 2003). This isolation of skills could also reduce ecological validity of the intervention as flow experiences, as qualitatively reported by athletes, are arguably most likely to occur throughout every aspect of one's performance.

4.3.4 *Qualitative Findings Regarding the Control and Manipulation of Flow*

In addition to intervention studies, researchers have explored athletes' perceptions regarding the controllability of flow (e.g., Jackson 1995; Chavez 2008). On average, 66 % of elite athletes perceive flow to be controllable, with an average of 26.5 % of participants perceiving flow to be difficult or impossible to control (see Swann et al. 2012a for a review). Although these findings are specific to the elite level, it is interesting that they seem to contradict the common suggestions that flow is an elusive and unpredictable state. In addition, Chavez (2008) reported that 81 % of athletes in his sample perceived that it was possible to restore or reinstate flow after disruption. Themes including positive thinking, relaxing, clearing the mind and building confidence were reported by these athletes as factors that can restore flow. Similarly, elite golfers reported that they could manage their flow states in order to maximise and prolong the experience (Swann et al. 2015a, b). Therefore, most research to date has focused on the *initiation* of flow, but there is also great potential (e.g., from an applied perspective) to understand if/how athletes from various sports and standards can manage and manipulate flow during performance. For example, professional golfers reported that positive distraction or dissociation from the task was important for prolonging their flow states (Swann et al. 2015b).

4.3.5 *Correlates of Flow in Sport*

Correlational research has also been conducted to explore constructs related to flow in sport. Studies have referred to specific concepts or personality traits which are suggested to increase an athlete's likelihood of experiencing flow. For example, associations have been found between dispositional flow and athlete engagement (Hodge et al. 2009), mental toughness (Crust and Swann 2013), mindfulness (e.g., Cathcart et al. 2014), confidence (e.g., Koehn 2013) and high perceived ability

(Jackson and Roberts 1992), psychological skill proficiency (Jackson et al. 2001), and mastery orientation (Kowal and Fortier 1999). Flow was also reported to significantly predict athletes' performance (Stavrou et al. 2007), while relationships between skill level and flow (Catley and Duda 1997) suggest that elite athletes may experience flow more frequently than those at recreational level. These correlations can be helpful in exploring the effects or consequences of flow (e.g., performance), as well as (indirectly) some of its possible antecedents (e.g., athlete engagement).

4.4 Discussion

The aim of this chapter was to review empirical research on flow in sport, in terms of methods commonly used, and empirical findings from studies into primary research themes in this area. Since the first studies emerged in 1992, this field has grown considerably and researchers have made important contributions to knowledge of these highly sought-after psychological states. Understanding how to help individuals gain such positive experiences from sport on a regular basis holds great importance for athletes ranging from young participants to elite performers. In turn, this field has great potential for athletes, coaches, practitioners, and even governing bodies (e.g., to encourage enjoyment and engagement in their sport). While important progress has been made, there are also a number of pressing issues should be addressed by researchers aiming to continue advancing this field.

4.4.1 Future Directions in the Study of Flow in Sport

4.4.1.1 Developing an Explanation of Flow Occurrence

Issues surrounding the occurrence of flow in sport are arguably most pressing, especially considering the current lack of a causal explanation for these states, which means that flow is still perceived to be elusive. Researchers should start moving beyond identification of factors *associated* with flow, to develop understanding of *how* those factors influence its occurrence, the necessary and sufficient conditions for flow, and the mechanisms and processes through which flow occurs. This endeavour will benefit from the use of novel and innovative research designs aiming to collect "experience-near" data on flow – essentially a more practical alternative to the ESM within sport. Seifert and Hedderson (2010) could be a template for such work, as they observed participants at a skate park and then interviewed participants soon afterwards to explore whether they had experienced flow. Such a focus on specific, recent flow states holds promise in this area and could be useful for understanding flow occurrence in a way that moves beyond factors simply associated with these experiences. Preliminary support for this approach was reported using event-focused interviews with professional golfers (Swann et al. 2016), which provided a more chonological perspective of flow occurrence.

4.4.1.2 Refined Understanding of the Nature of Flow in Sport

It is also important to understand how the nature of flow may differ across sporting activities, with particular reference to a number of themes emerging in recent research. As discussed above, there is scope to develop refined understanding of how athletes experience flow in sport, including the possible expansion of Csikszentmihalyi's nine dimensions framework to encompass the heightened bodily awareness/perceptions reported in some qualitative studies (Bernier et al. 2009; Chavez 2008; Swann et al. 2015a). Researchers should seek to establish the extent to which such perceptions are reported across sports, or whether they are specific to activities of a certain type. For example, in swimming awareness of the body's state is highly relevant and almost part of the task itself, whereas other sports need reactions to changing external stimuli (e.g., tennis, soccer) and awareness of one's body could even hinder good performance.

Furthermore, elite golfers have reported awareness of being in flow as it occurs, and using specific strategies to manage and maximise their flow states (Swann et al. 2015a, b). Researchers should explore whether athletes in different types of activity report similar perceptions regarding awareness and management of flow, for example in sports with a much shorter duration (e.g., sprinting). Golfers have also reported being able to recognise flow in their competitors through factors such as body language, facial expression, and behaviour (Swann et al. 2015a). Further research on this issue with in other sports could be particularly useful from an applied perspective, and relevant to coaches and practitioners (e.g., sport psychologists). For example, if coaches can recognise when their athletes are in flow they may be able to respond accordingly in training and competition, in terms of knowing when to give advice, and when to avoid talking to (and possibly distracting) the athlete. In turn, effective management of flow by coaches has potential to enhance athletes' subjective experience, performance, and learning (i.e., during training).

Finally, there is increasing attention on team flow (e.g., Aubé et al. 2014; Walker 2010; see Chap. 15 by van den Hout at al. in this volume). Despite previous calls little attention has been placed on the possibility of team flow within sport as yet. Bakker et al. (2011) quantitatively assessed flow in soccer teams, reporting that flow at the team level is higher when the match results in a draw or a win than a loss. To supplement this initial study, qualitative exploration with athletes from team sports would provide detail and richer insights into the possibility of shared experiences of flow (e.g., using focus groups).

4.4.1.3 Flow Interventions in Sport

A multi-faceted intervention including psychological, physical and social factors may be the most appropriate approach for enhancing flow in sport, rather than testing the influence of certain mental skills on flow (as has been the case to date). The skills involved should be matched to the influencing factors and dimensions of flow, and the personality characteristics of the individual. Based on the studies reviewed in this chapter, such skills could target thorough preparation, task-focus, coping strategies, goal setting, motivational exercises, confidence building, and arousal manipulation. No such intervention appears to have been conducted as yet, presenting a further recommendation for researchers in this area.

4.4.1.4 Conclusion

Sport is a rich environment for individuals to experience flow, and for researchers to build understanding of these optimal states. While good progress has been made since the early 1990s, a number of issues remain in the study of flow in sport. The challenge for researchers in this field is to find ways of addressing them in order to help individuals flourish in sport and experience flow on a regular basis.

References

Aherne, C., Moran, A., & Londsale, C. (2011). The effect of mindfulness training on athletes' flow: An initial investigation. *The Sport Psychologist, 25*, 177–189.

Aubé, C., Brunelle, E., & Rousseau, V. (2014). Flow experience and team performance: The role of team goal commitment and information exchange. *Motivation and Emotion, 38*, 120–130.

Bakker, A., Oerlemans, W., Demerouti, E., Bruins Slot, B., & Karamat Ali, D. (2011). Flow and performance: A study among talented Dutch soccer players. *Psychology of Sport and Exercise, 12*, 442–450.

Bernier, M., Thienot, E., Codron, R., & Fournier, J. (2009). Mindfulness and acceptance approaches in sport performance. *Journal of Clinical Sports Psychology, 4*, 320–333.

Brewer, B. W., Van Raalte, J. L., Darwyn, E., & Van Raalte, N. S. (1991). Peak performance and the perils of retrospective introspection. *Journal of Sport and Exercise Psychology, 13*, 227–238.

Cathcart, S., McGregor, M., & Groundwater, E. (2014). Mindfulness and flow in elite athletes. *Journal of Clinical Sport Psychology, 8*, 119–141.

Catley, D., & Duda, J. (1997). Psychological antecedents of the frequency and intensity of flow in golfers. *International Journal of Sport Psychology, 28*, 309–322.

Chavez, E. (2008). Flow in sport: A study of college athletes. *Imagination, Cognition and Personality, 28*, 69–91.

Crust, L., & Swann, C. (2013). The relationship between mental toughness and dispositional flow. *European Journal of Sport Science, 13*, 215–220.

Csikszentmihalyi, M. (1975). *Beyond boredom and anxiety*. San Francisco: Jossey-Bass.

Csikszentmihalyi, M. (1992). A response to the Kimiecik & Stein and Jackson papers. *Journal of Applied Sport Psychology, 4*, 181–183.

Csikszentmihalyi, M., & Larson, R. (1987). Validity and reliability of the experience-sampling method. *The Journal of Nervous and Mental Disease, 175*, 526–536.

De Manzano, O., Theorell, T., Harmat, L., & Ullén, F. (2010). The psychophysiology of flow during piano playing. *Emotion, 10*, 301–311.

Delle Fave, A., Bassi, M., & Massimini, F. (2003). Quality of experience and risk perception in high-altitude rock climbing. *Journal of Applied Sport Psychology, 15*, 82–98.

Fournier, J., Gaudreau, P., Demontrond-Behr, P., Visioli, J., Forest, J., & Jackson, S. (2007). French translation of the flow state scale-2: Factor structure, cross-cultural invariance, and associations with goal attainment. *Psychology of Sport and Exericse, 8*, 897–916.

Harmat, L., de Manzano, O., Theorell, T., Högman, L., Fischer, H., & Ullén, F. (2015). Physiological correlates of the flow experience during computer game playing. *International Journal of Psychophysiology, 97*, 1–7.
Haworth, J. (1993). Skills-challenge relationships and psychological well-being in everyday life. *Society & Leisure, 16*, 115–128.
Hodge, K., Lonsdale, C., & Jackson, S. (2009). Athlete engagement in sport: An exploratory investigation of antecedents and consequences. *The Sport Psychologist, 23*, 186–202.
Jackman, P., Van Hout, M., Lane, A., & Fitzpatrick, G. (2014). Experiences of flow in jockeys during flat-race conditions. *International Journal of Sport and Exercise Psychology*. doi:10.1080/1612197X.2014.956327.
Jackson, S. (1992). Athletes in flow: A qualitative investigation of flow states in elite figure skaters. *Journal of Applied Sport Psychology, 4*, 161–180.
Jackson, S. (1995). Factors influencing the occurrence of flow state in elite athletes. *Journal of Applied Sport Psychology, 7*, 138–166.
Jackson, S. (1996). Toward a conceptual understanding of the flow experience in elite athletes. *Research Quarterly for Exercise & Sport, 67*, 76–90.
Jackson, S., & Csikszentmihalyi, M. (1999). *Flow in sports: The keys to optimal experiences and performances*. Champaign: Human Kinetics.
Jackson, S., & Eklund, R. C. (2002). Assessing flow in physical activity: The flow state scale-2 and dispositional flow scale-2. *Journal of Sport and Exercise Psychology, 24*, 133–150.
Jackson, S., & Eklund, R. (2012). Flow. In G. Tenenbaum, R. Eklund, & A. Kamata (Eds.), *Measurement in sport and exercise psychology* (pp. 349–358). Champaign: Human Kinetics.
Jackson, S., & Kimiecik, J. (2008). Optimal experience in sport and exercise. In T. Horn (Ed.), *Advances in sport psychology* (3rd ed., pp. 377–399). Champaign: Human Kinetics.
Jackson, S., & Marsh, H. (1996). Development and validation of a scale to measure optimal experience: The flow state scale. *Journal of Sport and Exercise Psychology, 18*, 17–35.
Jackson, S., & Roberts, G. (1992). Positive performance state of athletes: Towards a conceptual understanding of peak performance. *Sport Psychologist, 6*, 156–171.
Jackson, S., Kimiecik, J., Ford, S., & Marsh, H. (1998). Psychological correlates of flow in sport. *Journal of Sport and Exercise Psychology, 20*, 358–378.
Jackson, S., Thomas, P., Marsh, H., & Smethurst, C. (2001). Relationships between flow, self-concept, psychological skills, and performance. *Journal of Applied Sport Psychology, 13*, 129–153.
Jackson, S., Martin, A. J., & Eklund, R. C. (2008). Long and short measures of flow: Examining construct validity of the FSS-2, DFS-2 and new brief counterparts. *Journal of Sport and Exercise Psychology, 30*, 561–587.
Kawabata, M., Mallett, C., & Jackson, S. (2007). The flow state scale-2 and dispositional flow scale-2: Examination of factorial validity and reliability for Japanese adults. *Psychology of Sport and Exercise, 9*, 465–485.
Keller, J., Bless, H., Blomann, F., & Kleinböhl, D. (2011). Physiological aspects of flow experiences: Skills-demand-compatibility effects on heart rate variability and salivary cortisol. *Journal of Experimental Social Psychology, 47*, 849–852.
Kent, M. (2006). *The Oxford dictionary of sports science and medicine* (3rd ed.). Oxford: Oxford University Press.
Kimiecik, J., & Stein, G. (1992). Examining flow experiences in sport contexts: Conceptual issues and methodological concerns. *Journal of Applied Sport Psychology, 4*, 144–160.
Koehn, S. (2013). Effects of confidence and anxiety on flow state in competition. *European Journal of Sport Science, 13*, 543–550.
Kowal, J., & Fortier, M. (1999). Motivational determinants of flow: Contributions from self-determination theory. *Journal of Social Psychology, 139*, 355–368.
Landhäußer, A., & Keller, J. (2012). Flow and its affective, cognitive, and performance-related consequences. In S. Engeser (Ed.), *Advances in flow research* (pp. 65–86). New York: Springer.

Lindsay, P., Maynard, I., & Thomas, O. (2005). Effects of hypnosis on flow states and cycling performance. *The Sport Psychologist, 19*, 164–177.

Martin, A., & Jackson, S. (2008). Brief approaches to assessing task absorption and enhanced subjective experience: Examining 'short' and 'core' flow in diverse performance domains. *Motivation and Emotion, 32*, 141–157.

Maxwell, J. (2011). *A realist approach for qualitative methods*. Thousand Oaks: Sage.

Nicholls, A., Polman, R., & Holt, N. (2005). The effects of individualized imagery interventions on golf performance and flow States. *Athletic Insight, 7*, 43–64.

Pain, M., Harwood, C., & Anderson, R. (2011). Pre-competition imagery and music: The impact on flow and performance in competitive soccer. *The Sport Psychologist, 25*, 212–232.

Pates, J., & Maynard, I. (2000). Effects of hypnosis on flow states and golf performance. *Perceptual and Motor Skills, 91*, 1057–1075.

Pates, J., Oliver, R., & Maynard, I. (2001). The effects of hypnosis on flow states and golf putting performance. *Journal of Applied Sport Psychology, 13*, 341–354.

Pates, J., Cummings, A., & Maynard, I. (2002). The effects of hypnosis on flow states and three-point shooting performance in basketball players. *The Sport Psychologist, 16*, 34–47.

Pates, J., Karageorghis, C., Fryer, R., & Maynard, I. (2003). Effects of asynchronous music on flow states and shooting performance among netball players. *Psychology of Sport and Exercise, 4*, 415–427.

Pates, J., Cowen, A. P., & Karageorghis, C. I. (2012). The effect of a client-centered approach on flow states and the performance of three elite golfers. *International Journal of Golf Science, 1*, 113–126.

Peifer, C., Schulz, A., Schächinger, H., Baumann, N., & Conny, H. A. (2014). The relation of flow experience and physiological arousal under stress – can u shape it? *Journal of Experimental Social Psychology, 53*, 62–6b9.

Russell, W. (2001). An examination of flow state occurrence in college athletes. *Journal of Sport Behaviour, 24*, 83–99.

Schüler, J., & Brunner, S. (2009). The rewarding effect of flow experience on performance in a marathon race. *Psychology of Sport and Exercise, 10*, 168–174.

Seifert, T., & Hedderson, C. (2010). Intrinsic motivation and flow in skateboarding: An ethnographic study. *Journal of Happiness Studies, 11*, 277–292.

Stavrou, N., & Zervas, Y. (2004). Confirmatory factor analysis of flow state scale in sports. *International Journal of Sport and Exercise Psychology, 2*, 161–181.

Stavrou, N., Jackson, S., Zervas, Y., & Karteroliotis, K. (2007). Flow experience and athletes' performance with reference to the orthogonal model of flow. *The Sport Psychologist, 21*, 438–457.

Stein, G., Kimiecik, J., Daniels, J., & Jackson, S. (1995). Psychological antecedents of flow in recreational sport. *Personality and Social Psychology Bulletin, 25*, 125–135.

Swann, C., Keegan, R., Piggott, D., & Crust, L. (2012a). A systematic review of the experience, occurrence, and controllability of flow in elite sport. *Psychology of Sport and Exercise, 13*(6), 807–819.

Swann, C., Keegan, R., Piggott, D., Crust, L., & Smith, M. F. (2012b). Exploring flow occurrence in elite golf. *Athletic Insight, 4*, 171–186.

Swann, C., Crust, L., Keegan, R., Piggott, D., & Hemmings, B. (2015a). An inductive exploration into the experience of flow in European Tour golfers. *Qualitative Research in Sport, Exercise and Health, 7*, 210–234.

Swann, C., Piggott, D., Crust, L., Keegan, R., & Hemmings, B. (2015b). Exploring the interactions underlying flow states: A connecting analysis of flow occurrence in European Tour golfers. *Psychology of Sport and Exercise, 16*, 60–69.

Swann, C., Keegan, R., Crust, L., & Piggott, D. (2016). Psychological states underlying excellent performance in professional golfers: "Letting it happen" vs. "making it happen". *Psychology of Sport and Exercise, 23*, 101–113.

Walker, C. (2010). Experiencing flow: Is doing it together better than doing it alone? *Journal of Positive Psychology, 5*, 3–11.

Yarrow, M. R., Campbell, J. D., & Burton, R. V. (1970). Recollections of childhood: A study of the retrospective method. *Monographs of the Society for Research in Child Development, 35*, 1–83.

Young, J. A. (2000). Professional tennis players in the zone. In S. J. Haake & A. Coe (Eds.), *Tennis science and technology* (pp. 417–422). Malden: Blackwell Science.

Chapter 5
Running and Flow: Does Controlled Running Lead to Flow-States? Testing the Transient Hypofontality Theory

Oliver Stoll and Jan M. Pithan

Abstract This chapter presents a summary of three studies, using treadmill running in a laboratory context, measuring flow-states via self-report data. To situate the theoretical context of the studies, Dietrich's (Conscious Cogn 12:231–256, 2003). Transient Hypofrontality Theory (THT) is outlined, to show that flow-states are theorized in this work as being as a result of a down-regulated prefrontal cortex. Also, other neuropsychological research into flow is summarized to build the justification of our three projects. Two non-experimental studies show that flow-states can be induced in a laboratory setting, using a specific workload approach on treadmill or bicycle ergometer. In the third, an experimental study, prefrontal tasks were manipulated while participants were running on a treadmill. The results show that the participants in the control condition (reacting to a visual stimulus) reported significant higher flow-scores than in the experimental-condition (calculating numbers). Participants showed no differences in verbal ability between the conditions. Individuals in the experimental condition showed a decreasing running pace on the treadmill compared to the control-group. The results indicated that down-regulated prefrontal cortex activity could be a possible underlying mechanism of flow-states, which might support the THT.

5.1 Introduction

Research into flow-states in sport has a long-standing tradition, since Csikszentmihalyi (1995) published studies in this field. Mostly, endurance sports like running have been used. Our previous research with runners sought empirical evidence for preconditions of flow-experiences (e.g. the demand-ability-fit) or a relationship between flow-experiences and performance (Stoll and Lau 2005). In two studies, we analysed one of the apparent conditions for flow-states, after Csikszentmihalyi et al. (2005) postulated that one must have a good balance between the perceived

O. Stoll (✉) • J.M. Pithan
Martin-Luther-University Halle-Wittenberg Halle (Saale), Halle, Germany
e-mail: oliver.stoll@sport.uni-halle.de

L. Harmat et al. (eds.), *Flow Experience*, DOI 10.1007/978-3-319-28634-1_5

challenges of the task at hand and one's own perceived skills, leading to confidence in one's ability to complete the task at hand.

In study 1, 160 runners who participated in a city marathon completed the Flow-Short-Scale (Rheinberg et al. 2003). We focused on 'flow' as a one-dimensional factor and related this to subjective and objective demand-ability-fit appraisals as well as to marathon-finishing times. The results could not confirm that the demand-ability fit is an obligatory circumstance to experience flow-states in marathon running. We found no correlations, either, between performance and flow for runners with marathon finishing-performances between 3 and 4 h.

In study 2 (Stoll and Lau 2005), we replicated the above design but also asked runners before the start to predict their finishing-time in the marathon, to compare that with their actual finishing time (to gauge their acuity in evaluating their performance). Results showed that there was no correlation between performance and flow-states in general, but that runners who anticipated their finishing time more accurately scored higher in flow than runners who were inaccurate. It seemed that it was not a simple subjective demand-ability fit in a specific situation that leads to flow, but rather the ability of runners' to accurately appraise their performance skills in relation to an expected result. We concluded that further research was needed into the trigger and the preconditions for flow-states need to be further understood.

With regard to explanatory theories, we found that not only cognitive approaches are relevant. Beside the endorphin-theory (Stoll 1997), which is highly debated in the scientific community as it may lack plausibility, other psychophysiological approaches have been proposed (e.g. the endocannabinoid-approach, Sparling et al. 2003). Neurotransmission in the dopaminergic system seems to play a role in flow disposition or proneness (de Manzano et al. 2013), while sympathetic arousal in the form of physiological stress shows a non-linear correlation with flow-experience (Peifer et al. 2014) with highest flow scores being reported under moderate stress. Ulrich et al. (2014) found correlations between activation in prefrontal, frontal cortex and amygdala and subjective flow-experience, supporting the idea that flow has a neurophysiological basis. However, the cortical oxygen level's relationship between flow and downregulation of the frontal cortex remains unclear (Harmat et al. 2015). All approaches that focus on just one mechanism fail to fully explain flow-states because they ignore related approaches from other disciplines. More holistic theoretical approaches like those from cognitive neuroscience might be helpful (Dietrich 2003, 2007).

This chapter therefore now summarises previous work in the cognitive neurosciences that might also account for the phenomenon of flow-experiences. One idea is that when the brain is under high effort, it may start to reserve its limited metabolic resources for operations that are critically needed at the time, which results necessarily in the downregulation of neural structures whose computations are not critical for the task at hand (Ferris et al. 2007; Goldstein and Kopin 2007). Dietrich (2006) supposes that, as the strain continues, the brain is forced to go ever deeper into a safe mode. Transient Hypofrontality Theory (THT) suggests that this decline progresses from brain areas that support the highest cognitive functions, down the functional hierarchy, one phenomenological subtraction at a time, to brain areas supporting the most basic ones (Brisswalter et al. 2002). The prefrontal cortex, being the most zenithal higher-order structure, is the first region whose computations may no longer be supported sufficiently to support self-consciousness. Prolonged, physical exercise is simply one example of a general neural mechanism that accounts for the phenomenology of various altered states of consciousness that involve the experience of timelessness, living in the here and now, reduced awareness of one's surroundings, and diminished analytical or attentional capacities (Larson and von Eye 2010).

Subtle modifications of mental functions that are typically ascribed to the prefrontal cortex, such as during meditation, are consistent with a state of frontal hypofunction (Brewer et al. 2011). To understand the neurocognitive mechanisms underlying flow-states it is required to accept the proposition that the brain runs two functionally and anatomically distinct information-processing systems, the explicit and implicit system (Dietrich and Stoll 2010) and that we rigorously apply the flexibility-efficiency tradeoff that exists between these two systems to the computational problem of skilled motor performance (Dietrich and Stoll 2010). These two systems operate on a continuum between flexibility (explicit) and efficiency (implicit).

In addition, the transient hypofrontality theory, which can account for the phenomenological features of autotelic experiences such as the merging of awareness and action, symptoms such as excluding of distractions, loss of the sense of time passing, or the lack of worry of possible failure are briefly outlined (Dietrich 2007, p. 275). These are all higher-order metacognitive processes that require, in order to be subtracted from consciousness, downregulation of relevant brain regions, primarily in the prefrontal cortex, that play a key role in the computation of these higher-order thoughts and feelings in the first place (Dietrich 2003). This hypothesis will now be described and analysed in more detail.

5.2 Transient Hypofrontality Theory (THT)

The Transient Hypofrontality Theory (THT) proposes a common neural mechanism for flow-states, especially related to at least three phenomenological descriptions of flow-states: sense of time becomes distorted, action and awareness are merged and focused attention is constant (Dietrich 2004). The theory is explicitly based on functional neuroanatomy and views consciousness as composed of various attributes, such as self-reflection, attention, memory, perception and arousal, which are ordered in a functional hierarchy with the frontal lobe necessary for the top attributes (Dietrich 2003, 2007). Although this implies a holistic view in which the entire brain contributes to consciousness, it is evident that not all neural structures contribute equally to conscious experience (Llinás et al. 1998; Shushruth 2013). This layering concept localizes the most sophisticated levels of consciousness in the higher, more explicit cognitive structures, the prefrontal cortex (Dietrich 2003, 2007).

From such considerations, the THT of altered states of consciousness can be formulated, which attempts to unify other reported altered states, such as long-distance running, meditation or hypnosis into a single theoretical framework. Because the prefrontal cortex is the neural substrate of the topmost layers, any change to conscious experience should affect, first and foremost, this structure (Knight and Grabowecky 2000). In this way the central nervous system manages to spare resources for necessary cognitive functions, like the reactivity to novel stimuli (Knight and Grabowecky 2000). Put another way, the highest layers of consciousness are most susceptible to change when brain activity changes/ shortage of resources is pending (Del Giorno et al. 2010). It follows from this "onion-peeling" principle that higher cognitive processes such as working memory, sustained and directed attention, and temporal integration are compromised first when an alteration to mental status occurs (Dietrich 2006). All altered states share phenomenological characteristics whose proper functions are regulated by the prefrontal cortex, such as time distortions, disinhibition from social norms, or a change in focused attention.

This suggests that the neural mechanism common to other altered states, as in a flow-experience (and seen and defined as: action and awareness are merged, distractions are excluded from consciousness, there is no worry of failure, Self-consciousness disappears, the sense of time becomes distorted) could be explained as the transient downregulation of functional networks in the prefrontal cortex (Dietrich 2004, 2007, p. 275). The reduction of specific contents to conscious experience is known as phenomenological subtraction. The deeper an altered state becomes, induced by the progressive downregulation of prefrontal regions, the more of those subtractions occur and people experience an ever greater departure from their normal phenomenology (Limb and Braun 2008). In altered states that are characterized by severe prefrontal hypoactivity – various drug states such as those induced by LSD or PCP, for instance – this change results in an extraordinarily bizarre phenomenology – hallucinations and delusions, most prominently. In altered states that are characterized by less prefrontal hypoactivity, such as long-distance running, meditation or hypnosis, the modification to consciousness is much more subtle (Dietrich 2003). In any event, the individual simply functions on the highest layer of phenomenological consciousness that remains fully operational. A consequence of the THT is that full-fledged consciousness is the result only of a fully operational brain.

5.3 Further Neuropsychological Research Into the THT

Dietrich and Sparling (2004) conducted two experiments to examine the possibility that different exercises selectively influence different types of cognition. These two experiments represented the first attempt to study higher-cognitive processes during exercise. Theoretically these studies are based on the central assumptions of the THT. In both experiments, athletes who exercised at a sustained, moderate pace (for

Table 5.1 Pearson correlations between the flow-dimensions and finishing time

1	2	3	4	5
Flow-sum	Smooth run	Feeling absorbed	Rumouring/concerns	Finishing time
1	0.87**	0.74**	0.12	−0.11
2	1	0.31**	0.01	−0.08
3		1	0.22*	−0.10
4			1	−0.05

*<.05, **<.01

65 min) were compared to sedentary controls on two neuropsychological tests, one that is generally regarded as heavily dependent on prefrontal cognition and one that is relatively irrelevant to prefrontal operation. To measure prefrontal-dependent cognition, they used the Paced Auditory Serial Addition Task (PASAT). This test consists of four series of 50 numbers from 1 to 9 presented at increasing speeds (2.4, 2.0, 1.6, and 1.2 s per digit). To measure prefrontal-independent cognition in Experiment 2, the Peabody Picture Vocabulary Test (PPVT-III) was administered. Results showed that during the exercise test, performances demanding prefrontal-dependent cognition were impaired, compared to the sedentary control group participants, while at the same time, cognitive processes requiring little prefrontal activity were unaffected.

We followed this idea, to conduct a series of studies in our own flow-research-program, seeking empirical evidence for the THT. As outlined in our introduction, in the first study, we tried to induce flow-experiences in runners on a treadmill (Reinhardt et al. 2006). For many decades, physical activity has been central to flow research, and continuous diagnostic studies of the flow construct have been needed. However, field studies that analyse the trigger mechanisms of flow experiences as well as the flow-performance correlation show inconsistent results (Stoll and Lau 2005).

In our first cross sectional study (Stoll and Lau 2005), flow-experiences and performance of 160 marathon-runners were investigated. In this study we used the Flow Short-Scale (Rheinberg et al. 2003) to measure flow-experiences (as self-report). This scale can be analysed as a sum-score, or divided in the subscales "feeling absorbed" and "smooth run". Furthermore three further items measure "Rumouring/Concerns" and "Optimal fit between demands and abilities". If an athlete e.g. responded with a "5" in 1–9 Likert-scale, he reported an optimal demand-ability fit. We divided the sample into two groups: (1) Optimal Fit-Reporters and (2) Non-Optimal-Fit Reporters. Flow-Sum-Score acted as dependant variable. A t-test showed no significant differences in flow between Optimal- and Non-Optimal-Fit-Reporters ($t=1.53$, $p=0.69$). Nevertheless, a comparison between OptimalFit-Reporters and Non-Optimal-Fit-Reporters and Finishing Times as dependant variable showed a significant difference ($t=3.54$, $p=0.04$). OptimalFit-Reports run faster than Non-Optimal-Fit Reporters. Furthermore we correlated flow-experiences and finishing-time. The result can be seen in Table 5.1.

Flow correlates with its subdimensions quite high, but not with "Rumouring/Concerns" and also not with performance.

Table 5.2 Descriptives: flow-sum-scores, demand, ability, and demand-ability-fit (D.-A.-Fit) over the running time

Dimension	Value	10 min	20 min	30 min	40 min	Total
Flow-score	M	5.67	5.71	5.64	5.24	5.57
	SD	0.77	1.03	1.01	0.73	0.79
Demand	M	5.53	5.63	5.83	5.83	5.70
	SD	1.72	1.40	1.34	1.32	1.18
Ability	M	5.33	5.17	5.20	5.27	5.24
	SD	1.40	1.49	1.47	1.51	1.41
D.-A.-Fit	M	5.03	5.23	5.20	5.27	5.18
	SD	1.52	1.14	1.27	1.37	1.16

Note: Flow-score ranges from 1 (low) to 7 (high). Demand, Ability and D.-A-Fit ranges from 1 to 9, 5 = "optimal demand", "optimal ability" and "optimal demand-ability-fit"

Since absolute running performance is not necessarily a good predisposition for an optimal demand-ability fit, because planned finishing times differ very much in a marathon runners field, we conducted a second study (also in Stoll and Lau 2005). Seventy-four runners completed the Flow-Short-Scale, but we asked them predict their planned finishing-times pre-race. Some were reliable performance-estimater and some were not reliable (either under or over-estimating their finishing times). Using the analysis-steps of the first study, we found in the second study a significant difference between "Optimal-Fit-Reporter" and "Non-Optimal-Fit-Reporter" and Flow-Sum-Score as dependent variables, due to the fact that the "Optimal-Fit-Reporter" scored higher in the Flow-Sum-Score ($t=3.04$, $p=0.003$). We replicated the result that flow and absolute finishing times are not related ($r=-0.08$, $p=ns$), and we could not find an effect of "under-, over- or optimal finishing-time-estimator", using flow-sum-score as a dependant variable ($F=0.01$, $p=0.93$).

For this reason, we conducted further research, the aim of which was (1) to analyse if the postulated demand-ability-fit (Csikszentmihalyi 1995) of runners under laboratory conditions is a precondition for the development of flow-experiences and (2) to document the dynamics of flow-experiences in a continuous performance situation as well as the correlation of flow experiences with physiological variables.

Using the demand-oriented speed regulation of the treadmill, we succeeded to get all runners ($n=30$) to run to an individually above average demand-level and let them run in this condition for 40 min. We used a specific treadmill that is able to regulate individually the speed of the runners based on a pre-test in heart-rate variability (Pulsar, h/p/Cosmos 30). The target workload zone was individually calculated up to 80 % of the maximal heart-rate capacity of each individual runner (Laukkanen et al. 1998; Tulppo et al. 1996). Summarizing the main results of this study, it could be shown that runners report a continuous deep and stable flow-experience, as measured with the *Flow-Short-Scale*, (Rheinberg et al. 2003) every 10 min while running in the calculated target workload zone (Table 5.2). Flow-Scores were above 5 (Maximum-Score = 7) while the individuals were running.

Table 5.3 Pearson product moment correlations (*p<0.5) of the flow sub-scales and demand-ability-fit over the running time

Dimension	10 min	20 min	30 min	40 min
Flow sum-score	0.127	0.272	0.248	0.230
Smooth run	0.025	0.155	0.237	0.180
Feeling absorbed	0.227	0.366*	0.206	0.207

Table 5.4 Physiological parameters over the running time (descriptives)

Parameter	Values	10 min	20 min	30 min	40 min
Lactate (mmol/l)	M	4.21	3.36	3.13	2.99
	SD	1.62	1.24	1.08	0.68
Running speed (km/h)	M	10.30	9.81	9.51	9.16
	SD	2.10	1.85	1.98	1.75
Heart rate (beat per minute, BPM)	M	171.10	171.10	171.10	171.10
	SD	8.70	8.70	8.70	8.70

Table 5.5 Pearson product moment correlations (*p<0.5) of the dimension "Demand" of the flow-short scale and lactate and running speed

Parameter	N	10 min	20 min	30 min	40 min
Lactate (mmol/l)	30	0.333	0.425*	−0.228	−0.083
Running speed (km/h)	30	0.026	0.106	0.086	0.029

These flow-experiences experiences were independent from subjective reports of a demand-ability fit. This D-A-Fit correlates with low positively with Feeling Absorbed after 20 min continuous running in the heart-rate target zone. All other correlations are even lower and not significant (see Table 5.3). Our analysis showed furthermore that the correlations between the physiological parameters (e.g. lactate) and the subjective demand-appraisal support the research paradigm that runners can be led into an individually controlled "demand-ability-situation" under laboratory conditions. While running, the lactate of participants is close to the aerobic-anaerobic threshold, which shows that the individuals ran with high intensively (Table 5.4) and the Demand-subdimension from the Flow-Short-Scale correlates positively with lactate, which again shows that flow-experiences need a high intensive running workload (Table 5.5).

In a further study, we tried to replicate these results in a clinical setting. If flow-experiences are the consequence of a downregulated prefrontal cortex and if this downregulation can be induced by high-intensive endurance workload, this approach could be effective in a running therapy context for the treatment of depression. One symptom of depression is that patients suffer from rumination, which is dependent on prefrontal-cortex- activity.

Reinhardt et al. (2008) ran a study using the above-mentioned work-load-regulation to induce flow to 31 adult volunteers with moderate depressive disorders. Using a load-oriented and speed regulating bicycle-ergometer, the participants were kept within an individual demand-level and cycled in this condition for 40 continuous minutes. Flow-state was measured using the Flow-Short Scale (Rheinberg et al. 2003) during the activity. Effects of mood variations were assessed immediately before and after the training using a profile of mood-questionnaire (BFS; Abele and Brehm 1986). According to the main results, the participants reported (confirming study 1) a continuous, deep and stable flow-experience. The effects of mood variation can thus be illustrated in the form of an iceberg profile, which means that negative emotions decreased and positive emotions increased.

A third study, using this paradigm was conducted by Saad Al Youssef (2012). Using a within-subjects design and two different neuropsychological tests, a comparable pattern of impairment emerged in this experiment. Thirty-three participants (11 female, 22 male) had to run on a treadmill, again following our workload paradigm for 30 min in a given, individual demand-level. The determination of the heart-rate target zone (OwnZone) was based on the calculation of the individual heart-rate-variability (Laukkanen et al. 1998; Tulppo et al. 1996). For this study, we used the already above mentioned treadmill (Pulsar 30/h/p Cosmos) which adjusts the velocity speed on the individual calculated heart-rate-variability to a given time. The area of the *OwnZone* was chosen "hard", which is approximately 80–90 % of the maximal heart rate. In the experimental condition participants had to fulfill a prefrontal-dependent cognition-test, while running. In a control condition (on another day), participants had to complete a prefrontal-independent test, while running. We expected that the participants would score lower on flow-experiences in experimental condition compared to the control condition.

To measure prefrontal-dependent cognition, we used a sub-test of the Wechsler-Intelligence-Test (Wechsler 2008), in detail the sub-test *Mathematical Thinking*. The test consists of given numbers, which have to be down-calculated in steps of three-number-blocks in a given time (22 calculation-tasks). To measure prefrontal-independent cognition participants had to react to a given visual stimulus (a red cross) on a monitor fixed to the treadmill. Performance on *Mathematical Thinking*, which measures sustained attention and working memory ability, was impaired in subjects when running, but not when tested in the control condition (not prefrontal-dependent task, the stimulus-reaction-test). In 30 min the experimental-test condition (or the control-test-condition) flow-experiences were also measured three times (using the Flow-Short-Scale; Rheinberg et al. 2003). The results showed that the participants in the control condition (just reacting on a visual stimulus) reported significantly higher flow-scores than in the experimental-condition (calculating numbers). Participants showed no differences in verbal ability between the conditions. Furthermore individuals in the experimental condition showed a decreasing running pace, while running on the treadmill compared to the control-group-individuals.

5.4 Discussion

The results reported here provide indirect evidence in favour of the hypothesis that prolonged exercise might result in a state of transient hypofrontality. Only a few studies reported indirectly a downregulation of the prefrontal cortex during exercise (e.g. Dietrich and Sparling 2004). However, the cognitive testing in these studies was limited to either basic choice reaction time and/or visual recognition tasks. These tasks represent comparatively simple decisional paradigms that are not sufficiently selective to evaluate changes in specific higher-cognitive abilities that may occur during exercise. Our results that higher-cognitive functioning is selectively impaired during exercise do not run counter to the findings that performance on simpler cognitive tasks is enhanced during exercise. Nevertheless these findings, even considering methodological limitations, may suggest that flow-experiences are due to a down-regulated prefrontal cortex. At the very least, these results indicate that during endurance exercise different cognitive functions are affected to different degrees.

The converging evidence from several psychometric tests that are widely accepted as indicative of specific cognitive impairments, multiple exercise modes, various exercise lengths, and different experimental designs permit the more advanced conclusion that endurance exercise selectively compromises prefrontal-dependent executive functions such as working memory, sustained attention, and the ability to inhibit habitual responses (Dietrich and Sparling 2004). The failure of concomitant deficits on two cognitively taxing prefrontal-independent tasks, coupled with the fact that physiological measures were carefully controlled, argues strongly against a general cognitive decline, general arousal, and/or fatigue explanation. Future research will have to address a number of issues related to the finding that endurance exercise selectively and transiently impairs prefrontal-dependent psychological processes.

Although several EEG studies have already demonstrated that treadmill running of the same intensity used in the present study reduces prefrontal activity (for a review, see Kubitz and Pothakos 1997), it would be highly desirable to replicate the present results in a study that also makes use of physiological measures. Additionally, other neuro-imaging measures such as optical imaging or EEG combined with other selective neuropsychological measures in a sports- and exercise-setting are needed to further explore the complex interaction between exercise and mental function.

Recent advances in psychology and neuroscience have greatly enhanced our understanding of the contribution of the prefrontal cortex to cognition. In the future, this knowledge will allow exercise scientists to ask more specific questions regarding the effects of exercise on cognition and furthermore its function to altered states of consciousness. Using a novel methodology that makes use of this knowledge, the data of Dietrich and Sparling (2004) and our data (Saad Al Youssef 2012) are the first to show changes in higher-cognitive functions during an actual exercise bout and thus represent a possible start in that direction.

References

Abele, A., & Brehm, W. (1986). Zur Konzeptualisierung und Messung von Befindlichkeit. Die Entwicklung der Befindlichkeitsskalen (BFS) [Conceptualization and measurement of mood – the development of a mood-profile (BFS)]. *Diagnostica, 32*, 209–228.

Brewer, J. A., Worhunsky, P. D., Gray, J. R., Tang, Y., Weber, J., & Kober, H. (2011). Meditation experience is associated with differences in default mode network activity and connectivity. *Proceedings of the National Academy of Science of the United States of America, 108*(50), 20254–20259.

Brisswalter, J., Collardeau, M., & René, A. (2002). Effects of acute physical exercise characteristics on cognitive performance. *Sport Medicine, 32*(9), 555–566.

Csikszentmihalyi, M. (1995). *Beyond boredom an anxiety*. San Francisco: Jossey-Bass.

Csikszentmihalyi, M., Abuhamdeh, S., & Nakamura, J. (2005). Flow. In A. Elliot (Ed.), *Handbook of competence and motivation* (pp. 598–698). New York: The Guilford Press.

de Manzano, Ö., Cervenka, S., Jucaite, A., Hellenäs, O., Farde, L., & Ullén, F. (2013). Individual differences in the proneness to have flow experiences are linked to dopamine D2- induced flow experiences. *NeuroImage, 86*, 194–202.

Del Giorno, J. M., Hall, E. E., O'Leary, K. C., Bixby, W. R., & Miller, P. C. (2010). Cognitive function during acute exercise A test of the transient hypofrontality theory. *Journal of Sports and Exercise Psychology, 32*, 312–323.

Dietrich, A. (2003). Functional neuroanatomy of altered states of consciousness. The transient hypofrontality hypothesis. *Consciousness and Cognition, 12*, 231–256.

Dietrich, A. (2004). Neurocognitive mechanisms underlying the experience of flow. *Consciousness and Cognition, 13*, 746–761.

Dietrich, A. (2006). Transient hypofrontality as a mechanism for the psychological effects of exercise. *Psychiatry Research, 145*, 79–83.

Dietrich, A. (2007). *Introduction to consciousness*. London: Palgrave Macmillan.

Dietrich, A., & Sparling, P. B. (2004). Endurance exercise selectively impairs prefrontal-dependent cognition. *Brain and Cognition, 55*, 516–524.

Dietrich, A., & Stoll, O. (2010). Effortless attention in sports performance. In B. J. Bruya (Ed.), *Effortless attention: A new perspective in the cognitive science of attention and action* (pp. 159–178). Cambridge: MIT Press.

Ferris, L. T., Williams, J. S., & Shen, C. L. (2007). The effect of acute exercise on serum brain-derived neurotrophic factor levels and cognitive function. *Medicine and Science in Sports and Exercise, 39*(4), 728–734.

Goldstein, D., & Koppin, I. J. (2007). Evolution of concepts of stress. *Stress, 10*(2), 109–120.

Harmat, L., de Manzano, Ö., Theorell, T., Fischer, H., & Ullén, F. (2015). Physiological correlates of the flow experience during computer game playing. *International Journal of Psychophysiology, 97*, 1–7.

Knight, R. T., & Grabowecky, M. (2000). Prefrontal cortex, time and consciousness. In M. S. Gazzaniga (Ed.), *The new cognitive neurosciences* (pp. 1319–1339). Cambridge, MA: MIT Press.

Kubitz, K. A., & Pothakos, K. (1997). Does aerobic exercise decrease brain activation? *Journal of Sport & Exercise Psychology, 19*, 291–301.

Larson, E., & von Eye, A. (2010). Beyond flow: Temporality and participation in everyday activities. *American Journal of Occupational Therapy, 64*, 152–163.

Laukkanen, R. M. T., Maijanen, S., & Tulppo, M. P. (1998). Determination of heart rates for training using Polar Smartedge heart rate monitor. *Medicine and Science in Sports and Exercise, 30*(5), 1430.

Limb, C. J., & Braun, A. R. (2008). Neural substrates of spontaneous musical performance: An fMRI study of jazz improvisation. *PloS One*. doi:10.1371/journal.pone.0001679.

Llinás, R., Ribary, U., Contreras, D., & Pedroarena, C. (1998). The neuronal basis for consciousness. *Philosophical Transactions Royal Society London Biological Science, 353*, 1841–1849.

Peifer, C., Schukz, A., Schächinger, H., Baumann, N., & Antoni, C. H. (2014). The relation of flow-experience and physiological arousal under stress – can u shape it? *Journal of Experimental Social Psychology, 52*, 62–69.

Rheinberg, F., Vollmeyer, M. & Engeser, S. (2003). Die Erfassung des Flow-Erlebens [The diagnostic of flowexperience]. In I. Steinsmeyer-Pelster & F. Rheinberg, (Eds.). *Diagnostik von Motivation und Selbstkonzept* [Diagnostics of motivation and self-concept]. (S.261–279), Göttingen: Hogrefe.

Reinhardt, C., Lau, A., Hottenrott, K., & Stoll, O. (2006). Flow-Erleben unter kontrollierter Beanspruchungssteuerung [Flow-experiences under controlled workload-regulation]. *Zeitschrift für Sportpsychologie, 13*, 140–146.

Reinhardt, R., Wiener, S., Heimbeck, A., Stoll, O., Lau, A., & Schliermann, R. (2008). Flow in der Sporttherapie der Depression – ein beanspruchungsorientierter Ansatz [Flow in sports therapy with depressed patients – a work-load oriented approach]. *Bewegungstherapie und Gesundheitssport, 24*, 147–151.

Saad Al Youssef, H. (2012). *Transient hypofrontality and flow-experiences*. Doctoral thesis, Martin-Luther-University Halle-Wittenberg, Department of Sports Science, Halle (Saale), Germany.

Shushruth, S. (2013). Exploring the neural basis of consciousness through anesthesia. *The Journal of Neuroscience, 33*(5), 1757–1758.

Sparling, P. B., Giuffrida, A., Piomelli, D., Rosskopf, L., & Dietrich, A. (2003). Exercise activates the endocannabinoid system. *Cognitive Neuroscience, 14*, 959–965. doi:10.1097/01.wnr.0000097048.56589.47.

Stoll, O. (1997). Endorphine, Laufsucht und Runner's High. Aufstieg und Niedergang eines Mythos [Endorphins, running addiction and runner's high. Rise and decline of a myth]. *Leipziger Sportwissenschaftliche Beiträge, 28*(1), 102–121.

Stoll, O., & Lau, A. (2005). Flow-Erleben beim Marathonlauf – Zusammenhänge mit Anforderungspassung und Leistung [Flow-experiences while marathon running – correlations with demand-fitting and performance]. *Zeitschrift für Sportpsychologie, 12*(3), 75–82.

Tulppo, M. P., Makikallio, T. H., Takala, T. E., Seppanen, T., & Huikuri, H. V. (1996). Quantitative beat-to-beat analysis of heart rate dynamics during exercise. *American Journal of Physiology, 271*, 244–252.

Ulrich, M., Keller, J., Hönig, K., Waller, C., & Grön, G. (2014). Neural correlates of experimentally induced flow experiences. *NeuroImage, 86*, 194–202.

Wechsler, D. (2008). *Wechsler Adult Intelligence Scale (WAIS-IV) – German Version by F. Petermann*. Frankfurt/M.: Pearson.

Part III
Flow, Creativity and Productivity

Chapter 6
Flow in Creativity: A Review of Potential Theoretical Conflict

Genevieve M. Cseh

Abstract This chapter reviews both qualitative and experimental research, arguing that some theories surrounding flow are potentially contradictory to theories of creativity. Dual-process thought systems and hypofrontality theories are discussed in relation to creativity and flow, highlighting omissions in research to date, and the need for further empirical investigation of creativity in flow. Four specific areas for future research are proposed: (1) a more in-depth understanding of self-evaluative mechanisms during flow, and the relevance of clear goals and feedback within creative domains; (2) whether flow during deliberate forms of creativity is possible and whether this contradicts hypofrontality theories; (3) the complex relationship between creativity, affect, and flow; and (4) whether and how flow relates to creative achievement.

6.1 Introduction

Csíkszentmihályi reports that the first inklings of flow theory came to him while he was a graduate student, studying creativity in the visual arts (Nakamura and Csíkszentmihályi 2005). While observing artists hard at work, he noted that they worked feverishly on artworks that, when finished, were often abandoned and then never thought of again. This led him to wonder what it might be about the subjective experience of creating, rather than the external rewards – e.g., fame and fortune from selling a finished product – that drove artists to create. This question and his initial qualitative work triggered the discovery of flow, which has now become a cornerstone concept in the field of motivation psychology (Csíkszentmihályi et al. 2005; Deci and Ryan 1985; Eccles and Wigfield 2002). Flow and creativity have therefore been closely intertwined from the very beginning. Since creativity is arguably the force behind all human progress, and flow is a significant force driving creativity, this close relationship makes the study of creative flow especially

G.M. Cseh (✉)
School of Art, Design & Fashion, University of Central Lancashire,
223 Victoria Building, Preston, Lancashire, PR1 2HE England, United Kingdom
e-mail: genevieve@gcseh.com

L. Harmat et al. (eds.), *Flow Experience*, DOI 10.1007/978-3-319-28634-1_6

important. Nonetheless, of all the activities that can potentially inspire flow, the creative domain remains relatively underexplored.

Since the traditional nine components of flow experience (e.g., skill-challenge balance, effortless sense of control, clear goals and feedback: see Csíkszentmihályi 2002) seem to be reported universally in qualitative studies of people engaged in a variety of activities (Massimini et al. 1988), it has been largely assumed that flow differs little between activities in terms of prerequisites, consequences, or correlates. However, there are some suggestions to the contrary (Delle Fave et al. 2011) as well as noticeable gaps in flow research that need to be addressed before such a universality of the theory can truly be confirmed. Additionally, studying the unique factors that contribute to flow development during creativity can provide new layers of information about both flow and creativity, separately and together.

The majority of flow research to date has focused on regimented activities, ones which can become automated with practice, where performance can be monitored and controlled easily, and which therefore have clear goals and standards of success. Of all the components of flow, clarity of goals and unambiguous feedback have received the least critical attention from researchers, perhaps in part because they are straightforward aspects in these more frequently studied, systematic activities.

Flow research has been particularly strong in the domain of athletics (Engeser and Schiepe-Tiska 2012; Jackson and Csíkszentmihályi 1999; Jackson and Kimiecik 2008; Jackson et al. 2001), where the colloquial phrase 'in the zone' has long been used synonymously for flow, with perhaps more emphasis on peak performance in addition to the subjective flow experience (Murphy 1996; Young and Pain 1999). Video and computer games are most frequently used to examine flow experimentally (Chen 2007; Rheinberg and Vollmeyer 2003; Sweetser and Wyeth 2005), as the task difficulty can be easily controlled and manipulated and these games are therefore an ideal experimental tool for following the learning curve of ever-increasing skill with practice in relation to increasing task demands.

However, there are potentially important differences between creative activities and those mentioned above, on which the majority of flow theory has been founded: i.e., the act of creating can never be learned to the point of rote automaticity, since it depends – by definition – on the creation of something novel each time, and the careful assessment of that novelty. The standards by which creative actions are judged are also inherently much more ambiguous and complex than they often are in other domains (Csíkszentmihályi 1996; Simonton 2000), and creative activity requires a good deal of conscious cognitive processing (Allen and Thomas 2011), which is to an extent at odds with theories that suggest flow is mainly experienced during unconscious/automated processing of highly practiced actions (e.g., Dietrich 2004a).

This chapter will argue that more research is required specifically on flow within creative activity, and particularly using more experimental methods. Previous work on flow during creativity and the methodologies utilised thus far are reviewed, and four possible areas for future research are proposed: (1) the clear goals/unambiguous feedback components of flow; (2) the feeling of effortless automaticity and control during flow in relation to hypofrontality theory (Dietrich 2004a) and dual-process systems of creative thought (Allen and Thomas 2011); (3) links between creativity, flow, and affect; and (4) whether/how flow relates to creative performance.

6.2 Methods Used in Previous Research

Although artists may have been the original inspiration for flow, and the subject of several qualitative studies, there has been a lack of experimental research focusing on flow in creative activities. In some ways this is surprising, given that it was artists who inspired the theory and therefore seem to be prime subjects for the study of flow. On the other hand, it is perhaps unsurprising, as both flow and creativity are concepts that have been notoriously difficult to quantify and define (Moneta 2012; Mumford 2003); it is possible that, when tackled together, they have so far been considered scientifically unmanageable.

There have been numerous qualitative studies on flow in relation to creativity, using interview techniques. Csíkszentmihályi (1975, 1996) interviewed artists, musicians, and other creators (e.g., scientists) to explore creativity in relation to the known components of flow previously proposed, where he acknowledged that some components, including feedback, were more complex in creative domains. Reynolds and Prior (2006) explored how flow could benefit women suffering from cancer, finding it helped to reduce stress by reducing intrusive thoughts about illness. They also noted that clear goals did not seem to feature very highly in the accounts of the women while creating. Similarly, Chilton (2013) reviewed the relevance of flow to art therapy practice. Banfield and Burgess (2013) investigated the importance of embodiment in creative flow development, focusing on haptic input from the chosen medium (2D and 3D media artists) and how this influences engagement, a rare re-examination of the components that contribute to flow during creativity.

However, these were all qualitative case studies which, while rich in phenomenological detail, come with the usual caveats associated with qualitative data, e.g., that they have been interpreted subjectively, are based on anecdotal recall abilities temporally removed from the phenomenon they are reporting, and lack generalisability. Therefore more experimental work is needed, for the sake of rigorous control of extraneous influences, to examine the flow experience directly after it happens, and to determine factors that can be manipulated to show measurable effects on flow. When the arts are examined experimentally, it tends to be in the context of musical performance (Bakker 2005; de Manzano et al. 2010) or other *performing* arts (Gruzelier et al. 2010). The emphasis has therefore been on actions that are (like athletics and video games) learned, highly practiced, and which are then more or less automatically executed, rather than novelty-producing actions. This has left the flow of conscious thought and cognitive processes like creativity disproportionately unexplored.

The only experimental studies found to date on flow during specifically creative actions (visual synthesis: Cseh et al. 2015a; or group musical composition: MacDonald et al. 2006), found mixed results about the link between creator flow and its relationship to creative performance. In a novel adaptation of the task, Cseh et al. used the *creative mental synthesis task* (originally designed to explore mental imagery in creativity: Finke and Slayton 1988) to experimentally simulate the creative visual design process using non-artist participants, and measuring flow post-task using the Flow State Scale (Jackson et al. 2010), alongside pre-post-task mood measures and performance ratings. The synthesis task involves presenting participants with sets of simple geometric and alphanumeric shapes (e.g., circle, triangle, X, J, 8), then asking them to combine these symbols into a new, recognizable composite picture of an object or scene. This study was designed to determine whether experiencing flow during a simple creative task would be associated with a positive change in affect, and whether flow was associated with both self-perceived and external measures of performance. Findings showed that experiencing creative flow was related to an improvement in affect (increased positive/decreased negative) over the course of the creative task, and to self-perceived performance, but not to externally rated subjective and objective measures of performance.

In MacDonald et al. (2006), on the other hand, groups of music students were tasked with composing pieces of music. Mean group flow measures were taken using a form of the Experience Sampling Form (ESF: Csíkszentmihályi and Csíkszentmihályi 1988), to determine if higher group flow during composition could be linked to better performance reviews of compositions by various levels of instructors. They found a link between group flow and superior creative performance as rated by postgraduate tutors, but not with ratings by senior lecturers.

These experimental findings, therefore, show equivocal links between flow and objective or externally rated creative performance. No other experimental work was found specifically in relation to novelty-producing actions and flow. This shows an area of flow research which has been underexplored to date. The two existing experimental studies also suggest some specific methods for future research on flow in at least visual and musical creativity, and with individual creators vs. groups.

6.3 Discussion: Theoretical Conflicts and Future Research

The scant experimental work on creative flow has so far focused on the links between experiencing flow and level of creative performance achieved. Qualitative research has mainly been used to explore the subjective experience of creating and flow, and how this may help in clinical settings. Qualitative methods are indeed most suited for exploring an individual creator's phenomenology, especially in the case of flow, which is a highly personal, subjective phenomenon. However, not much work has been done to re-examine the theories and assumptions surrounding creative flow, such as the unique components that may help facilitate flow during creativity specifically, its neural underpinnings, and its consequences in terms of affect and performance outcomes. This section highlights some theoretical conflicts between flow theories and theories of creativity, as well as factors which remain unknown, and which require closer scrutiny in future research.

6.3.1 Clear Goals and Unambiguous Feedback Components

"Coherent, non-contradictory demands for action and clear, unambiguous feedback" (Csíkszentmihályi 1975, p. 46) are considered essential components for flow development, the assumption being that in order to attain the skill-demand balance that is thought to lead to flow, one needs to be monitoring one's own skill and be certain that it is adequate to handle the challenges of the task to achieve an identified goal through a clear action plan. This is a reasonable, theory-based assumption and an uncomplicated issue when standards of success in an activity are clear-cut. For example, the athlete knows she has been successful when she wins a game with specific rules, or crosses a finish line before her competitors. The video game player knows he is doing well when he manages to 'level up' in a game after shooting a requisite number of targets. The flute player knows she is hitting all the correct notes of a highly practiced piece of music because she does not hear a jarring note. Feedback and goals are clear in all these examples, because judgment is based on objective criteria. But even researchers who have made the study of creativity their life's work have been struggling to find a conclusive definition of what should be considered creative and what is not (Mumford 2003), and how best to assess creativity. In other words, how does a painter, a writer, a composer know while they are creating that their idea or the final product are of a high quality when judgment of creativity is subjective and changeable?

Csíkszentmihályi (1996) acknowledged that the issue of feedback is not as straightforward for creators as it is in other domains because there is a shared social aspect to the judgment of creative work, which often operates on a lengthy timescale between creation and dissemination. The creative arts hinge on a dialogue between an individual creator, cognitive and material processes, a product, and an audience in a wider social context (Glăveanu 2013). Whether a work is considered creative or not by either creators themselves or their peer community is a complicated, subjective, and imprecise matter. The ultimate judgment of how creative a work is deemed to be can take a long time and depend on who is evaluating it, and when and where, and is still open to personal opinions. Because the experience of flow theoretically depends on having clear, immediate feedback, Csíkszentmihályi argued that creators deal with this ambiguity of feedback by "internalizing the field's criteria of judgment to the extent that they can give feedback to themselves, without having to wait to hear from experts" (1996; p. 116), which they learn to do through experience; i.e., they learn to encode a prediction system based on previous experiences and observations, intuitively knowing which factors the audience will respond to well and which they will not. This is what provides them with the instant and clear self-feedback to facilitate flow. However, Simonton (1988) argued that many artists – even famous and experienced masters such as Beethoven – were not always good predictors of which of their works would be popular with their audience (i.e., their 'field').

Simonton (2000) also disputed that this sort of predictive expertise in the creative arts can ever be learned. First, unlike other fields where the principles of a first success can add to and build onto the next success, this is untrue of creative endeavours, where the next creative endeavour in fact benefits from being different to the preceding success, due to novelty being a defining factor of creativity. Secondly, artworks are often very complex and the judgment of their merit is based on a wide variety of factors – e.g., in the visual arts: colour, composition, style, subject matter, historical influences, personal preferences, emotional tone – that it is impossible for anyone, no matter their experience, to be able to make a 100 % correct assessment of all the necessary factors involved to predict how an audience will respond to all of them.

These are not factors with which most athletes, for instance, have to contend, at least not to the same degree. The success or failure of one performance can inform and build toward the outcome of the next, as novelty is not often the end goal in athletic growth, but rather improvement of previous speed, strength, etc. In other words, athletes' successes are progressive, while creators' are self-contained to each individual performance. As athletes also have clear goals to work towards, self-perceptions and external, objective success judgments mesh easily. Therefore it is easy to see why flow is often confused with objective peak performance, though this is not always true (Landhäußer and Keller 2012): all that theoretically matters to flow development is the athlete's own perception, and this will likely match objective reality as there is little room for error or bias. This is not necessarily the case for creators.

Since flow only theoretically depends on perceived skill and demand, it could be argued that for flow to develop, it does not matter whether a creator has an objectively accurate assessment of their skill, only that they are pleased with and certain of the progress of their work, even if that assessment is skewed in some way. However, the theory that goals and feedback need only be based on personally-defined criteria assumes that creators are always able to give themselves unambiguous feedback about how well they are attaining at least their own personal goals, and that they never end up misleading or surprising themselves. However, anecdotal accounts by historical creative masters (e.g., see Beveridge 1957; Ghiselin 1952; Koestler 1964) frequently show a mixed sense of certainty during the self-evaluation phases of the creative process. There are many instances of creators noting that there can be a disconnect between initial ideas and their practical application or execution, which can lead to a high skill rating in one stage (e.g., when they have their initial idea) and a low one in another (e.g., when they execute that idea), illustrating the ambiguity inherent in self-monitoring of skill within the continuum of the creative process. This means that there are potentially cognitive faults or limitations in the self-feedback system, which can add an additional layer of ambiguity to an already ambiguous domain.

This begs the question: are the prerequisites of clear goals and unambiguous feedback (which can be considered two sides of the same coin: Keller and Landhäußer 2012) as vital to the development of flow in the creative domain as has been previously suggested in relation to less subjective domains? These factors may in some ways be undesirable components, both to creativity and to flow. Tolerance of ambiguity is a common personality variable of creative people (Comadena 1984; Merrotsy 2013; Zenasni et al. 2008), and the creative process is an iterative process that is believed to necessarily change its goals on a continual basis in dialogue with the physical world (Dewey 1934; Glăveanu 2013; Suwa and Tversky 1997). It is adaptability to the vagaries of chance that defines and drives the creative process.

Since creative criteria are subjective (as evidenced by frequent public controversy over avant-garde art), creative individuals need to be more tolerant of this factor than others in other fields may be. Tolerance of ambiguity may therefore be another factor in Csíkszentmihályi's (2002) proposed *autotelic* personality, i.e., the personality type most likely to experience flow, particularly in creative pursuits. Those who choose to go into creative professions seem to see ambiguity as a chance for exploration and discovery rather than uncomfortable uncertainty, and therefore a lack of clear goals and feedback during the process may not so much impede flow as feed it.

However, even if ambiguity and clear goals are necessary for creators, the way that creators achieve clarity in a profession with ever-changing and subjective standards of success requires further study. Many of the creative scientists Csíkszentmihályi (1996) spoke to mentioned that an important form of self-feedback was the ability to tell the difference between fruitful and unfruitful ideas early in the creative process. Likewise, Perkins (1981) identified the ability to be critical and discerning as a more important skill for creative success than being able to simply generate novel ideas. If unambiguous self-feedback is in fact essential to both creativity and flow, it would stand to reason that those creators who possess and make use of certain cognitive abilities and tools which allow them to examine their initial ideas as vividly and as accurately as possible will be more likely to experience creative flow throughout the creative process. These cognitive tools will help translate ideas into successful physical reality and to filter unfeasible concepts early, before expending energy on executing ideas that will not work.

However, what are these cognitive skills that enable an artist to achieve these goals and thereby, perhaps, flow? This is a question that needs to be addressed and could begin to explain how the processes of self-evaluation help to facilitate or hinder flow. Some work has been done recently, showing that mental and physical self-feedback, and differences between expectations and outcomes, may affect flow differentially. For example, access to perceptual feedback through sketching may help to clarify mental imagery self-feedback during the conceptual phases of visual creativity. Additionally, the consistency of self-feedback – for instance, whether expectations match outcomes, and self-surprise – may also play an important role in flow (Cseh et al. 2015b). However, more work needs to be done to understand the reasons behind the links and to explore other cognitive feedback processes important for flow to occur.

6.3.2 *Self-Feedback and Dual-Process Thought*

Perkins (1981) argued that evaluation during creativity is neither explicit nor implicit, but a combination of the two. Perkins carried out experiments with artists, poets, etc., asking them to give a running verbal commentary about their process as they created a piece of work. He found that creators referred to intuitive evaluative feelings about why things were good or bad about their work, but then tended to localize the reason for that judgment in more analytic terms 50–80 % of the time, such as 'good because this colour unifies the whole' or 'bad because the ending is clichéd', implying that there is conscious analysis mixed with intuitive feelings about why an artwork is deemed successful or not.

According to Csíkszentmihályi (2002), evaluating skill in flow must be implicit, because a characteristic of flow is the loss of conscious self-reflection, and focusing on the self would interrupt concentration on the task. The validity of this assumption is questionable, however; Delle Fave et al. (2011) noted that in fact many people show more self-consciousness than usual during flow. Confusion about this flow dimension might arise from the fact that self-monitoring is not always seen by respondents as negative, and that it is an essential contributor to the unambiguous feedback component, which requires analysis of how an idea or action relates to both the self and the external world.

This leads to a conflict in theories of creativity and flow. Allen and Thomas (2011) suggest that creative thought is always a combination of type 1 (intuitive, spontaneous, unconscious) thought processes and type 2 (deliberate, conscious, analytical). This is reflected in the current twofold definition of creativity: something is creative if it is novel (generating uninhibited, unusual ideas and associations; i.e., type 1 thought), but checked by its usefulness and practicality (analysis of appropriateness to a purpose, i.e., type 2 thinking: Mumford 2003; Sawyer 2006; Sternberg et al. 2005). Flow, however, is mainly characterised as solely type 1 thought.

6.3.3 Automaticity, Hypofrontality Theory, and Dual-Process Thinking

Dietrich (2004a) proposes that many of the experiential 'symptoms' of flow, such as lost self-consciousness and time distortion, are a result of a temporary hypofrontality that occurs in the brain – executive and deliberate (type 2) functions like self-awareness or conscious decision-making are inhibited. The automatic nature of flow is considered a result of highly practiced skills being deployed without needing to invest much conscious thought on decision-making, allowing intuitive, unconscious systems to take over. If creativity is always achieved in eureka moments of sudden insight (type 1 thought), then this hypofrontal neural pattern of flow makes sense. There is a plethora of research and anecdotal accounts that suggest many creative insights happen spontaneously without prior conscious work (Ghiselin 1952; Gilhooly 1996; Perkins 1981) – the basis for the 'divine inspiration' myth of creative genius (Sawyer 2006) – and certainly there are technical aspects to creating that are practiced to the point of becoming automatic. It could therefore be argued that flow is more likely to occur during these moments of creating that are spontaneous rather than deliberate. However, this dismisses the fact that although some parts of creativity happen automatically, outside the conscious control of the creator, there are other equally important stages and processes that cannot happen without higher-order executive processing, such as evaluation, decision-making, working memory, cognitive control, and so on, at least in some forms of creativity (Allen and Thomas 2011; Dietrich 2004b).

In ancient times, creativity was considered a gift from the Muse, a divine inspiration passively received from a mysterious external source, rather than actively pursued and generated by the creator (Plato, 380 B.C.E./2009). Today we know better; we are aware of the unconscious and its ability to produce thoughts without the creator having conscious knowledge of their origin. Science now considers creativity part of everyday cognition, simply a form of problem-solving that humans are universally capable of to varying extents (Finke et al. 1992). Yet the generation of creative ideas is still spoken of in terms of impromptu and passive experience, though this is at least in many circumstances a myth (Sawyer 2006). When flow during creativity is described, it is the unconscious side of creativity that is highlighted. The painter looks up from her painting hours later only to think 'did I do that?' The sculptor feels as though he is one with the clay, not separate or thinking about what to do next, but simply melting into the activity without awareness of acting upon his medium.

However, some forms of creativity are more deliberate, which Dietrich himself acknowledges (2004b), and these creative actions rely more heavily on type 2 analysis and conscious trial-and-error processing. For example, the 9-to-5 workaday designer or engineer must produce work on demand and to deadlines, and it is possible that they still experience flow under these conditions – flow is, after all, often experienced in the workplace. Does experiencing flow while consciously generating and evaluating ideas preclude the hypofrontality theory of flow? Oliverio (2008) has argued that novelty-production in the creative process may follow the implicit cortical systems in regions like the basal ganglia, but that the flipside of the creativity coin – the analytical selection of an idea that is also appropriate to a purpose – or the deliberate synthesis of ideas requires high activation of the prefrontal cortex, and that this appears to contradict the notion of creative flow as simply a period of hypofrontality. After all, some executive processes (such as attentional focus) are highly functional during flow, while others are not.

Flow is also believed to require a sense of autonomy and intrinsic motivation (autotelic experience/reward), suggesting that having conscious control over the details of an activity could enhance flow. Having access to choices and exerting control during the creative process (and in general) can both enhance (Amabile and Gitomer 1984) and reduce creativity (Finke 1990), and may influence motivation and feelings of task difficulty and enjoyment in paradoxical ways (Iyengar and Lepper 2000; Schwartz 2004). Exerting choice requires cognitive effort (Payne 1976; Timmermans 1993), using higher order executive functions such as working memory, attention, self-referential analysis, and of course decision-making. Since creativity requires making decisions that have not been made before (novelty), from a practically infinite array of possibilities, the cognitive load during certain instances of creativity would also seem to contradict the view of a hypoactive prefrontal cortex. Additionally, research on frontotemporal dementia effects on creativity suggest that decline in executive regions of the brain – a more severe and permanent form of hypofrontality – can disinhibit rule-based and conventional processes to produce an initial boost in the novelty aspect of creativity, but that it can also inhibit planful behaviour and thereby impair the more formal, technical aspects of creativity and its appropriateness (Joy and Furman 2014).

Hence, flow during creativity and other cognitive pursuits may not hinge on unconscious automaticity due to practice to the same degree as it appears to in more regimented and physical activities, but may benefit from conscious decision-making and the deliberate exercising of control and choice. The hypofrontality theory of flow seems plausible for the majority of flow activities because it fits well in regards to the highly-practiced activities on which flow research usually focuses, but may not fit (at least not all) creative endeavours. Hypofrontality theory also seems at odds with the flow of thinking; however, Csíkszentmihályi (2002) devotes a chapter of his book to flow that occurs specifically in complex cognitive activities such as playing chess or solving difficult puzzles, which require extensive use of conscious, analytical, and executive functions.

Csíkszentmihályi alluded to the contradictory nature of flow by noting the paradox of control (2002) that occurs in flow. The person in flow feels in control of their actions and that their skills are adequate to meet the challenges of the task; but simultaneously, the experience feels automatic, as though it were happening outside of their control and with no effort on their part. Creativity too is dual in nature (Allen and Thomas 2011; Gilhooly and Murphy 2005). Examining these two paradoxical states together – flow during creativity – could potentially tell us more about the dual nature of consciousness and how implicit and explicit thought pathways may interact and complement one another to achieve the creative flow experience. An overemphasis on automated, mainly physical activities over less automated, mainly cognitive ones when researching flow runs the risk of over-generalising principles of flow to domains where it may not be appropriate to do so.

Furthermore, self-evaluation processes in creativity are complex and still poorly understood (Kozbelt 2007; Runco and Chand 1994). What is required is an in-depth understanding of the cognitive mechanisms that underlie the self-feedback system and creative cognition during flow. The specific pattern and degree of hypofrontality may differ significantly between different domains and activities, and result in subtle but essential differences between subjective flow experience in separate activity domains, and could also signal unique facilitating components and consequences.

6.3.4 Creative Flow and Affect

One of these purported consequences of flow is that it leads to greater happiness – both acute, short-term improvements to affective states (Cseh et al. 2015a; Rogatko 2007) and longer-term life satisfaction and wellbeing (Asakawa 2010). However, this warrants re-examination specifically in a creative context, particularly as the link between creativity and affect is still debated by researchers (Kaufmann and

Vosberg 1997). The literature on the relationship between flow and affect has been covered previously by Landhäußer and Keller (2012) and is discussed more fully in Cseh et al. (2015a). The consensus shows mostly significant links between flow and positive affect, though the causal direction of the link is unclear, and occasionally the link is not found.

Baas et al. (2008), in a meta-analysis of creativity-affect research, show that creativity can be facilitated by positive affective states, which is in line with Fredrickson's (2001) *broaden-and-build* theory. The affective consequences of creating are less clear, but some research suggests that the type of creative activity undertaken influences affect, with divergent thinking linked to increased positive affect, and convergent thinking linked to increased negative affect (Akbari Chermahini and Hommel 2012). Doubtless, there will be an enormous number of factors within the creative process that influence affect, but it is possible that experiencing flow is one of those factors; however, once again causal impacts of the variables on one another must still be determined. If creativity improves mood, is flow a mediator? Or does happiness facilitate not only creativity but also flow, a possibility proposed in Cseh et al. (2015a)? Although most flow-affect research has identified that flow is linked to post-task positive affect, more experimental evidence of a link to *changes* in affect (Cseh et al. 2015a; Rogatko 2007) and exploring how flow relates to more nuanced categorisations of emotion than simply the positive-negative polarity (e.g., activating vs. deactivating affective states: Baas et al. 2008) is necessary. Additionally, how both affect and flow relate to creative performance levels must be addressed to determine how flow factors into the cognition-emotion relationship.

6.3.5 Creative Flow and Enhanced Performance

Although self-perceived competence is a variable that is theoretically linked to flow (flow is only experienced when skills are thought adequate to cope with challenges), evidence of a direct causal impact of flow on enhanced objective performance is too often assumed and/or generalised to all activities (Nakamura and Csíkszentmihályi 2005), despite only correlational (Jackson et al. 2001; MacDonald et al. 2006) or lack of convincing supporting evidence (Cseh et al. 2015a; Keller and Bless 2008; Keller and Blomann 2008; Landhäußer and Keller 2012).

Landhäußer and Keller (2012) note that there is very little evidence to date about the flow-performance link in cognitive pursuits; therefore more work needs to be done to determine if and how flow contributes to cognitive achievement like creativity. Some research has shown that similar altered states such as those experienced during meditation can improve subsequent creative abilities (Colzato et al. 2012); electrical brain stimulation that induces a form of transient hypofrontality has also been shown to improve learning abilities (Clark et al. 2012) and mathematical problem-solving (Chi and Snyder 2011). However, it is not clear whether flow states (not necessarily the same phenomenon as hypofrontality or meditative states) would also have this effect on specifically creative cognition, and if so, why.

If this alleged flow-performance link truly exists, this too may differ between domains, and requires more empirical evidence either way. Privette and Bundrick (1991) and Csíkszentmihályi (1988) have cautioned that flow and objective peak performance do not always correspond and that the terms should not be used interchangeably, as they can be in sports research (Murphy 1996) or in popular accounts of flow (Adee 2012; Fox 2011; Kotler 2014). Even without immediate and acute influences on performance, flow may still be linked indirectly to performance over time, through its motivational influences. More longitudinal work should be conducted to determine whether flow leads to behaviours which contribute to greater achievement in a shorter amount of time, e.g., more time spent practicing, greater perseverance over obstacles, and so on. Assumptions that flow helps foster greater creativity are therefore premature and require much more experimental evidence.

6.4 Summary and Conclusion

This chapter has proposed that the conditions of flow are not uniform across activities and domains, despite previous qualitative research suggesting universality of the theory. In particular, the lack of clear goals and unambiguous feedback components of flow may not necessarily impede flow during creativity. Generally, the evaluative processes during both creativity and flow require further specific work.

The currently popular theory that flow is characterised by a period of hypofrontality (Dietrich 2004a) is at odds with a dual-systems view of cognition-intensive and deliberative activities like certain kinds of creative thought. More nuanced work to determine the neural patterns that help foster both creativity and flow at the same time should be explored, and whether different patterns distinguish flow during different activities – and why – should also be examined.

The affect and performance outcomes of flow also require more experimental evidence, and should examine more complex and subtle relationships, particularly since these are areas with which creativity researchers also continue to struggle.

It is my hope that more researchers will take up the reins to rigorously and specifically investigate which unique conditions of the creative process lead to flow within creativity, the neural patterns of different types of creative flow, and the long-term, meaningful outcomes of creative flow.

References

Adee, S. (2012, February 6). Zap your brain into the zone: Fast track to pure focus. *New Scientist, 2850.* http://www.newscientist.com/article/mg21328501.600-zap-your-brain-into-the-zone-fast-track-to-pure-focus.html?full=true&print=true. Accessed 15 Jan 2015.

Akbari Chermahini, S., & Hommel, B. (2012). Creative mood swings: Divergent and convergent thinking affect mood in opposite ways. *Psychological Research, 76*, 634–640. doi:10.1007/s00426-011-0358-z.

Allen, A. P., & Thomas, K. E. (2011). A dual process account of creative thinking. *Creativity Research Journal, 23*(2), 109–118. doi:10.1080/10400419.2011.571183.
Amabile, T. M., & Gitomer, J. (1984). Children's artistic creativity: Effects of choice in task materials. *Personality and Social Psychology Bulletin, 10*(2), 209–215. doi:10.1177/0146167284102006.
Asakawa, K. (2010). Flow experience, culture, and well-being: How do autotelic Japanese college students feel, behave, and think in their daily lives? *Journal of Happiness Studies, 11*(2), 205–223. doi:10.1007/s10902-008-9132-3.
Baas, M., De Dreu, C. K. W., & Nijstad, B. A. (2008). A meta-analysis of 25 years of mood-creativity research: Hedonic tone, activation, or regulatory focus? *Psychological Bulletin, 134*(6), 779–806. doi:10.1037/a0012815.
Bakker, A. B. (2005). Flow among music teachers and their students: The crossover of peak experiences. *Journal of Vocational Behavior, 66*, 26–44. doi:10.1016/j.jvb.2003.11.001.
Banfield, J., & Burgess, M. (2013). A phenomenology of artistic doing: Flow as embodied knowing in 2D and 3D professional artists. *Journal of Phenomenological Psychology, 44*(1), 60–91. doi:10.1163/15691624-12341245.
Beveridge, W. I. B. (1957). *The art of scientific investigation*. New York: W. W. Norton & Company.
Chen, J. (2007). Flow in games (and everything else). *Communications of the ACM, 50*(4), 31–34. doi:10.1145/1232743.1232769.
Chi, R. P., & Snyder, A. W. (2011). Facilitate insight by non-invasive brain stimulation. *PloS One, 6*(2), e16655. doi:10.1371/journal.pone.0016655.
Chilton, G. (2013). Art therapy and flow: A review of the literature and applications. *Art Therapy, 30*(2), 64–70. doi:10.1080/07421656.2013.787211.
Clark, V. P., Coffman, B. A., Mayer, A. R., Weisend, M. P., Lane, T. D. R., Calhoun, V. D., et al. (2012). TDCS guided using fMRI significantly accelerates learning to identify concealed objects. *NeuroImage, 59*(1), 117–128. doi:10.1016/j.neuroimage.2010.11.036.
Colzato, L. S., Ozturk, A., & Hommel, B. (2012). Meditate to create: The impact of focused-attention and open-monitoring training on convergent and divergent thinking. *Frontiers in Psychology, 3*, 116. doi:10.3389/fpsyg.2012.00116.
Comadena, M. E. (1984). Brainstorming groups: Ambiguity tolerance, communication apprehension, task attraction, and individual productivity. *Small Group Research, 15*(2), 251–264. doi:10.1177/104649648401500207.
Cseh, G. M., Phillips, L. H., & Pearson, D. G. (2015a). Flow, affect, and visual creativity. *Cognition and Emotion, 29*(2), 281–291. doi:10.1080/02699931.2014.913553.
Cseh, G. M., Phillips, L. H., & Pearson, D. G. (2015b). *Mental and perceptual feedback in the development of creative flow.* Manuscript submitted for publication.
Csíkszentmihályi, M. (1975). *Beyond boredom and anxiety*. San Francisco: Jossey-Bass.
Csíkszentmihályi, M. (1988). The future of flow. In M. Csíkszentmihályi & I. S. Csíkszentmihályi (Eds.), *Optimal experience: Psychological studies of flow in consciousness* (pp. 364–383). Cambridge: Cambridge University Press.
Csíkszentmihályi, M. (1996). *Creativity: Flow and the psychology of discovery and invention.* New York: Harper Perennial.
Csíkszentmihályi, M. (2002). *Flow: The classic work on how to achieve happiness* (Rev. ed.). London: Rider.
Csíkszentmihályi, M., & Csíkszentmihályi, I. S. (1988). Introduction to part IV. In M. Csíkszentmihályi & I. S. Csíkszentmihályi (Eds.), *Optimal experience: Psychological studies of flow in consciousness* (pp. 251–265). Cambridge: Cambridge University Press.
Csíkszentmihályi, M., Abuhamdeh, S., & Nakamura, J. (2005). Flow. In A. Elliot (Ed.), *Handbook of competence and motivation* (pp. 598–608). New York: The Guilford Press.
de Manzano, O., Theorell, T., Harmat, L., & Ullén, F. (2010). The psychophysiology of flow during piano playing. *Emotion, 10*(3), 301–311.
Deci, E. L., & Ryan, R. M. (1985). *Intrinsic motivation and self-determination in human behavior.* New York: Plenum.

Delle Fave, A., Massimini, F., & Bassi, M. (Eds.). (2011). The phenomenology of optimal experience in daily life. In *Psychological selection and optimal experience across cultures: Cross-cultural advancements in positive psychology 2* (Vol. 2, pp. 89–110). Dordrecht: Springer. doi:10.1007/978-90-481-9876-4

Dewey, J. (1934). *Art as experience*. New York: Putnam.

Dietrich, A. (2004a). Neurocognitive mechanisms underlying the experience of flow. *Consciousness and Cognition, 13*(4), 746–761. doi:10.1016/j.concog.2004.07.002.

Dietrich, A. (2004b). The cognitive neuroscience of creativity. *Psychonomic Bulletin and Review, 11*(6), 1011–1026.

Eccles, J. S., & Wigfield, A. (2002). Motivational beliefs, values, and goals. *Annual Review of Psychology, 53*, 109–132.

Engeser, S., & Schiepe-Tiska, A. (2012). Historical lines and an overview of current research on flow. In S. Engeser (Ed.), *Advances in flow research* (pp. 1–22). New York: Springer. doi:10.1007/978-1-4614-2359-1_1.

Finke, R. A. (1990). *Creative imagery: Discoveries and inventions in visualization*. Hillsdale: Laurence Erlbaum Associates.

Finke, R. A., & Slayton, K. (1988). Explorations of creative visual synthesis in mental imagery. *Memory and Cognition, 16*(3), 252–257.

Finke, R. A., Ward, T. B., & Smith, S. M. (1992). *Creative cognition: Theory, research, and applications*. Cambridge, MA: MIT Press.

Fox, D. (2011). Brain buzz. *Nature, 472*, 156–158. http://www.nature.com/news/2011/110413/full/472156a.html. Accessed 15 Jan 2015.

Fredrickson, B. L. (2001). The role of positive emotions in positive psychology: The broaden-and-build theory of positive emotions. *American Psychologist, 56*(3), 218–226. doi:10.1037/0003-066X.56.3.218

Ghiselin, B. (1952). *The creative process: A symposium*. Berkeley: University of California Press.

Gilhooly, K. (1996). *Thinking: Directed, undirected, and creative* (3rd ed.). San Diego: Academic.

Gilhooly, K., & Murphy, P. (2005). Differentiating insight from non-insight problems. *Thinking and Reasoning, 11*(3), 279–302. doi:10.1080/13546780442000187.

Glăveanu, V. P. (2013). Rewriting the language of creativity: The five A's framework. *Review of General Psychology, 17*(1), 69–81. doi:10.1037/a0029528.

Gruzelier, J., Inoue, A., Smart, R., Steed, A., & Steffert, T. (2010). Acting performance and flow state enhanced with sensory-motor rhythm neurofeedback comparing ecologically valid immersive VR and training screen scenarios. *Neuroscience Letters, 480*(2), 112–116. doi:10.1016/j.neulet.2010.06.019.

Iyengar, S. S., & Lepper, M. R. (2000). When choice is demotivating: Can one desire too much of a good thing? *Journal of Personality and Social Psychology, 79*(6), 995–1006.

Jackson, S. A., & Csíkszentmihályi, M. (1999). *Flow in sports: The keys to optimal experiences and performances*. Champaign: Human Kinetics.

Jackson, S. A., & Kimiecik, J. (2008). The flow perspective of optimal experience in sport and physical activity. In T. S. Horn (Ed.), *Advances in sport psychology* (3rd ed., pp. 377–399). Champaign: Human Kinetics.

Jackson, S. A., Thomas, P. R., Marsh, H. W., & Smethurst, C. (2001). Relationships between flow, self-concept, psychological skills, and performance. *Journal of Applied Sport Psychology, 13*, 129–153.

Jackson, S. A., Eklund, R. C., & Martin, A. (2010). *The flow manual: The manual for the flow scales*. Menlo Park: Mind Garden.

Joy, S. P., & Furman, L. (2014, August). *Progressive change in formal qualities of art produced over the course of frontotemporal dementia*. Paper presented at the annual meeting of the American Psychological Association, Washington, DC. https://www.researchgate.net/publication/264662859_Progressive_Change_in_Fomal_Qualities_of_Art_Produced_over_the_Course_of_Frontotemporal_Dementia. Accessed 15 Jan 2015.

Kaufmann, G., & Vosberg, S. K. (1997). 'Paradoxical' mood effects on creative problem-solving. *Cognition and Emotion, 11*(2), 151–170. doi:10.1080/026999397379971.
Keller, J., & Bless, H. (2008). Flow and regulatory compatibility: An experimental approach to the flow model of intrinsic motivation. *Personality and Social Psychology Bulletin, 34*, 196–209. doi:10.1177/0146167207310026.
Keller, J., & Blomann, F. (2008). Locus of control and the flow experience: An experimental analysis. *European Journal of Personality, 22*(7), 589–607. doi:10.1002/per.692.
Keller, J., & Landhäußer, A. (2012). The flow model revisited. In S. Engeser (Ed.), *Advances in flow research* (pp. 51–64). New York: Springer. doi:10.1007/978-1-4614-2359-1_3.
Koestler, A. (1964). *The act of creation*. London: Hutchinson.
Kotler, S. (2014, July 28). Innovation turbo-charge: How to train the brain to be more creative. *Forbes*. http://www.forbes.com/sites/stevenkotler/2014/07/28/the-innovation-turbo-charge-heightened-creativity-with-flow/. Accessed 15 Jan 2015.
Kozbelt, A. (2007). A quantitative analysis of Beethoven as self-critic: Implications for psychological theories of musical creativity. *Psychology of Music, 35*(1), 144–168. doi:10.1177/0305735607068892.
Landhäußer, A., & Keller, J. (2012). Flow and its affective, cognitive, and performance-related consequences. In S. Engeser (Ed.), *Advances in flow research* (pp. 65–86). New York: Springer. doi:10.1007/978-1-4614-2359-1_4.
MacDonald, R., Byrne, C., & Carlton, L. (2006). Creativity and flow in musical composition: An empirical investigation. *Psychology of Music, 34*(3), 292–306. doi:10.1177/0305735606064838.
Massimini, F., Csíkszentmihályi, M., & Delle Fave, A. (1988). Flow and biocultural evolution. In M. Csíkszentmihályi & I. S. Csíkszentmihályi (Eds.), *Optimal experience: Psychological studies of flow in consciousness* (pp. 60–81). Cambridge: Cambridge University Press.
Merrotsy, P. (2013). Tolerance of ambiguity: A trait of the creative personality? *Creativity Research Journal, 25*(2), 232–237. doi:10.1080/10400419.2013.783762.
Moneta, G. B. (2012). On the measurement and conceptualization of flow. In S. Engeser (Ed.), *Advances in flow research* (pp. 23–50). New York: Springer. doi:10.1007/978-1-4614-2359-1_2.
Mumford, M. D. (2003). Where have we been, where are we going? Taking stock in creativity research. *Creativity Research Journal, 15*(2–3), 107–120. doi:10.1080/10400419.2003.9651403.
Murphy, S. (1996). *The achievement zone*. New York: Berkley.
Nakamura, J., & Csíkszentmihályi, M. (2005). The concept of flow. In C. R. Snyder & S. Lopez (Eds.), *Handbook of positive psychology* (pp. 89–105). Oxford: Oxford University Press.
Oliverio, A. (2008). Brain and creativity. *Progress of Theoretical Physics Supplement, 173*, 66–78. doi:10.1143/PTPS.173.66.
Payne, J. W. (1976). Task complexity and contingent processing in decision making: An information search and protocol analysis. *Organizational Behavior and Human Performance, 16*(2), 366–387. doi:10.1016/0030-5073(76)90022-2.
Perkins, D. N. (1981). *The mind's best work*. Cambridge, MA: Harvard University Press.
Plato. (2009). *Ion* (trans: Jowett, B.). The internet classics archive (Original work published ca. 380 B.C.E.). http://classics.mit.edu/Plato/ion.html. Accessed 15 Jan 2015.
Privette, G., & Bundrick, C. M. (1991). Peak experience, peak performance, and flow: Correspondence of personal descriptions and theoretical constructs. *Journal of Social Behavior and Personality, 6*(5), 169–188.
Reynolds, F., & Prior, S. (2006). Creative adventures and flow in art-making: A qualitative study of women living with cancer. *British Journal of Occupational Therapy, 69*(6), 1–8.
Rheinberg, F., & Vollmeyer, R. (2003). Flow-erleben in einem Computerspiel unter experimentell variierten Bedingungen [Flow experience in a computer game under experimentally controlled conditions]. *Zeitschrift für Psychologie, 211*, 161–170.
Rogatko, T. P. (2007). The influence of flow on positive affect in college students. *Journal of Happiness Studies, 10*(2), 133–148. doi:10.1007/s10902-007-9069-y.

Runco, M. A., & Chand, I. (1994). Problem finding, evaluative thinking, and creativity. In M. A. Runco (Ed.), *Problem finding, problem solving, and creativity* (pp. 40–76). Norwood: Ablex.
Sawyer, R. K. (2006). *Explaining creativity: The science of human innovation*. Oxford: Oxford University Press.
Schwartz, B. (2004). *The paradox of choice: Why more is less*. New York: Harper Collins.
Simonton, D. K. (1988). *Scientific genius: A psychology of science*. Cambridge: Cambridge University Press.
Simonton, D. K. (2000). Creative development as acquired expertise: Theoretical issues and an empirical test. *Developmental Review, 20*(2), 283–318. doi:10.1006/drev.1999.0504.
Sternberg, R. J., Lubart, T. I., Kaufman, J. C., & Pretz, J. E. (2005). Creativity. In K. J. Holyoak & R. G. Morrison (Eds.), *Cambridge handbook of thinking and reasoning* (pp. 351–369). Cambridge: Cambridge University Press.
Suwa, M., & Tversky, B. (1997). What do architects and students perceive in their design sketches? A protocol analysis. *Design Studies, 18*, 385–403.
Sweetser, P., & Wyeth, P. (2005). GameFlow: A model for evaluating player enjoyment in games. *ACM Computers in Entertainment, 3*(3), 1–24.
Timmermans, D. (1993). The impact of task complexity on information use in multi-attribute decision making. *Journal of Behavioral Decision Making, 6*, 95–111.
Young, J. A., & Pain, M. D. (1999). The zone: Evidence of a universal phenomenon for athletes across sports. *Athletic Insight The Online Journal of Sport Psychology, 1*(3), 21–30.
Zenasni, F., Besançon, M., & Lubart, T. (2008). Creativity and tolerance of ambiguity: An empirical study. *Journal of Creative Behavior, 42*(1), 61–73. doi:10.1002/j.2162-6057.2008.tb01080.x.

Chapter 7
Intuition and Flow

Lauri Järvilehto

Abstract Intuition is the capacity to make decisions and create new ideas without conscious deliberation. Flow is the optimal experience where action becomes automatic and conscious thought seems to meld together with the action itself. Both intuition and flow concern our capacity to cognition and action without heavy input from reflective and conscious cognitive mechanisms. Dual process theories of cognition offer a compelling position to explain the functioning of both intuition and flow. In the dual process theories of cognition, two separate cognitive systems are suggested: the non-conscious System 1 and the conscious System 2. Intuition and flow engage to a great extent the same cognitive mechanisms, at the same time without being reduced to definitions in terms of one another. Both intuition and flow involve ontogenetic System 1 processing that enables us to function very well in a culturally evolving, changing environment. In summary, flow can be construed as intuitive action, whereas intuition can be thought of as cognition in flow.

7.1 Introduction

Intuition is the capacity to make decisions and create new ideas without conscious deliberation. Flow is the optimal experience made famous by Mihály Csikszentmihályi, where action becomes automatic and conscious thought seems to meld together with the action itself. Both intuition and flow concern our capacity to cognition and action without heavy input from reflective and conscious cognitive mechanisms.

Both intuition and flow can be studied fruitfully in the context of the dual process theories of cognition. These theories, most prominently advocated by Keith Stanovich, Jonathan Evans and Daniel Kahneman, posit the existence of two largely separate cognitive systems. (Evans 2003, 2009, 2010; Stanovich 2004, 2009; Kahneman 2011) Stanovich has coined the now standard distinction into the non-conscious System 1 and the conscious System 2 (Stanovich and West 2000).

In terms of the dual process theories, both intuition and flow can be construed as relying a great deal on non-conscious processes taking place in System 1. The two

L. Järvilehto (✉)
Helsinki Academy of Philosophy, Aalto University, Espoo, Finland
e-mail: lauri.jarvilehto@gmail.com

L. Harmat et al. (eds.), *Flow Experience*, DOI 10.1007/978-3-319-28634-1_7

have, in other words, a degree of cognitive similarity. However, there is a significant differentiating factor between the two. Namely, while intuition concerns thinking and generating ideas, flow concerns action. Therefore, it can be roughly argued that intuition is System 1 thinking, whereas flow is System 1 doing.

7.2 Dual Process Theories of Cognition

Human cognition has often been thought of as primarily rational and conscious. The role of the non-conscious mind started surfacing into prominence by the latest in the nineteenth century, and broke through to mainstream theorizing in the early twentieth century works of Sigmund Freud. After Freud's work, various theories positing the existence of non-conscious cognition have surfaced, with eventually the dual process theories initiated in the 1960s and 1970s by Keith Stanovich, Jonathan Evans and others. In the recent years, dual processing theories have become a very prominent research paradigm in cognitive psychology.

The dual process theories of cognition quite literally propose the existence of two separate cognitive systems. System 1 is thought of as non-conscious, evolutively old, fast, capable of massive parallel processing and typical to all higher animals. System 2 is, in contrast, thought of as conscious, evolutively rather new, slow, capable of only processing a small amount of information serially and typical only to humans and possibly some higher primates. Sometimes the two are referred to as the implicit and explicit system, respectively.

It should be noted that there is no one single dual process theory of cognition, but rather a group of theories that address the intricacies of conscious and non-conscious cognition with a variety of emphases (See e.g. Evans 2009; Stanovich 2009; Evans and Stanovich 2013.) In fact, in the recent years, Evans and Stanovich in particular have moved from advocating a more fixed Systems view towards a more dynamic Types view, where System 1 and 2 are replaced with a single cognitive system in charge of dealing with non-conscious Type 1 and conscious Type 2 cognitive processes (Evans and Stanovich 2013.) However, for the purposes of the present discussion, System 1 and System 2 suffice as abstractions that differentiate non-conscious and conscious thought processes.

While there are various interpretations of dual processes, practically all dual process theories agree on the existence of two cognitive systems, or two types of cognition. One is dedicated to various conscious operations such as algorithmic reasoning and reflection. This is typically referred to as System 2. The other is, in turn, dedicated to non-conscious operations, such as associative thinking, emotional reactions and autonomous cognitive processes.

Evans formulates the bedrock of dual processing as follows:

> Dual-process theories of thinking and reasoning quite literally propose the presence of two minds in one brain. The stream of consciousness that broadly corresponds to System 2 thinking is massively supplemented by a whole set of autonomous subsystems in System 1

> that post only their final products into consciousness and compete directly for control of our inferences, decisions and actions. (Evans 2003, p. 458.)

While System 2 is the cognitive system distinctive to human beings, it is slow and its capacity is quite constrained. While System 2 enables clarity of thought and conscious manipulation of symbols, its constraints require also active participation from the habit-driven and autonomous System 1. System 1 is fast, parallel and concerns autonomous thought processes. Where System 2 is phenomenologically describable as "stream of thought," System 1's phenomenology can be described as the "things that pop into your head." As Evans (2003, p. 458) points out, System 1 processes "post only their final products into consciousness." While measuring the precise capacity of either cognitive system is difficult, if not impossible, most of the literature agrees on the fact that System 1 has a massive processing capacity, whereas System 2 is dramatically limited in contrast.

George Miller famously showed that the human conscious information processing capacity is dramatically lower than we intuitively think, at around seven units, give or take two (Miller 1956). This number has since been adjusted downwards. The consensus of most present-day memory researchers is that conscious processing concerns only about three to five items of information at a time (Dietrich 2004, p. 752).

Mihály Csikszentmihályi (1990, p. 29) argues, based on Herbert Simon (1978) and Daniel Kahneman (1973), among others, that human conscious capacity is at its upper limit 126 bits per second. Djiksterhuis, Aarts and Smith are more pessimistic, and posit a range of 30–50 bits per second (Djiksterhuis et al. 2006, p. 82.). Manfred Zimmermann (1989) is one of the few scientists to have presented a measurement for both conscious and non-conscious processing. Zimmermann argues, well in line with the above, that the conscious mind processes about 40 bits per second. The afferent nervous system of the human cognitive apparatus in turn processes 11.2 million bits per second.

The constraints of System 2 can be tested by various working memory tests as well as attention tests that have shown that human beings can typically hold on to only a very few items of information or points of attention at a time. In contrast, while the processing power of System 1 is harder to test, it appears to be in a completely different order of magnitude compared to System 2. To demonstrate this discrepancy, Zimmermann's research works as a satisfactory heuristic. System 1 is evolutionally old and shared with most higher animals. It concerns cognitive phenomena such as emotions and instinct that are shared throughout animalkind. These processes are generated by System 1 and only their end results, such as feelings and reactions, are posted to System 2 for reflection. System 2 is, in turn, evolutionally new and typical to humans. It concerns cognitive phenomena such as reflection and algorithmic processes. Keith Stanovich (2009) has also suggested that System 2 should in fact be split into two subsystems, namely the reflective and the algorithmic minds. Both concern conscious processing, but their nature is quite different. Reflective mind concerns evaluation and affecting ongoing thought processes. Algorithmic mind concerns manipulations of symbols and analytic thought.

While there is a great discrepancy between Systems 1 and 2, their arrangement is actually quite optimal for many cognitive processes. Once a skill has been learned sufficiently well, it can be performed again and again by System 1 without the need for conscious intervention. Conscious intervention, i.e. using volition, is highly taxing (See e.g. Baumeister et al. 1998; Baumeister and Tierney 2011). To this end, the ability to commit thought processes and skills to a non-volitional non-conscious cognitive system releases the scarce resources to address situations where the present skill-set is found lacking. As Daniel Kahneman points out, "Constantly questioning our own thinking would be impossibly tedious, and System 2 is much too slow and inefficient to serve as a substitute for System 1 in making routine decisions" (Kahneman 2011, p. 28).

7.3 On the Nature of Intuition

Throughout the history of thought, intuitive thinking has perplexed thinkers. It is, after all, quite astonishing how some individuals have time and again such "a-ha!" moments of inspiration where it seems that a new wonderful idea or a solution to a difficult problem appears out of nowhere. There have been numerous attempts at defining intuition, roughly divisible into two subgroups of intuition as immediate apprehension and intuition as immediate insight. The former group concerns theories presented by such thinkers as Immanuel Kant (1998) and George Bealer (1996). It is, in particular, a popular position in philosophical schools of thought. The latter group concerns theories advocated by various psychologists, such as Gerd Gigerenzer (2007) or Daniel Kahneman (2011). In the context of the present paper, our interests are geared towards the latter kind of intuition: the ability to generate viable insight without conscious effort. (For a more detailed analysis of the two positions, see Järvilehto 2015.)

Based on dual processing theories (Evans 2003, 2009, 2010; Stanovich and West 2000; Stanovich 2004, 2009), as well as work on automaticity and unconscious thought (see e.g. Bargh et al. 1996; Bargh and Chartrand 1999; Djiksterhuis 2004; Djiksterhuis and Nordgren 2006) and intuitive decision making (Gigerenzer 2007; Klein 1998; Kahneman 2011), I define intuition here as an expertise- and experience-based capacity to produce viable results by System 1 autonomous and non-conscious thought processes. It is important to draw the distinction between System 1 processes that are driven by experience and expertise, and System 1 processes that are driven by the phylogenetic structures typical to our species. In other words, we must differentiate intuition and instinct.

While instinctual processes have been streamlined by evolution to work well in a natural environment, our cultural evolution has forced us into a situation where many genetically determined processes – what Stanovich (2004) calls the "short leash" goals of genes – may not have a viable function. Aggressive protective behavior or the maximizing of energy intake do not function well in a civilized society with an abundance of foodstuff on offer. In order to generate viable insight by

System 1 processes, System 1 must first be structured so that its processes are well aligned with our culturally evolved environment. This requires both experience and expertise. Not all System 1 inputs are viable ones. They involve also instincts and many kinds of ideas that have no applicability at all. While the massive capacity of System 1 goes a long way to explain how intuitive decisions can be better than conscious ones, differentiating intuitive and instinctive inputs is very difficult. In fact, intuitive and instinctive inputs are often phenomenologically so similar that some kinds of demarcation criteria are required.

To this end, differentiating System 1 processes by their evolutive basis goes a long way to help us identify viable intuitions from non-viable System 1 inputs. Phylogenetic System 1 processes are such processes are based on our evolutionary history. They concern processes that drive physical reactions (like sudden fright or the knee-jerk), emotional reactions, protective parental behavior, fight or flight reactions, sexual reactions and the tendency to maximize energy intake. They are common across the entire species, determined by our genetic code and mostly autonomous throughout the entire life of the person, if not checked by reflective thought or ontogenetic System 1 processes. Ontogenetic System 1 processes are, in turn, generated by experience and practice. As much of research has shown, expertise requires a considerable amount of deliberate practice to develop new skills. (See e.g. Ericsson et al. 1993, 2007; Dane and Pratt 2007.) A great deal of the literature focused on intuition also supports the idea of intuition as driven by expertise and skills. (See e.g. Klein 1998; Gladwell 2005; Gigerenzer 2007; Dane and Pratt 2007; Kahneman and Klein 2009; Kahneman 2011).

Intuition has been sometimes attributed almost magical properties – how some people "just know by their gut feeling." In the light of the recent research, it appears rather to be simply a form of skilled cognition that is driven by ontogenetic System 1 processes acquired by experience and practice. As I have written elsewhere, "Intuition is about utilizing past experiences and the associative nature of System 1 to produce viable insight in various situations" (Järvilehto 2015).

The rough guideline for identifying the viability of System 1 generated inputs is to evaluate their evolutionary background. While phylogenetic processes work well in a natural environment, ontogenetic processes have in turn been tailored by experience and practice to meet the demands of our present culturally evolved environment. In addition to these constraints, there are other demarcation criteria pertinent in identifying viable intuitions, such as the evaluation of the validity of the environment in which the skill set has been generated and the effect of known cognitive biases (See e.g. Kahneman 2011; Kahneman and Klein 2009; for discussion, see Järvilehto 2015). The distinction between ontogenetic and phylogenetic System 1 processes goes, however, a long way to differentiate viable and non-viable System 1 inputs. If you work in a field you know you have a great deal of experience and expertise in, it is likely that your experience has generated a sufficient amount of System 1 processes that enable highly sophisticated decision-making without the intervention of the conscious mind. In turn, if you operate in a field that is unknown to you, even a very pressing intuition may be likely to be unviable. In other words, if you know what you are doing, trust your gut. Otherwise, think it through.

7.4 Flow in the Context of Dual Processing

Flow is the optimal state of experience where action and awareness meld together and doing becomes practically autonomous (Csikszentmihályi 1975, 1990; for a review of flow research, see Nakamura and Csikszentmihályi 2002). According to Mihály Csikszentmihályi (1990, p. 49), who introduced the concept of flow into the scientific literature, there are several typical conditions to flow:

- The chance of completing the task at hand.
- Concentration on the task at hand.
- Clear goal.
- Immediate feedback.
- Deep but effortless involvement.
- A sense of control.
- Concern for the self disappears.
- The sense of the duration of the task is altered.

The chance of completing the task at hand means that no immediate obstacles exists to prevent the completion of the task. Concentration on the task at hand means that the entire attention, or System 2 capacity, of the agent is dedicated to the task at hand. A clear goal means that there is a distinct and unambiguous end state towards which the action is intended. Immediate feedback means that the agent is aware of her progress with the task at hand.

Effortless involvement means that the task at hand has been practiced to a degree of automaticity where no System 2 reflection or interventions are needed. In Stanovich's terms, this could be described as System 2's reflective mind being offline. This in turn leads to the disappearance of the concern for the self. And finally, the sense of duration of the task is distorted: time just seems to "fly by." While in much of the literature flow state is characterized as independent of conscious thought, it is by no means an *unconscious* state. The agent is, after a fact, very much aware of what is going on. It is, in fact, conscious *effort* – the need to analyze and guide action – that is missing, due to the high level of automaticity of the action. The conditions of flow can be broken down to *task-related* and *cognition-related* parameters and the *indicators* of flow. The task related parameters are the chance of completing the task at hand, having a clear goal and getting immediate feedback. The cognition related parameters are automaticity and effortless involvement and the sense of control. Finally, indicators of flow are the concern of the self disappearing and the distortion of time perception.

Flow requires a sufficient degree of skill. In fact, one of the demarcation criteria Csikszentmihályi (1975) offers for determining the flow state is the balancing of challenges and skills. If the task at hand is too easy in relation to present skills, the agent is bored. And if the task is too hard, the agent is stressed and anxious. But a properly balanced task first requires the entire attention of the conscious System 2, but does not cause too many anomalies or problems to require System 2 to engage in reflection and problem solving. In a way, System 2 can, indeed, be thought of as a kind of a problem-solving function. When System 1 is capable enough of automatically producing desired effects, System 2, or at least the reflective part thereof, can remain offline and let System 1 processes carry out. But if an anomaly or a problem is encountered – if System 1 processes run afoul – then System 2 reflection is brought online to assess and evaluate the situation and to take conscious action.

To achieve flow, it is often important to have the chance of completing the task at hand. The chance of completion, together with a clear goal, gives System 2 a target to orient towards. This enables concentration on the task at hand. If the task is not clearly defined, it is very hard to orient towards a given course of action, and attention is prone to wander. Immediate feedback works as an indicator of whether the ongoing System 1 processes work in desired ways or not. If the expected feedback is not met (for example, if a given score in a game is not reached), System 2 is engaged and an alternative strategy of action is sought.

In summary, flow is a state where System 1 processes are carried away automatically, without the intervention of reflective System 2. As is the case with intuition, it is also typically the case that ontogenetic System 1 processes are required to reach flow. Only once a sufficient skill level is reached, can flow be attained, and more forcibly so in a culturally evolved environment, where many of our phylogenetic System 1 processes are not only dysfunctional but clearly detrimental to our well-being, such as aggressive tendencies or maximizing energy intake. In this sense, flow can be construed as an action-oriented counterpart for intuition.

7.5 The Relationship Between Intuition and Flow

Intuition is the capacity to make decisions and create new ideas without conscious deliberation. Flow is the optimal experience, where conscious thought seems to meld together with the action itself. Both intuition and flow involve ontogenetic System 1 processes that have been acquired through experience and practice. While flow can also involve instinctive processes – phylogenetic System 1 processes –, in a culturally evolved environment this is not typically the case. It could be surmised that a jaguar running through the savannah is in a state of phylogenetic flow, but such a state would no doubt be quickly cut short on the interstate. As Csikszentmihályi points out,

> Living exclusively by genetic and social instructions is fine as long as everything goes well. But the moment biological or social goals are frustrated – which in the long run is inevitable – a person must formulate new goals, and create a new flow activity for himself, or else he will waste his energies in inner turmoil. (Csikszentmihályi 1990, p. 207.)

To this end, while intuition is more clearly defined through the requirement of ontogeny of the involved System 1 processes, also flow, for the relevant parts in a culturally evolved environment, is most emphatically generated by ontogenetic System 1 processes.

Flow can be thought of as intuitive action, where as intuition in turn can be construed as cognition in flow. In both cases, we need to have first acquired a sufficient skill level to be able to reach the desired action or insight, and then to commit the process to the automatic System 1. Both intuition and flow enable us to adapt very well to a quickly changing, culturally evolving environment. While our genetic code may direct us to predefined patterns of behavior and action, we can affect this to a great deal by both System 2 based reflective cognition (overriding System 1 where needed), as well as by practicing and generating new System 1 capacities and skills.

To summarize, intuition is System 1 thinking and flow is System 1 doing. Both stem from the same source of ontogenetic System 1 processes that we have generated by experience and practice. Both intuition and flow enable us to rely more on the massive parallel capacity of System 1 in a culturally evolving and changing environment and thus to function better than if we had only our instincts and our rational minds to go by.

7.6 Concluding Remarks

At a first glance, both intuition and flow appear to be similar states in the sense that they both involve a great degree of automaticity and seem, at least to an extent, to be a form of non-conscious cognition or action. In the context of dual processing theories of cognition, both intuition and flow can be explained as functions of the non-conscious massively parallel processing of System 1, demarcated by the ontogeny of System 1 processes involved in producing intuitions and enabling flow. According to the dual processing theories of cognition, we have not just one mind, but in fact two. The non-conscious System 1 enables us to carry out massively parallel processing, but is fuzzy and mostly inaccessible to conscious direction. The conscious System 2 is, in turn, capacity-constrained and mostly serial processing, but enables us to interrupt ongoing cognitive processes and actions and to volitionally direct action and attention. While the parallel processing of System 1 goes a long way to explaining the sometimes wondrous phenomenology of both intuition and flow, it alone does not suffice. More forcibly so, because there are also many cognitive processes whose phenomenology is almost indiscernible from intuitive processes, but whose viability is poor. To this end, the division between ontogenetic and phylogenetic System 1 processes is needed to differentiate intuitions from instincts, and flow in a culturally evolved environment from flow in a natural environment.

While intuitive System 1 processes are, by definition, of ontogenetic nature, it could be argued that flow can also be reached by phylogenetic processes in a natural environment. However, also flow requires almost without exception ontogenetic System 1 processes. In the natural environment there may still be anomalous situations where new learning is required to be able to function properly. And in a culturally evolved environment ontogenetic System 1 processes are a necessity for flow.

Without sufficient skills to meet present challenges, System 2 is constantly engaged in reflection and problem solving, and reaching the flow state is practically impossible.

Intuition and flow engage to a great extent the same cognitive mechanisms, at the same time without being reduced to definitions in terms of one another. Both intuition and flow involve ontogenetic System 1 processing and enable us to function very well in a culturally evolving, changing environment. In a sense, flow can be thought of as intuitive action, whereas intuition can be thought of as cognition in flow. To recapitulate, intuition is System 1 thinking, and flow is System 1 doing.

References

Bargh, J. A., & Chartrand, T. L. (1999). The unbearable automaticity of being. *American Psychologist, 54*(7), 462–479.

Bargh, J. A., Chen, M., & Burrows, L. (1996). Automaticity of social behavior: Direct effects of trait construct and stereotype activation on action. *Journal of Personality and Social Psychology, 71*(2), 230–244.

Baumeister, R. F., & Tierney, J. (2011). *Willpower: Rediscovering the greatest human strength* (Kindle Edition). New York: The Penguin Press.

Baumeister, R. F., Bratlavsky, E., Muraven, M., & Tice, D. M. (1998). Ego depletion: Is the active self a limited resource? *Journal of Personality and Social Psychology, 74*(5), 1252–1265.

Bealer, G. (1996). A priori knowledge and the scope of philosophy. *Philosophical Studies, 81*, 121–142.

Csikszentmihályi, M. (1975). *Beyond boredom and anxiety: Experiencing flow in work and play*. San Francisco: Jossey-Bass.

Csikszentmihályi, M. (1990). *Flow: The psychology of optimal performance*. New York: Harper Perennial.

Dane, E., & Pratt, M. G. (2007). Exploring intuition and its role in managerial decision making. *Academy of Management Review, 32*(1), 33–54.

Dietrich, A. (2004). Neurocognitive mechanisms underlying the experience of flow. *Consciousness and Cognition, 13*, 746–761.

Djiksterhuis, A. (2004). Think different: The merits of unconscious thought in preference development and decision making. *Journal of Personality and Social Psychology, 87*(5), 586–598.

Djiksterhuis, A., & Nordgren, L. F. (2006). A theory of unconscious thought. *Perspectives on Psychological Science, 1*, 95–106.

Djiksterhuis, A., Aarts, H., & Smith, P. K. (2006). The power of the subliminal: On subliminal persuasion and other potential applications. In *The new unconscious* (pp. 77–105). New York: Oxford University Press.

Ericsson, K. A., Krampe, R. T., & Resch-Römer, C. (1993). The role of deliberate practice in the acquisition of expert performance. *Psychological Review, 100*(3), 363–406.

Ericsson, K. A., Prietula, M. J., & Cokely, E. T. (2007). The making of an expert. *Harvard Business Review, 85*(7–8), 114–121.

Evans, J. S. B. T. (2003). In two minds: Dual-process accounts of reasoning. *Trends in Cognitive Sciences, 7*(10), 454–459.

Evans, J. S. B. T. (2009). How many dual-process theories do we need? One, two, or many? In J. S. B. T. Evans & K. Frankish (Eds.), *In two minds: Dual processes and beyond* (pp. 33–54). Oxford: Oxford University Press.

Evans, J. S. B. T. (2010). *Thinking twice*. Chippenham: Oxford University Press.

Evans, J. S. B. T., & Stanovich, K. (2013). Dual process theories of higher cognition: Advancing the debate. *Perspectives on Psychological Science, 8*(3), 223–241.
Gigerenzer, G. (2007). *Gut feelings: The intelligence of the unconscious* (Kindle Edition). Londan: Allen Lane.
Gladwell, M. (2005). *Blink: The power of thinking without thinking*. London: Penguin.
Järvilehto, L. (2015). *The nature and function of intuitive thought and decision making*. Cham: Springer.
Kahneman, D. (1973). *Attention and effort*. Englewood Cliffs: Prentice-Hall.
Kahneman, D. (2011). *Thinking, fast and slow* (Kindle Edition). London: Penguin.
Kahneman, D., & Klein, G. (2009). Conditions for intuitive expertise: A failure to disagree. *American Psychologist, 64*(6), 515–526.
Kant, I. (1998). *Critique of pure reason* (P. Guyer & A. W. Wood, Trans.). New York: Cambridge University Press.
Klein, G. (1998). *Sources of power: How people make decisions*. Cambridge: The MIT Press.
Miller, G. (1956). The magical number seven, plus or minus two: Some limits on our capacity for processing information. *Psychological Review, 63*, 81–97.
Nakamura, J., & Csikszentmihályi, M. (2002). The concept of flow. In *Handbook of positive psychology* (pp. 89–105). New York: Oxford University Press.
Simon, H. A. (1978). Rationality as process and as product of thought. *The American Economic Review, 68*(2), 1–16.
Stanovich, K. (2004). *Robot's rebellion: Finding meaning in the Age of Darwin*. Chicago: University of Chicago Press.
Stanovich, K. (2009). Distinguishing the reflective, algorithmic, and autonomous minds: Is it time for a tri-process theory? In J. S. B. T. Evans & K. Frankish (Eds.), *In two minds: Dual processes and beyond* (pp. 55–88). Oxford: Oxford University Press.
Stanovich, K. E., & West, R. F. (2000). Individual differences in reasoning: Implications for the rationality debate? *Behavioral and Brain Sciences, 23*, 646–726.
Zimmermann, M. (1989). The nervous system in the context of information theory. In R. F. Schmidt & G. Thews (Eds.), *Human physiology* (pp. 166–173). Berlin: Springer.

Chapter 8
Flow at Work as a Moderator of the Self-Determination Model of Work Engagement

Daniela De Fraga and Giovanni B. Moneta

Abstract This study extends the self-determination model of work engagement. Based on flow theory and self-determination theory, it was hypothesised that the extent to which workers experience flow at work would moderate the positive association between perceived managerial autonomy support and work engagement, in such a way that for employees with more flow the association would be weaker (H1), and the positive associations between autonomy support and satisfaction of intrinsic psychological needs, in such a way that for employees with more flow these associations would be weaker (H2). A sample of 177 workers completed the Work Climate Questionnaire, Basic Need Satisfaction at Work Scale, Utrecht Work Engagement Scale, and Flow Short Scale. Moderated mediation modelling supported hypothesis 1 and hypothesis 2 limitedly to the needs for competence and relatedness. The findings indicate that workers with more flow at work are more likely to engage in the job regardless of autonomy support.

8.1 Introduction

Workers' psychological connection with their jobs has become the core research theme in the field of organisational psychology (Leiter and Bakker 2010). One of the reasons is that workers who are engaged have a propensity for working to their full potential, perform to a high standard, are committed, and interested in the company's success (Harter et al. 2002). Moreover, work engagement has benefits for the employee, as it entails a positive and fulfilling job-related state of mind (Sonnentag et al. 2010), which is characterised by a sense of energetic, effective, and enthusiastic connection with the activities in the job (Leiter and Bakker 2010).

This chapter was adapted from an undergraduate thesis written by the first author and supervised by the second author.

D. De Fraga • G.B. Moneta (✉)
School of Psychology, London Metropolitan University,
Room T6-20, Tower Building, 166-220 Holloway Road, London N7 8DB, UK
e-mail: g.moneta@londonmet.ac.uk

L. Harmat et al. (eds.), *Flow Experience*, DOI 10.1007/978-3-319-28634-1_8

Work engagement is a cognitive-affective state that involves employees' perception of being able to deal successfully with the demands of their work with vigour, dedication, and absorption (Schaufeli and Bakker 2003). This state is theorised to contribute to employees' overall well-being, which in turn helps to prevent undesired outcomes such as job burnout (Leiter and Bakker 2010).

Where does work engagement come from? The self-determination model of work engagement (Deci et al. 2001) states that the primary factors influencing work engagement are perceived managerial autonomy support and satisfaction of the intrinsic psychological needs for autonomy, competence, and relatedness. However, nothing is known about individual factors that may influence the extent to which contextual factors, such as perceived managerial autonomy support, are conducive to need satisfaction and work engagement. The aim of the present study is to gain a better understanding of when perceived managerial autonomy support leads to need satisfaction and work engagement. In particular, this study proposes and tests an extended self-determination model of work engagement (Deci et al. 2001) that includes flow (Csikszentmihalyi 1975/2000) as a moderating variable.

8.1.1 The Self-Determination Model of Engagement

Self-determination theory (SDT; Deci and Ryan 1985; Ryan and Deci 2000) defines need satisfaction in terms of cognitions, emotions, and behaviour. Autonomy need satisfaction involves performing with a sense of volition and initiation of one's own actions (Deci et al. 2001), as well as the feeling of having choice (Gagné and Deci 2005). Competence need satisfaction entails succeeding at tasks which are challenging and the accomplishment of desired results. Relatedness need satisfaction relies on a sense of mutual respect, care, and consideration with others (Deci et al. 2001).

Although there are various facets of work autonomy (e.g., work schedule autonomy or work criterion autonomy) that are associated with more work commitment and work satisfaction (Sadler-Smith et al. 2003), the self-determination model of work engagement (Deci et al. 2001) posits that the main contributor to both work engagement and fulfillment of the intrinsic needs is managerial autonomy support (Deci et al. 2001). A worker's perception of managerial autonomy support can be achieved when managers or most immediate supervisors understand and recognise the viewpoint of their employees (Deci and Ryan 1985), offer information which is meaningful, and allow for choice (Baard et al. 2004).

The self-determination model of work engagement posits that perceived managerial autonomy support fosters satisfaction of intrinsic psychological needs and, in turn, satisfaction of these needs fosters work engagement. Several studies found that perceived autonomy support (e.g., Deci and Ryan 1985; Ryan and Deci 2000; Deci and Vansteenkiste 2004) and perceived managerial autonomy support (e.g., Deci et al. 2001; Baard et al. 2004) explain satisfaction of the intrinsic psychological needs. Moreover, Deci et al. (2001) found in two workers samples, one from the

U.S.A. and the other from Bulgaria, that satisfaction of the intrinsic psychological needs explains work engagement and mediates the positive relation between perceived managerial autonomy support and work engagement. Therefore, perceived managerial autonomy support appears to be a core promoter of both intrinsic psychological need satisfaction and work engagement.

However, the relations between perceptions of managerial autonomy support in the job, intrinsic need satisfaction, and engagement might be more complex. Task enjoyment, experience during the activity, and challenge intensity also seem important for workers' optimal functioning and engagement. In particular, as captured by the term autotelic experience (Csikszentmihalyi 1992/2002), individuals may engage in an activity purely by its own sake because they provide inner rewards for themselves by developing the ability to find enjoyment in the task regardless of external encouragements such as perceptions of autonomy support in the work climate.

8.1.2 *Flow as a Moderator of the Self-Determination Model of Engagement*

Flow is an optimal experience wherein the person acts with total involvement in an intrinsically motivated activity; the experience is characterised by a state of complete absorption in the task (Nakamura and Csikszentmihalyi 2005), profound intrinsic enjoyment and enriched cognitive efficiency (Moneta 2014). The flow state involves deep and undivided concentration and low self-awareness, which is often accompanied by a distorted perception of time (Ullen et al. 2012). Flow is expected to occur more often when the person identifies greater opportunities for action and has the necessary skills to engage in them (Nakamura and Csikszentmihalyi 2005) and hence experiences a balance between perceived challenges and skills (Csikszentmihalyi 1975/2000; Loubris et al. 1995). Moreover, flow is more likely to occur when goals are clear and feedback from the activity is immediate (Csikszentmihalyi 1975/2000).

Although flow appears to be easier to achieve in supportive work contexts, some employees may be able to enjoy their work and experience flow even in an austere and limited work climate by viewing environmental constraints as opportunities to express their creativity and self-determination (Csikszentmihalyi 1990). These individuals possibly have developed an autotelic personality, tend to be more resilient than others when faced with non-supportive work contexts, and are particularly active in pursuing challenging tasks in which they can see themselves as very skilled (Csikszentmihalyi 1990). Furthermore, autotelic persons are capable of converting pressure into enjoyable challenges and control their minds so as to continually perceive anything as a potential motive of joy (Csikszentmihalyi 1990). Accordingly, autotelic workers may experience flow more frequently and intensely than others (Csikszentmihalyi 1990) particularly in poor work climates.

Bakker (2005) has defined flow in the work context as a short-term peak experience that is characterised by absorption, enjoyment, and intrinsic motivation. The element of absorption refers to a state of profound concentration in which workers are completely immersed in their job (Bakker 2005), entirely forget what is happening around them, and have a sensation that time is flying (Csikszentmihalyi 1990). As such, flow in the job may work as a buffer that isolates employees from the environment, making them less sensitive to perceptions of the work context. In turn, workers' perception of managerial autonomy support may be less predictive of work engagement for employees with more flow in the job. Therefore, the following hypothesis is proposed:

H1: The positive association between perceived managerial autonomy support and work engagement will be moderated (buffered) by flow at work, in such a way that the association will be weaker for those with higher levels of flow.

The enjoyment element of flow stems from the employees performing a work-related task purely because they find it intrinsically rewarding, as flow makes the activity inherently rewarding (Csikszentmihalyi 1990), with no need for external recompenses. Because the flow experience is self rewarding, entails a sense of freedom during the task, and involves the feeling of achievement in carrying out challenging tasks to the best of one's abilities, it should facilitate the satisfaction of intrinsic psychological needs on its own, independent of contextual factors such as perceived managerial autonomy support. Therefore, the following hypothesis is proposed:

H2: The positive association between perceived managerial autonomy support at work and intrinsic needs satisfaction for (a) autonomy, (b) competence, and (c) relatedness will be moderated (buffered) by flow at work, in such a way that the association will be weaker for those with higher levels of flow.

8.1.3 Goals of the Study

The two research hypotheses in combination constitute the moderated mediation model shown in Fig. 8.1, which illustrates the proposed moderating role of flow on the path from perceived managerial autonomy support to work engagement, as well as on the paths from perceived autonomy support to intrinsic needs satisfaction for autonomy, competence, and relatedness. The model posits that flow at work will buffer the effect of perceived autonomy support on work engagement (*H1*) and on intrinsic needs satisfaction for autonomy (*H2a*), competence (*H2b*), and relatedness (*H2c*). The goal of the present study is to test this extended self-determination model of work engagement.

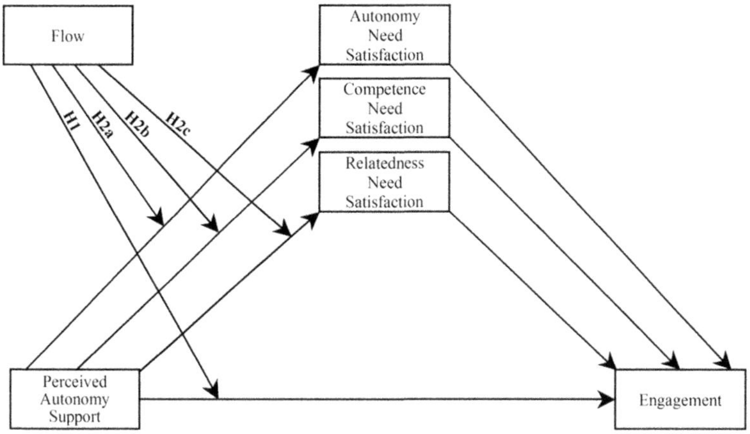

Fig. 8.1 Conceptual diagram of the hypothesised moderating effects of flow on the self-determination model of work engagement (Deci et al. 2001)

8.2 Method

8.2.1 Participants

A convenience sample of 177 workers participated in the study. There were 67 males (37.9 %) and 110 females (62.1 %) with ages ranging from 19 to 74 ($M = 37.33$; $SD = 13.21$). There were 120 (67.8 %) Whites, 24 (13.6 %) Blacks, 3 (1.7 %) Chinese, 5 (2.8 %) Indians, 1 (0.6 %) Japanese, 12 (6.8 %) from other ethnic backgrounds, and 12 (6.8 %) participants of mixed ethnicity. The nationality distribution was 67 (37.9 %) British citizens and 110 (62.1 %) participants from other nationalities. In relation to educational background, 111 (62.7 %) participants earned an undergraduate degree, and 57 (32.2 %) also held a postgraduate degree.

Participants were from a wide variety of occupations, such as engineer, customer services assistant, care worker, recruiter, and lecturer. The employment type distribution was 102 full-time workers (57.6 %), 63 part-time workers (35.6 %), and 12 workers who had special working arrangements (6.8 %). The weekly working hours average was 42.57 ($SD = 13.67$) for full-time employees, 19.51 ($SD = 10.86$) for part-time employees, and 27.04 (SD = 14.53) for employees with other types of working hours. The majority of the participants were employed by a company ($n = 150$; 84.7 %), whilst the others were self-employed ($n = 20$; 11.3 %) or owned their own company or business ($n = 7$; 4 %). Job tenure varied from 0 to 52 years ($M = 5.42$ years, $SD = 7.40$).

8.2.2 Measures

This research was approved by a university ethics panel and the data were collected through an online survey, which contained the following questionnaires.

8.2.2.1 Perceived Autonomy Support Scale (PAS); Also Called Work Climate Questionnaire (WCQ)

The PAS measures perceptions of the degree of autonomy supportiveness of workers' most immediate supervisor or manager (Baard et al. 2004) through 15 self-report items (e.g., "I feel that my manager provides me choices and options") rated on a scale ranging from 1 ("strongly disagree") to 7 ("strongly agree"). The scale score was calculated by averaging all the items, with higher scores indicating more perceived autonomy support. The Cronbach's alpha of the scale ranged from 0.92 to 0.96 in previous studies in which the target person (e.g., doctor, instructor, or manager) varied (Williams et al. 1996; Williams and Deci 1996).

8.2.2.2 Basic Need Satisfaction at Work Scale (BNSW; Also Named Intrinsic Need Satisfaction Scale)

The BNSW measures the extent to which workers experience satisfaction of their three intrinsic needs (autonomy, competence, and relatedness) at work (Kasser et al. 1992) through 21 self-report items (e.g., "I feel like I can make a lot of inputs to deciding how my job gets done" [autonomy], "I have been able to learn interesting new skills on my job" [competence], and "I really like the people I work with" [relatedness]) on a scale ranging from 1 ("not at all true") to 7 ("very true"). The subscale scores were calculated by averaging their constituent items, with higher scores indicating more need satisfaction. The Cronbach's alpha reported in previous studies ranged between 0.62 and 0.79 for autonomy, between 0.73 and 0.81 for competence, and between 0.57 and 0.84 for relatedness (Leone 1995; Deci et al. 2001; Baard et al. 2004).

8.2.2.3 Utrecht Work Engagement Scale 9 (UWES-9)

The UWES-9 measures work engagement (Schaufeli et al. 2006) through 9 self-report items (e.g., "At my work, I feel bursting with energy") on a scale ranging from 0 ("never") to 6 ("always/every day"). The scale score was calculated by averaging all the items, with higher scores indicating more work engagement. In the original validation study, the Cronbach's alpha ranged between 0.85 and 0.92 across ten investigated countries (Schaufeli et al. 2006).

8.2.2.4 Flow Short Scale (FSS)

The FSS measures levels of flow experienced during an activity (Engeser and Rheinberg 2008) through 10 self-report items (e.g., "I am totally absorbed in what I am doing") on a scale ranging from 0 ("not at all") to 6 ("very much"). In this study, participants were instructed to complete the scale thinking of their experience at work. The scale score was calculated by averaging all the items, with higher scores indicating more flow at work. In the original validation study, the Cronbach's alpha was 0.92 (Engeser and Rheinberg 2008).

8.2.3 Overview of Statistical Analyses

The analysis used Hayes' (2013) regression modelling approach to multiple and moderated mediation, which is robust to non-normality, and Hayes' (n.d.) PROCESS Macro for SPSS. Hayes's model 4 (multiple mediation model) was used to partially replicate Deci and co-workers' (2001) self-determination model of engagement. Hayes' model 8 (multiple moderated mediation model) was used to test the hypothesised extension of the self-determination model of engagement.

In order to reduce collinearity, the scores of all variables were standardised prior to fitting the models; so that, all the estimated coefficients are standardised regression coefficients. The models were estimated using 50,000 bootstrap permutations for bias correction. The indirect effects were tested using 95 % confidence intervals.

The proposed extension of the self-determination model of engagement includes four hypothesised interactions. These were simultaneously estimated in a single run. Nevertheless, for the sake of clarity, the results are presented separately by each specific path. The standard convention is used to identify the various paths of the models: *a* represents paths from the predictors to the mediators, *b* represents paths from the mediators to the outcome variable, and *c* represents paths from the predictors to the outcome variable.

8.3 Results

8.3.1 Data Description

Table 8.1 shows the descriptive statistics of the study variables. With the exception of competence need satisfaction, Cronbach's alpha of the scales exceeded 0.7, reflecting satisfactory to good internal consistency (e.g., Kline 2013). As expected, all the variables were positively correlated with one another.

Table 8.1 Means, standard deviations, correlation coefficients and Cronbach's alpha coefficients (in parentheses) of the study variables

Variables	M	SD	1.	2.	3.	4.	5.	6.
1. Perceived autonomy support[a]	4.87	1.49	(0.97)					
2. Autonomy need satisfaction[a]	4.54	1.15	0.68**	(0.78)				
3. Competence need satisfaction[a]	5.26	1.00	0.49**	0.61**	(0.64)			
4. Relatedness need satisfaction[a]	4.98	1.05	0.47**	0.57**	0.54**	(0.82)		
5. Engagement[b]	4.08	1.16	0.47**	0.63**	0.64**	0.48**	(0.91)	
6. Flow[b]	3.59	0.98	0.38**	0.48**	0.52**	0.36**	0.66**	(0.85)

N=177, **p<0.01 (1-tailed)
[a]Range of the scale = 1–7
[b]Range of the scale = 0–6

8.3.2 Replication of the Self-Determination Model of Work Engagement

In accordance with Deci and co-workers' (2001) model, engagement was the outcome variable (Y), perceived autonomy support was the predictor variable (X), and the three intrinsic needs – (M_1) autonomy, (M_2) competence, and (M_3) relatedness – were the mediating variables. Table 8.2 shows the estimated regression coefficients, their standard errors, the significance levels of each direct effect and the overall model summary.

The estimated coefficients for paths a_1 and b_1 were both positive. The indirect effect of perceived autonomy support on engagement through autonomy need satisfaction was positive (0.227) and significant (95 % CI: 0.118–0.351). Likewise, the estimated coefficients for paths a_2 and b_2 were both positive. The indirect effect of perceived autonomy support on engagement through competence need satisfaction was positive (0.193) and significant (95 % CI: 0.111–0.297). The estimated coefficients for paths a_3 and b_3 were both positive. However, the indirect effect of perceived autonomy support on engagement through relatedness need satisfaction was positive (0.031) but not significant (95 % CI: –0.036 to 0.115). Finally, the total indirect effect of perceived autonomy support on engagement through the three needs satisfaction was positive (0.450) and significant (95 % CI: 0.317–0.610). In all, the analysis replicated the self-determination model of engagement, with the caveat that relatedness need satisfaction did not turn out to be a mediator.

Table 8.2 Standardised regression coefficients, standard errors, and model summary information for the self-determination mediation model of engagement

	Outcome															
	M_1 (autonomy)				M_2 (competence)				M_3 (relatedness)				Y (engagement)			
Predictor		Coeff.	SE	*p*		Coeff.	SE	*p*		Coeff.	SE	*p*		Coeff.	SE	*p*
X (PAS)	a_1	0.676	0.056	<0.001	a_2	0.493	0.066	<0.001	a_3	0.468	0.067	<0.001	c'	0.020	0.074	0.789
M_1 (autonomy)		–	–	–		–	–	–		–	–	–	b_1	0.336	0.084	0.001
M_2 (competence)		–	–	–		–	–	–		–	–	–	b_2	0.391	0.072	<0.001
M_3 (relatedness)		–	–	–		–	–	–		–	–	–	b_3	0.066	0.069	0.342
	$R^2=0.457$				$R^2=0.243$				$R^2=0.219$				$R^2=0.501$			
	$F(1, 175)=147.373, p<0.001$				$F(1, 175)=56.160, p<0.001$				$F(1, 175)=49.044, p<0.001$				$F(4, 172)=43.125, p<0.001$			

N = 177

PAS perceived autonomy support, *Autonomy* autonomy need satisfaction, *Competence* competence need satisfaction, *Relatedness* relatedness need satisfaction

8.3.3 *Test of the Moderated Mediation Model of Work Engagement*

8.3.3.1 Moderation of the Path from Perceived Autonomy Support to Engagement (H1)

In this part of the model, engagement was the outcome variable, perceived autonomy support was the predictor variable (X), and flow (W) was the moderator and predictor variable. Table 8.3 shows the regression estimates. Flow and the interaction of flow and perceived autonomy support were significant predictors of engagement, whereas perceived autonomy support was not a significant predictor.

Figure 8.2 shows the interaction between perceived autonomy support and flow in the prediction of engagement. The negative association for high flow illustrated in

Table 8.3 Regression of work engagement on perceived autonomy support and flow: Estimated standardised regression coefficients, their standard errors and significance levels, and model summary

	Coeff	Std. error	t	p
Perceived autonomy support (X) c_1	−0.007	0.066	−0.108	0.914
Flow (W) c_2	0.390	0.058	6.684	<0.001
Perceived autonomy support × flow (XW) c_3	−0.099	0.046	−2.132	0.035
$R^2=0.609$				
$F(6,170)=44.087, p<0.001$				

N = 177

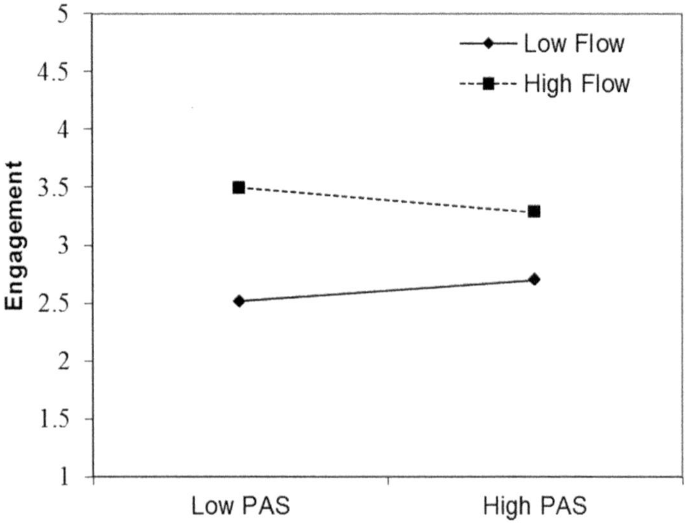

Fig. 8.2 Interaction plot of engagement as a function of PAS (perceived autonomy support) for low (−1SD) and high (+1SD) levels of flow

Table 8.4 Regression of autonomy need satisfaction on perceived autonomy support and flow: estimated standardised regression coefficients, their standard errors and significance levels, and model summary

	Coeff	Std. error	t	p
Perceived autonomy support (X) a_1	0.560	0.058	9.606	<0.001
Flow (W) a_2	0.267	0.057	4.700	<0.001
Perceived autonomy support × flow (XW) a_3	−0.061	0.050	−1.236	0.218
$R^2 = 0.522$				
$F(3,173) = 63.016, p < 0.001$				

N = 177

the figure was not significant. The figure shows that flow moderates the association between perceived autonomy support and engagement in such a way that perceived autonomy support is positively associated with engagement for low flow, and it is not associated with engagement for high flow. These findings indicate that perceived autonomy support predicts engagement only for those with low levels of flow in the job, and hence support hypothesis 1. Moreover, the figure shows that the effect of perceived autonomy support on engagement was way weaker than that of flow.

8.3.3.2 Moderation of the Path from Perceived Autonomy Support to Autonomy Need Satisfaction (H2a)

In this part of the model, autonomy need satisfaction was the outcome variable, perceived autonomy support was the predictor variable (X), and flow was the moderator and predictor variable (W). Table 8.4 shows the regression estimates. Flow and perceived autonomy support were significant predictors of autonomy need satisfaction, whereas the interaction of flow and perceived autonomy support was not a significant predictor. These findings indicate that flow does not moderate the relationship between perceived autonomy support and autonomy need satisfaction, and hence do not support hypothesis 2a.

8.3.3.3 Moderation of the Path from Perceived Autonomy Support to Competence Need Satisfaction (H2b)

In this part of the model, competence need satisfaction was the outcome variable, perceived autonomy support was the predictor variable (X), and flow was the moderator and predictor variable (W). Table 8.5 shows the regression estimates. Flow, perceived autonomy support, and the interaction of flow and perceived autonomy support were significant predictors of competence need satisfaction.

Figure 8.3 shows the interaction between perceived autonomy support and flow in the prediction of competence need satisfaction. The figure shows that flow moderates the association between perceived autonomy support and competence need satisfaction in such a way that perceived autonomy support is positively associated

Table 8.5 Regression of competence need satisfaction on perceived autonomy support and flow: estimated standardised regression coefficients, their standard errors and significance levels, and model summary

	Coeff	Std. error	t	p
Perceived autonomy support (X) a_1	0.307	0.065	4.698	<0.001
Flow (W) a_2	0.395	0.064	6.199	<0.001
Perceived autonomy support × Flow (XW) a_3	−0.141	0.056	−2.530	0.012
$R^2 = 0.398$				
$F(3,173) = 38.150, p < 0.001$				

N = 177

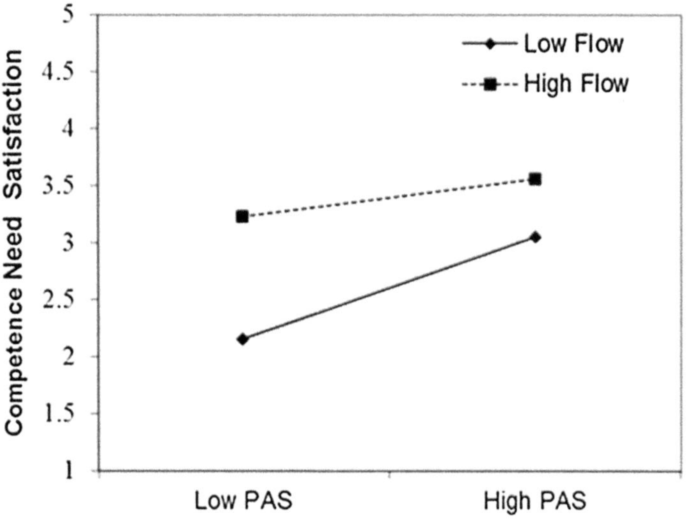

Fig. 8.3 Interaction plot of competence need satisfaction as a function of PAS (perceived autonomy support) for low (−1SD) and high (+1SD) levels of flow

with competence need satisfaction for low flow, and it is less associated with competence need satisfaction for high flow. These findings indicate that perceived autonomy support is a better predictor of competence need satisfaction for those with low levels of flow in the job, and hence support hypothesis 2b.

8.3.3.4 Moderation of the Path from Perceived Autonomy Support to Relatedness Need Satisfaction (H2c)

In this part of the model, relatedness need satisfaction was the outcome variable, perceived autonomy support was the predictor variable (X), and flow was the moderator and predictor variable (W). Table 8.6 shows the regression estimates.

Table 8.6 Regression of relatedness need satisfaction on perceived autonomy support and flow: estimated standardised regression coefficients, their standard errors and significance levels, and model summary

	Coeff.	Std. Error	*t*	*p*
Perceived autonomy support (X) a_1	0.347	0.071	4.864	<0.001
Flow (W) a_2	0.217	0.070	3.124	0.002
Perceived autonomy support × Flow (XW) a_3	−0.148	0.061	−2.446	0.015
$R^2 = 0.284$				
$F(3,173) = 22.835$, $p < 0.001$				

N = 177

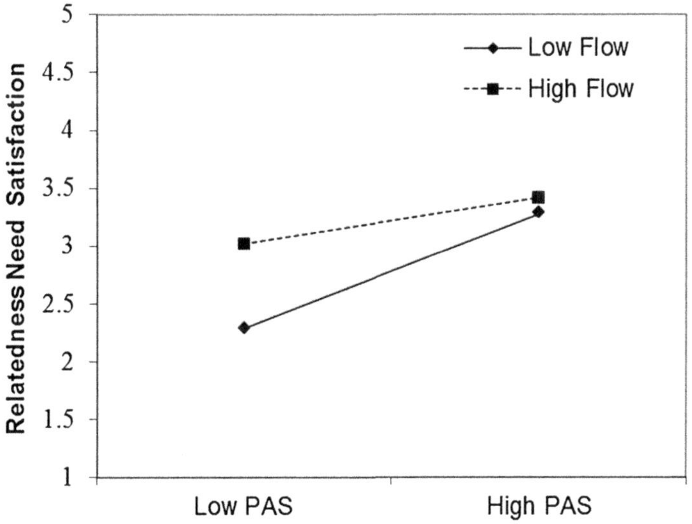

Fig. 8.4 Interaction plot of relatedness need satisfaction as a function of PAS (perceived autonomy support) for low (−1SD) and high (+1SD) levels of flow

Flow, perceived autonomy support, and the interaction of flow and perceived autonomy support were significant predictors of relatedness need satisfaction.

Figure 8.4 shows the interaction between perceived autonomy support and flow in the prediction of relatedness need satisfaction. The figure shows that flow moderates the association between perceived autonomy support and relatedness need satisfaction in such a way that perceived autonomy support is positively associated with relatedness need satisfaction for low flow, and it is less associated with relatedness need satisfaction for high flow. These findings indicate that perceived autonomy support is a better predictor of relatedness need satisfaction for those with low levels of flow in the job, and hence support hypothesis 2c.

8.4 Discussion

This study examined the buffering role of flow on the self-determination mediation model of work engagement (Deci et al. 2001) using a multicultural sample of workers from a variety of professions. Mediation analysis substantially replicated Deci and co-workers' findings. Moderated mediation analysis fully supported hypothesis 1, and partially supported hypothesis 2. These findings provide preliminary support for an extended model of work engagement, and suggest that flow functions as a personal resource that isolates employees from the work environment and hence helps them to engage in work independently of perceptions of managerial autonomy support.

8.4.1 Replication of the Self-Determination Model of Engagement

The patterns of correlations between variables from this study were consistent with those in Deci and co-workers' (2001) study. The analysis of the mediation model of engagement revealed that all the hypothesised paths were significant except for that from relatedness need satisfaction to engagement, which was not significant. This difference in findings between the two studies may be due to either chance or small differences in the research methods used. In all, the self-determination mediation model of work engagement worked well on the sample of the present study, indicating that perceived managerial autonomy support promotes work engagement through the satisfaction of intrinsic psychological needs.

8.4.2 The Extended Moderated Mediation Model of Work Engagement

The moderated mediation analysis fully supported hypothesis 1, revealing that there was no association between perceived managerial autonomy support and work engagement for employees with high levels of flow in the job. Consistent with flow theory (e.g., Csikszentmihalyi 1990; Bakker 2005), this finding suggests that employees who experience high levels of flow in the job are less reliant on their work atmosphere due to a state of profound task absorption and heightened concentration that makes them more self-motivated and less aware of the environment.

In particular, once in flow, individual's attention is freely invested in accomplishing the task at hand (Csikszentmihalyi 1990), and the concentration is so intense that the person is less able to detect and take in consideration contextual cues (Moneta 2014). A plausible explanation is that the nervous system has a limited capacity of how much information can be processed at each time. For example, it is estimated that individuals can process a maximum of 126 bits of information per second (Csikszentmihalyi 1990). Given that to understand what another person is saying involves processing about 40 bits of information per second (Csikszentmihalyi 1990), it seems almost impossible for employees high in flow to keep track of what is happening in the work environment due to limits in attentional resources. As a result, workers who experience high levels of flow are more likely to remain engaged in work independently of the degree of autonomy supportiveness in their job.

The moderated mediation analysis supported hypothesis 2 for the needs of competence and relatedness, but not for the need of autonomy. On the one hand, the analysis revealed that the positive relations between perceived managerial autonomy support and competence need satisfaction and relatedness need satisfaction were weaker for workers with more flow in the job. On the other hand, the analysis revealed that the positive relation between perceived managerial autonomy support and autonomy need satisfaction had virtually the same strength for workers with different levels of flow in the job.

The finding that flow buffers the association between perceived managerial autonomy support and competence need satisfaction has a straightforward interpretation within flow theory. As competence need satisfaction involves mastering tasks (Gagné 2003), flow is likely to facilitate the satisfaction of this need through workers' sense of capability in carrying out challenging tasks (Csikszentmihalyi 1990) and perceptions of greater opportunities for action when holding the basic skills to engage in them (Nakamura and Csikszentmihalyi 2005). Through either path, flow is likely to foster satisfaction of the need for competence independent of external rewards and conditions.

The finding that flow buffers the association between perceived managerial autonomy support and relatedness need satisfaction requires a more speculative interpretation. Undertaking pleasant and intrinsically motivated activities can help to enhance relatedness feelings (Reis et al. 2000). As such, workers high in flow are likely to benefit from this optimal experience in satisfying their need for relatedness without relying as much as those low in flow in social activities and the provision of contextual cues.

The finding that flow does not buffer the positive relation between perceived managerial autonomy support and autonomy need satisfaction is somewhat at odds with flow theory but is congruent with self-determination theory (Deci and Ryan 1985; Ryan and Deci 2000), which posits that perceived autonomy support is a key facilitator for autonomy need satisfaction. Although flow entails a sense of freedom during the absorption in intrinsically rewarding work activities, and hence can predict autonomy need satisfaction on its own, perceived managerial autonomy support is the strongest predictor of autonomy need satisfaction, and its predictive power is unaffected by flow.

What does cause work flow-ers to be more independent from environmental influences in their work engagement? Two complementary answers can be suggested. On the one hand, work flow-ers may have had developmental experiences that helped them to learn how to self regulate flow in achievement contexts.

In particular, they may have developed a metacognition of flow (Wilson and Moneta 2012, 2016), meant as knowledge and beliefs about the flow experience and one's own ability to make it happen at will, through, for example, vicarious learning derived from the observation of successful role models. On the other hand, work flow-ers may be predisposed genetically to develop an autotelic personality. In particular, research on twins found that flow pronness has a sizeable heritability of 41 % (Mosing et al. 2012), and individuals who are genetically predisposed for experiencing flow also tend to have personality traits such as low neuroticism, high conscientiousness (Ullén et al. 2012), openness to experience (Butkoviæ et al. 2015), and internal locus of control (Mosing et al. 2012), which are likely to support volitional behaviour and task focus in achievement contexts. As such, genetic factors may influence both flow in work and independence from the work environment. Moreover, even perceptions of the work environment were found to have fairly large heritability (Butkovic et al. 2015; Mosing et al. 2012). Therefore, work flow-ers' genetic makeup may help them simultaneously to reach flow in work and to perceive the work environment as being more flow-conducive or less flow-disruptive than deemed by their colleagues. In all, it is likely that environmental and genetic factors interact in the development of the autotelic independence from the work environment found in this study.

8.4.3 Limitations

The present study is limited by the small sample size with mixed occupations, the correlational design, and the total reliance on self-reported measures. Moreover, this study did not consider individual differences that are known to influence both flow and work engagement, such as Big Five personality traits (Ullen et al. 2012) and autotelic traits (Baumann 2012). Finally, this study ignored potentially relevant work environment factors. For instance, the occurrence of both flow and work engagement is likely to be facilitated by environmental circumstances such as adequate levels of difficulty in the job, clarity of goals, and opportunity for creativity in the job (Moneta 2012). The investigation of individual and environmental factors could bring a more thorough understanding of the moderating roles of flow on the self-determination model of work engagement.

8.4.4 Theoretical and Practical Implications

Although self-determination theory (Ryan and Deci 2000) and flow theory (Csikszentmihalyi 1992/2002) share various common goals, such as the interest in human strengths and their positive development (Deci and Vansteenkiste 2004), they have somewhat different theoretical tenets. For example, self-determination theorists argue that for individuals to actualise and be optimally active they need nutriments from the social environment (e.g., perceived autonomy support) in order to fulfill their intrinsic needs (Ryan and Deci 2000; Deci et al. 2001; Deci and Vansteenkiste 2004), whereas flow theorists posit that there need to be a balance between challenges and capabilities, and focus on the involvement of individuals with their tasks (Csikszentmihalyi 1990; Loubris et al. 1995; Bakker 2005). The present study contributes to the integration of these theoretical frameworks.

The main finding of the present study is that there is no relationship between perceived managerial autonomy support and work engagement for those with high flow in work, suggesting that the contextual factor of perceived managerial autonomy support is less important, or even irrelevant, in fostering work engagement for this particular group of workers. Therefore, this study shows that synergism between flow theory and self-determination theory can lead to more insightful and comprehensive models of engagement with potential applications to work settings.

In particular, for those companies that are unable to provide adequate levels of managerial autonomy support for their workers, the provision of clear goals and optimally challenging tasks may be the key for keeping employees intrinsically satisfied and engaged in their jobs. In turn, workers high in flow may be good candidates for companies lacking resources or model managements (Moneta in press).

8.4.5 Conclusions

This pilot study provides preliminary evidence in support of an extended self-determination model of work engagement that includes flow as a buffer to poor managerial autonomy support. The findings from this study indicate that workers with higher levels of flow at work are less reliant on their work conditions and more likely to engage in the job regardless of work environment factors that fall under the umbrella of autonomy support. These findings are consistent with the notions of autotelic self and autotelic experience, which imply that external forces do not rule whether the person will be able to find enjoyment and task focus in adverse situations, and that what matters most is the way a person perceives challenges. Because autotelic persons are more resilient in challenging situations, they may be ideal candidates for startup and other companies facing shortness of resources and unpredictability. Future research should assess the robustness of the extended self-determination model of work engagement across a range of work environments and its sensitivity to individual and cultural differences.

References

Baard, P. P., Deci, E. L., & Ryan, R. M. (2004). Intrinsic need satisfaction: A motivational basis of performance and well-being in two work settings. *Journal of Applied Social Psychology, 34*(10), 2045–2068.

Bakker, A. B. (2005). Flow among music teachers and their students: The crossover of peak experiences. *Journal of Vocational Behavior, 66*(1), 26–44.

Baumann, N. (2012). Autotelic personality. In S. Engeser (Ed.), *Advances in flow research* (pp. 165–186). New York: Springer.
Butkovic, A., Ullén, F., & Mosing, M. A. (2015). Personality and related traits as predictors of music practice: Underlying environmental and genetic influences. *Personality and Individual Differences, 74*, 133–138.
Csikszentmihalyi, M. (1975/2000). *Beyond boredom and anxiety: Experiencing flow in work and play* (2nd ed.). San Francisco: Jossey-Bass.
Csikszentmihalyi, M. (1990). *Flow: The psychology of optimal experience*. New York: Harper & Row.
Csikszentmihalyi, M. (1992/2002). *Flow: The psychology of happiness* (2nd ed.). Kent: Mackays of Chatham.
Deci, E. L., & Ryan, R. M. (1985). *Intrinsic motivation and self-determination in human behavior*. New York: Plenum.
Deci, E. L., & Vansteenkiste, M. (2004). Self-determination theory and basic need satisfaction: Understanding human development in positive psychology. *Ricerche di Psicologia, 1*(27), 23–40.
Deci, E. L., Ryan, R. M., Gagné, M., Leone, D. R., Usunov, J., & Kornazheva, B. P. (2001). Need satisfaction, motivation, and well-being in the work organizations of a former eastern bloc country: A cross-cultural study of self-determination. *Personality and Social Psychology Bulletin, 27*(8), 930–942.
Engeser, S., & Rheinberg, F. (2008). Flow, performance and moderators of challenge-skill balance. *Motivation and Emotion, 32*(3), 158–172.
Gagné, M. (2003). The role of autonomy support and autonomy orientation in prosocial behavior engagement. *Motivation and Emotion, 27*(3), 199–223.
Gagné, M., & Deci, E. L. (2005). Self-determination theory and work motivation. *Journal of Organizational Behavior, 26*(4), 331–362.
Harter, J. K., Schmidt, F. L., & Hayes, T. L. (2002). Business-unit-level relationship between employee satisfaction, employee engagement, and business outcomes: A meta-analysis. *Journal of Applied Psychology, 87*(2), 268.
Hayes, A. F. (2013). *Introduction to mediation, moderation, and conditional process analysis: A regression-based approach*. New York: Guilford Press.
Hayes, A. F. (n.d.). *SPSS PROCESS macro syntax reference*. Accessed 3 July 2011.
Kasser, T., Davey, J., & Ryan, R. M. (1992). Motivation and employee-supervisor discrepancies in a psychiatric vocational rehabilitation setting. *Rehabilitation Psychology, 37*(3), 175–187.
Kline, P. (2013). *Handbook of psychological testing*. London: Routledge.
Leiter, M. P., & Bakker, A. B. (2010). Work engagement: Introduction. In M. P. Leiter & A. B. Bakker (Eds.), *Work engagement: A handbook of essential theory and research* (pp. 1–9). New York: Psychology Press.
Leone, D. R. (1995). *The relation of work climate, higher order need satisfaction, need salience, and causality orientations to work engagement, psychological adjustment, and job satisfaction*. Unpublished doctoral dissertation. University of Rochester, Rochester.
Loubris, S., Crous, F., & Schepers, J. (1995). Management by objectives in relation to optimal experience in the workplace. *Journal of Industrial Psychology, 2*(21), 12–17.
Moneta, G. B. (2012). Opportunity for creativity in the job as a moderator of the relation between trait intrinsic motivation and flow in work. *Motivation and Emotion, 36*(4), 491–503.
Moneta, G. B. (2014). *Positive psychology: A critical introduction*. Hampshire: Palgrave Macmillan.
Moneta, G. B. (in press). Applications of flow to work. In C. Fullagar, & A. Delle Fave (Eds.), *The positive psychology of flow at work*. New York: Basic Books.
Mosing, M. A., Cesarini, D., Johannesson, M., Magnusson, P. K. E., Pedersen, N. L., Nakamura, J., Madison, G., & Ullén, F. (2012). Genetic and environmental influences on the relationship between flow proneness, locus of control and behavioral inhibition. *PLoS ONE, 7*, e47958.

Nakamura, J., & Csikszentmihalyi, M. (2005). The concept of flow. In C. R. Snyder & S. J. Lopez (Eds.), *Handbook of positive psychology* (pp. 89–105). New York: Oxford University Press.

Reis, H. T., Sheldon, K. M., Gable, S. L., Roscoe, J., & Ryan, R. M. (2000). Daily well-being: The role of autonomy, competence, and relatedness. *Personality and Social Psychology Bulletin, 26*(4), 419–435.

Ryan, R. M., & Deci, E. L. (2000). Self-determination theory and the facilitation of intrinsic motivation, social development, and well-being. *American Psychologist, 55*(1), 68–78.

Sadler-Smith, E., El-Kot, G., & Leat, M. (2003). Differentiating work autonomy facets in a non-Western context. *Journal of Organizational Behavior, 24*(6), 709–731.

Schaufeli, W. B., & Bakker, A. B. (2003). *UWES–Utrecht work engagement scale: Test manual.* Unpublished Manuscript. Utrecht: Department of Psychology, Utrecht University

Schaufeli, W. B., Bakker, A. B., & Salanova, M. (2006). The measurement of work engagement with a short questionnaire: A cross-national study. *Educational and Psychological Measurement, 66*(4), 701–716.

Sonnentag, S., Dormann, C., & Demerouti, E. (2010). Not all days are created equal: The concept of state work engagement. In M. P. Leiter & A. B. Bakker (Eds.), *Work engagement: A handbook of essential theory and research* (pp. 25–38). New York: Psychology Press.

Ullén, F., de Manzano, Ö., Almeida, R., Magnusson, P. K., Pedersen, N. L., Nakamura, J., et al. (2012). Proneness for psychological flow in everyday life: Associations with personality and intelligence. *Personality and Individual Differences, 52*(2), 167–172.

Williams, G. C., & Deci, E. L. (1996). Internalization of biopsychological values by medical students: A test of self-determination theory. *Journal of Personality and Social Psychology, 70*(4), 767–779.

Williams, G. C., Grow, V. M., Freedman, Z., Ryan, R. M., & Deci, E. L. (1996). Motivational predictors of weight loss and weight-loss maintenance. *Journal of Personality and Social Psychology, 70*(1), 115–126.

Wilson, E. E., & Moneta, G. B. (2012). Flow as a way of coping: A qualitative study of the metacognitions of flow. In B. Molinelli & V. Grimaldo (Eds.), *Handbook of the psychology of coping: New research* (pp. 133–150). Hauppauge: Nova.

Wilson, E. E., & Moneta, G. B. (2016). *The Flow Metacognitions Questionnaire (FMQ): A two factor model of flow metacognitions. Personality and Individual Differences, 90*, 225–230.

Part IV
Flow in Education

Chapter 9
The EduFlow Model: A Contribution Toward the Study of Optimal Learning Environments

Jean Heutte, Fabien Fenouillet, Jonathan Kaplan, Charles Martin-Krumm, and Rémi Bachelet

Abstract The intention of the following chapter is to shed light on primary factors that play a role in defining what we coin as an *optimal learning environment*, an environment that buttresses an experience of flow for learners (see Chap. 10 by Andersen in this volume). The chapter begins with an overview of flow related research reframed for the purpose of measuring the experience of flow in learning. A longitudinal study of flow experienced by students undertaking a Massive Open Online Course (MOOC) is described. The Flow in Education scale (EduFlow Scale) used in the study is described and the results of the study presented. The results illustrate the potential value and relevance of measuring flow in learning as well as the relation to the extended concept of cognitive absorption. We conclude the chapter with a presentation of a model of heuristic learning: the *Individually Motivated Community* model. The model builds upon three major theories of the self: Self-Determination, Self-Efficacy and Autotelism-Flow.

J. Heutte (✉)
Univ. Lille, EA 4354 – CIREL (Centre Interuniversitaire de Recherche en Education de Lille), Lille 59000, France
e-mail: jean.heutte@univ-lille1.fr

F. Fenouillet
Chart-UPON - EA 4004, University of Nanterre, Nanterre, France

J. Kaplan
Chart-UPON - EA 4004, University of Nanterre, Nanterre, France

ECP-EA 4571, ISPEF, Université Lumière Lyon 2, Lyon, France

C. Martin-Krumm
APEMAC EA 4360 UDL, Metz, France

Institut de Recherche Biomédicale des Armées (IRBA), Brétigny, France

IFEPS Angers Les Ponts de Cé, Les Ponts de Cé, France

R. Bachelet
Centrale Lille, Université Lille Nord de France, Lille, France

L. Harmat et al. (eds.), *Flow Experience*, DOI 10.1007/978-3-319-28634-1_9

9.1 Introduction

Flow or autotelic experience (providing well-being through the task activity itself) is "the experience of complete absorption in the present moment" (Nakamura and Csikszentmihalyi 2009, p. 195). Heutte et al. (2013), during their work within the Positive Psychology movement that was recently initiated with Seligman and Csikszentmihalyi (2000) and in accordance with Gable and Haidt's definition (2005), proposed that Positive Educational Psychology could be designated as the scientific study of the conditions and processes that contribute to the flourishing or optimal functioning of:

- Learners, people working in education or training and all players who are part of the educational community;
- Actual or virtual communities in which the above-mentioned people learn or work;
- Education and training systems, organizations or arrangements.

New prospects for research in the domain open when considering these three levels: people, groups, and institutions. On each of these levels the intimate and social dimensions of pleasure associated with understanding and making oneself understood are explored in a quest for optimal learning environments. Optimal learning environments are defined by Heutte (2014) as environments that support a state of flow in the process of learning.

According to Nakamura and Csikszentmihalyi (2009, p. 195) conditions for reaching a state of flow include:

1. A balance between perceived skills and perceived task demands,[1] or opportunities for action, that stretch but do not overmatch existing skills;
2. Clear proximal goals;
3. Immediate feedback.

In consideration of these conditions, Autotelism-Flow is a subjective experience that is characterized by the combination of distinct (experiential) states that co-occur during engagement in a skill-related activity (see Chap. 11 by Freire et al. in this volume) (Nakamura and Csikszentmihalyi 2009), specifically including:

1. An intense and focused concentration on the present moment;
2. The merging of action and awareness;
3. The loss of self-consciousness (i.e. loss of awareness of oneself as a social player);

[1]According to Keller and Landäußer (2012) and Rheinberg (2008), the term 'demands' is more appropriate than the term 'challenge'. Keller and Landäußer argue that "the propositions regarding the boundary conditions of flow experience can be simplified and reduced [...to] the antecedent factor 'Perceived fit of skill and task demands'" (2012, p. 53). "In any case, a sense of control is definitely one of the most important components of the flow experience, whether or not an 'objective' assessment justifies such feelings" (Csikszentmihalyi 1975, p. 46).

4. A strong feeling of control, specifically over one's actions, characterized by a feeling of ability to deal with the situation and a feeling that one knows how to deal with whatever comes next;
5. Distortion of the temporal experience, or a modified experience of time (typically, a sense that time has passed faster than usual);
6. Experience of the activity as intrinsically rewarding (enjoyment and well-being rooted in the activity itself) such that often the end-goal is just an excuse for the process (the *autotelic experience*).

This chapter offers to present a model of flow in educational contexts, referred to as the EduFlow Model (Heutte et al. 2014a). The chapter begins with a description of the conceptual dimensions of flow. A subgroup of these dimensions was used in the Flow in Education Scale (EduFlow Scale). The dimensions are then presented. What follows is the description of a study that used the EduFlow Scale derived from the model. This study explored the relations between the EduFlow Model dimensions using Structural Equation Modelling (SEM) to analyze learners' flow in a Massive Open Online Course (MOOC).

Most researchers concur with the conceptualization of flow as an autotelic experience (see Chap. 11 by Freire et al. in this volume). The intuitive understanding of the concept requires an operational definition nevertheless; an operation somewhat more complicated with varying results (see Hoffman and Novak 2009, for a review). Engeser and Schiepe-Tiska (2012) pointed out that there is a certain level of disagreement among researchers as to how flow should be measured. "Indeed, over the past 35 years, researchers have kept developing and validating new measurement instruments for flow, and modifying and revalidating established ones, which indicates that a gold measurement standard for flow has yet to be achieved" (Moneta 2012, p. 23).

Having analyzed 30 different flow categorizations, Hoffman and Novak (2009) found significant disparities concerning both (1) the definition/conceptualization of flow dimensions, and (2) the antecedents, the experience of flow and its effects. A challenge for researchers lies with building adequate measurement instruments for both the experience and its effects. The difficulty is related to the fact that the experience of flow is described as one in which the subject loses self-awareness as a result of being highly focused and absorbed in the activity at hand. This makes self-reports of flow effects difficult. Furthermore, due to fluctuation in the state, there is a risk of disturbing the fine balance needed to achieve or sustain the state by intruding upon the subject if intervening. This would be the case if micro-interventions during the subject's activity were used to observe the state and its effects. To date, various measurement instruments have been created and used to study the highly unstable and subjective phenomenon of flow in an attempt to overcome the challenges posed by its measurement. Qualitative methods have been applied using interviews, questionnaires and the Experience Sampling Method (ESM; Csikszentmihalyi and Larson 1984; Csikszentmihalyi and LeFevre 1989; Nakamura and Csikszentmihalyi 2009).

Mayers' flow scale (1978) is one of the first self-administered questionnaires designed to estimate the frequency at which a person feels each one of the nine flow dimensions initially described (Csikszentmihalyi 1990). The instrument was frequently used for repeated-measures designs (e.g. Delle Fave and Massimini 1992) in order to assess differences in the state of flow depending on the activity being carried out and at various moments during that activity. More recently, a general flow scale was developed on the basis of existing questionnaires to be applied in specific contexts such as during sport activities (Jackson and Marsh 1996; Jackson and Eklund 2002) and psychotherapy (Parks 1996).

According to Rheinberg et al. (2003), the intrusive nature and the time expenditure associated with using the ESM put the flow process itself at risk of being interrupted. Using other common measurement instruments presents the same inconvenience. It is hence recommended to use flow measurement instruments that use short questionnaires such as the Flow-Kurzskala Scale (see Chap. 10 by Andersen in this volume) (FKS, Rheinberg et al. 2003). Vollmeyer and Rheinberg (2006) estimated that FKS is a measurement scale that could be adapted to numerous contexts. In order to facilitate the measurement of flow in studies in which flow is not the central concept, Jackson et al. (2008)) validated a shorter version of FKS containing only nine items, one for each dimension. However, this does not enable researchers to structurally separate dimensions from observed data. More recently, Bakker (2008) developed a 13-item flow at work scale, the Work-Related Flow Inventory (WOLF). This scale includes three dimensions: work absorption, work enjoyment, and intrinsic work motivation. The scale does not account for the conditions of flow occurrences.

9.2 Choice of Dimensions to Include in Measures of Autotelism-Flow in Educational Contexts

Delle Fave et al. (2011) affirm that it is extremely important that the measurement instruments adhere strictly to the nine original dimensions of flow. This is the position that many have adopted. The Flow-State Scale (FSS2), a nine dimensions scale originally elaborated by Jackson and Eklund (2002, 2004) for sports activities, has been tested and used in various contexts: theater; creative or performing arts; work and music; online shopping; and, video gaming.

Procci et al. (2012) nevertheless identify limits to strictly and systematically applying the framework of the nine original dimensions. For Procci and colleagues flow differences observed in latent factor correlations are due to contextual contingencies and variations in activities. Heutte et al. (2014b) observe that barely half of the nine dimensions of FFS2 are actually perceived by learners in educational context. Flow perception appears to vary and is context bound. For example, in activities that are less physically strenuous or demanding, cognitive aspects are more salient and more inter-related. Variations in context do not invalidate the theoretical framework comprised of the nine components of flow. It is plausible that the nine components are simply not equally prominent in all contexts.

Hoffman and Novak (2009) noted that researchers have been confronted with the dilemma between privileging a short unidimensional scale that enables to quickly capture a general state of flow; and, to include all flow components. In the former the trade-off is losing resolution; in the latter, overburdening respondents, which may lead to loss of accuracy and incomplete responses. This may explain why numerous flow researchers have chosen to collapse dimensions, or drop some in a quest for more compact questionnaires to suit specific research contexts or when focusing on particular dimensions of interest.

When constructing the Flow in Education Scale (EduFlow Scale), Heutte et al. (2014a) were confronted with a similar dilemma. They chose to select some of the nine dimensions while leaving seemingly less relevant ones out. The dimensions that were retained are:

- *Cognitive absorption* (related concepts include: focused immersion (Agarwal and Karahanna 2000; Fu et al. 2009); work absorption (Bakker 2008); and concentration (Jackson and Eklund 2002; Novak et al. 2000; Shernoff et al. 2003)).
- *Time transformation* (Jackson and Eklund 2002; also referred to as temporal dissociation Agarwal and Karahanna 2000; Novak et al. 2000);
- *Autotelic activity and well-being* (related to the concept of enjoyment: Agarwal and Karahanna 2000; Bakker 2008; Novak et al. 2000; Shernoff et al. 2003).

9.3 Cognitive Absorption: When Nothing Can Disturb an Activity Centered on Understanding

According to Csikszentmihalyi, an autotelic activity or experience of flow is characterized by numerous persons as one of the best moments in their lives. These are experiences in which actions unfold with an extraordinary impression of fluidity, painless effort and a strong sense of ease. Descriptions include being completely engaged in the activity to a degree that nothing external could disturb the subject. The pleasure of being engaged in the activity and persistence in it, both related to the intrinsic nature of the subject's engagement, are characteristic of total immersion, a hallmark of flow (Nakamura and Csikszentmihalyi 2009).

Autonomous motivation is not the only type related to activity that produces an experience of flow. Many activities are engaged in voluntarily even when motivation is extrinsically controlled (Deci and Ryan 2000). Once engaged in these, one often reaches a state of deep concentration as a result of embracing the activity fully in an attempt to do as best as one can.

Different types of extrinsic motivation affect regulations with various degrees of autonomy. Introjected regulation can ensue from internal prods and pressures such as threats of guilt or self-esteem-relevant contingencies. When internalization of externally controlled regulations are higher, such as when social values are espoused and acquire value, integration by the subject can lead to identified regulation, or when identification with the values is full, lead to integrated regulation (Deci and Ryan 2000, 2008).

We suggest that the central concept of Cognitive Absorption (CA) can be expanded to any activity related to comprehension. After discussion with Ruy Agarwall and Elena Karahanna, and with their permission, we extended the concept of CA (Agarwal and Karahanna 2000) to include a state of deep involvement in an activity focused on understanding with—or without—software (Heutte 2014). CA corresponds to a deep state of commitment connected to a total-focus episode (optimal experience). The cognitive activity entirely absorbs (or focuses) cognitive resources, to the point that nothing but understanding matters. It has an immediate consequence: nothing can disrupt concentration as it is exclusively committed to the process of understanding. Thus, we define CA as an exclusive focus of attention, extreme in intensity and peaceful, related to a state of total concentration during an activity (Heutte 2011). CA can be portrayed as an *invading* interest for the activity. It can in some way be said to occur beyond the subject's will when the subject is caught up in the activity.

9.4 Loss of Self-Consciousness: The Social Dimension of Flow

Heutte and associates (2014a) and Heutte (2011, 2014) retained the dimension Loss of Self-Consciousness (LSC) while regarding it as a social dimension. Here the interest lies in the role that other persons are playing in personal agency. This interest includes the role of individual motivation in collective activity (see Chap. 11 by Freire et al. in this volume). Considering controlled motivation, social factors need to be accounted for in processes of internalization and integration of regulations. Social factors include learners' socialization, feelings of belonging and relatedness (Deci and Ryan 2000; Heutte 2011, 2014; Richer and Vallerand 1998).

LSC produces serenity together with no concern with oneself. It is characterized by a feeling of growing beyond the boundaries of ego. The blurring occurs when "one needs to step out of the cocoon of personal goals and confront larger issues in the public arena" (Csikszentmihalyi 1993, p. 293). The following descriptions are relevant too: LSC «marks the fading of Mead's 'me' from awareness» (Nakamura and Csikszentmihalyi 2002, p. 92). Nakamura and Csikszentmihalyi (2009, p. 195) describe this as a «loss of awareness of oneself as a social actor». We suggest that this dimension of flow brings the dynamic relationship between the social world and cognitive development to the fore (Mead 1934).

Blending egos (Sawyer 2007) occurs when people recognize that ingenuity results from the performance of the entire group. Ingenuity is not attributable to the sole performance of any one of the group's individual members. In their studies on the effects of flow in educational context, Shernoff and Csikszentmihalyi (2009) demonstrated that students experiencing flow were more likely to perceive their classmates as friends. Peers also spent more time in academic activities such as individual and group work (Rathunde and Csikszentmihalyi 2005), demonstrated more cooperation (Andersen 2005), as well as had a higher sense of belongingness (Johnson 2004). The works of these authors led Heutte et al. (2014a) to conclude that LSC represents the social dimension of flow. In reference to social developmental psychology, which considers social interaction as key to individual cognitive development (e.g., Vygotsky 1962; Bandura 1997), LSC emerges as an essential criterion in relation to environmental and personal factors. Among factors that influence learner engagement are school contexts that may foster to varying degrees optimal learning experiences (See Chap. 10 by Andersen in this volume) (Shernoff et al. 2003).

9.5 The EduFlow Scale: An Instrument in the Service of Studying Optimal Learning Environments

Heutte et al. (2014a) opted to study four dimensions for the assessment of optimal learning environments i.e. environments that support learners' flow. To this end the EduFlow Scale was developed. The four dimensions it measures are:

- FlowD1: *Cognitive absorption*—increased concentration and immersion in the task.
- FlowD2: *Time transformation*—alteration in the perception of time, sometimes leading to a lengthened duration of immersion in the task.
- FlowD3: *Loss of self-consciousness*—lack of self-concern related to an increase in importance of the psycho-social dimension of learning.
- FlowD4: *Autotelic experience*—well-being during task performance resulting from purpose in the task itself that enhances persistence and the desire to engage in the activity again.

The EduFlow Scale has been tested in various educational contexts with students ranging from primary school to university including face-to-face learning (Heutte 2011; Fenouillet et al. 2014) and online learning (Caron et al. 2014; Heutte et al. 2014b, 2014c). From these studies the EduFlow Model was derived (cf. Fig. 9.1).

The EduFlow Scale has several advantages: it can be used in different educational contexts; it is a 12-item scale reducing respondent burden; and, it differentiates four dimensions of flow that are relevant to cognitive processes (there are three items per dimension).

9.6 Personal and Collective Self-Efficacy: The Power of Believing You Can

Drawing upon inspiration from Bandura (1986, p. 391), we contend that personal as well as collective self-efficacy refer to people's judgments of their personal and collective capabilities to organize and execute courses of action required to attain

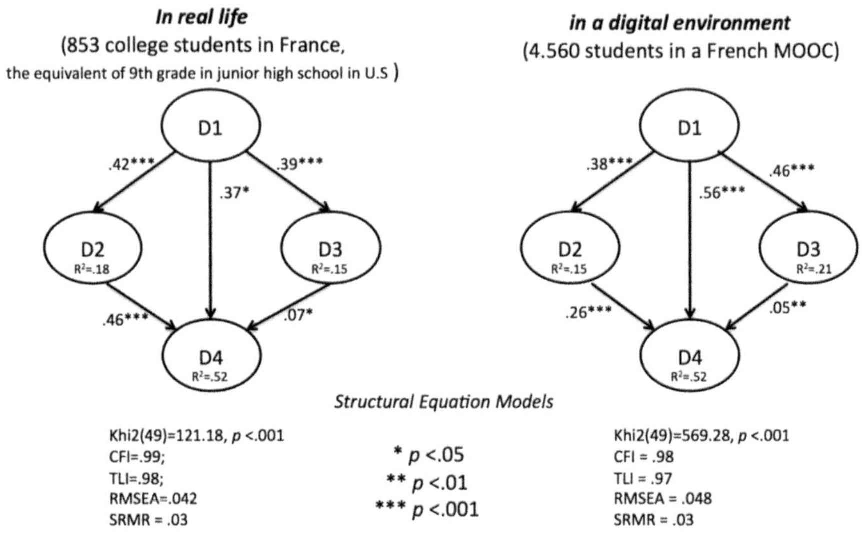

Fig. 9.1 Ecological validity of the EduFlow model. Relationships between different dimensions of flow in education (Heutte et al. 2014a). Note: *D1* FlowD1—cognitive absorption. *D2* FlowD2—time transformation. *D3* FlowD3—loss of self-consciousness. *D4* FlowD4—autotelic experience—well-being

designated goals (Heutte 2011). Self-efficacy beliefs are central to human agency. Strongly perceived self- and collective efficacy mediate human accomplishment and contribute to personal and collective well-being. People who are confident in their capabilities approach difficult tasks as challenges to be mastered rather than as threats to be avoided. Of course, personal efficacy and collective efficacy go hand-in-hand because a «collection of inveterate self-doubters is not easily forged into a collectively efficacious force» (Bandura 1997, p. 480). Individuals are socially embedded and are rarely alone in facing problems, difficulties, or challenges. «Simply stated, collective efficacy is the extent to which we believe that we can work together effectively to accomplish our shared goals» (Maddux 2002, p. 284).

A high sense of personal and collective self-efficacy increases learner readiness to invest effort, and supports persistence and willingness to face difficulties. It helps learners recover volition after an experience judged as negative. Heutte (2011) demonstrated that *Cognitive Absorption* (CA), autotelic activity and well-being are linked to personal and collective self-efficacy beliefs. Under certain circumstances when learners interact, a feeling of collective self-efficacy can more saliently affect CA than individual self-efficacy can (cf. Perceived Self and Collective Efficacy Flow Contributions Model [PSCEFC], Heutte 2011, p. 184). Heutte (2011, 2014) named the Volitional Loop of Perceived Collective-Efficacy (VLPCE) a virtuous loop in which Perceived Collective Efficacy (PCE) leads to CA which leads to an autotelic experience—well-being, leading again to PCE and so on. The VLPCE may well be one of the best drivers of persistence in working or learning with others.

9.7 Project Management MOOC

Project Management MOOC Session 1 was the first xMOOC to be organized in France. It was developed from a preexisting open courseware website. Enrollment opened January 11, 2013. Courses began March 18 the same year and offered two individual tracks: Basic and Advanced. A Team Project track was later opened too. Voluteers ran the MOOC and support was provided by École Centrale de Lille who sponsored the project. Technical support for the MOOC application—Canvas was provided by Unow, a French startup company.

Project Management MOOC Session 3 followed the same principles, but added seven optional modules (see Fig. 9.2). Basic and advanced tracks were launched in March 2014. The tracks lasted 5 weeks each with an extra week for final exams.

There were 11,827 enrollees out of which 5,899 completed at least one quiz of the Basic track.

Success rates (Bachelet 2014) were:

- Entry rate 50 %. The ratio is the number of students who submitted at least one short quiz divided by the total number of enrollees.
- Basic track success rate: 38 %. The ratio is calculated by dividing the number of students who submitted at least one short quiz by the number of students successfully terminating the Basic track. Basic track success was determined from an average score made up of at least a 70 % success score on course material tests plus at least a 60 % success score on the final examination.

The MOOC required 25 h of study for the Basic track and 45 for the Advanced track. These included assignments and peer assessments. The additional Team track required at least 25 extra hours of study. Students were entitled to European Credit Transfer and Accumulation System (ECTS) credits, awarded by École Centrale Lille after the final assessment.

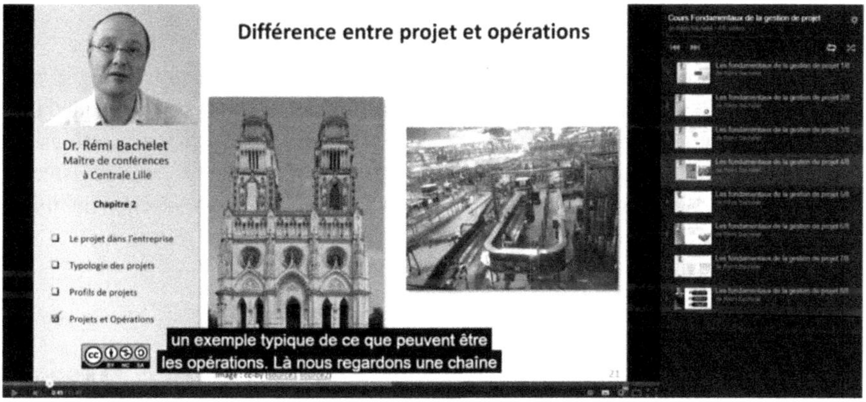

Fig. 9.2 Video courses on the Project Management MOOC

9.7.1 *Procedure*

Data collection was carried out between March and May 2014. Two online questionnaires using LimeSurvey (version 2.05) were administered:

- Questionnaire One (Q1) contained 33 groups of questions spread over three screen-pages.
- Questionnaire Two (Q2) contained 42 groups of questions spread over three screen-pages.

Q1 was administered just after the MOOC began, during the first week. A reminder e-mail was sent 2 weeks later. Q2 was administered 6 weeks after the MOOC began with a reminder e-mail following 1 week later.The two questionnaires contained questions from the following scales:

- EduFlow Scale containing its four dimensions.
- PSE: Perceived Self-Efficacy beliefs in university courses (Heutte 2011, adapted from Schwarzer and Jerusalem 1995)
- PCE: Perceived Collective-Efficacy beliefs in university courses (Heutte 2011, adapted from Schwarzer and Jerusalem 1995)
- For each questionnaire, 7-point Likert-type items were used ranging from *strongly disagree* to *strongly agree*.

Distractors questions were also included to ensure that respondents paid attention (e.g. Do not answer this question. Move on to the next).

Eleven thousand eight hundred and twenty seven invitation e-mails were sent out to invite MOOC students to participate.

9.8 Results

9.8.1 *Data Analysis*

- Q1 (Mean response time 23 min.): Access to the questionnaire was registered 7,313 times. Four thousand seven hundred twenty seven respondents reached the third screen-page of the questionnaire without answering distractor questions.
- Q2 (Mean response time 25 min.): Access to the questionnaire was registered 3,410 times. Two thousand one hundred thirty five respondents reached the third screen-page of the questionnaire without answering distractor questions.

9.8.2 *Flow Change*

Between the first and the second questionnaire, all of the flow dimensions were exhibited by students who persisted in the course for more than 6 weeks (see Table 9.1).

Table 9.1 Flow change over time in the Project Management MOOC

Factor	Survey	M	SE	F	P	η^2	N
Flow D1	Q1	4.93	0.92	F(11,847) = 63.67	<0.001	0.03	1,848
	Q2	5.08	0.84				
Flow D2	Q1	4.92	1.22	F(11,840) = 36.84	<0.001	0.02	1,841
	Q2	5.09	1.15				
Flow D3	Q1	4.06	1.54	F(11,841) = 56.13	<0.001	0.03	1,842
	Q2	4.32	1.44				
Flow D4	Q1	5.06	1.11	F(11,833) = 8.51	<0.01	0.01	1,834
	Q2	5.13	1.07				

There is an increase of flow that is statistically significant in all dimensions with a slightly stronger increase for Loss of self-consciousness. The effects (η^2 /ETA-squared) nevertheless remain very small (see Table 9.1):

- $\eta^2=0.03$ for FlowD1-Cognitive absorption;
- $\eta^2=0.02$ for FlowD2-Time transformation;
- $\eta^2=0.03$ for FlowD3-Loss of self-consciousness;
- $\eta^2=0.01$ for FlowD4-Autotelic experience—well-being.

The analysis suggests that student volition during the MOOC is linked to relative stability over time in all flow dimensions. Results also suggest that the MOOC enabled an optimal learning experience for those students who responded to the questionnaires, but this may have not been the case for those who dropped out.

9.8.3 *Self and Collective Efficacy: Flow Contributions (PSCEFC) Model*

The analysis of data using SEM enabled validation of the Self and Collective Efficacy—Flow Contributions (PSCEFC) Model for Cognitive Absorption and Autotelic Experience—Well-Being dimensions (D1 and D4). The following omnibus chi-square tests and fit indices were used: Comparative Fit Index (CFI; Bentler 1990), Tucker Lewis Index (TLI; Tucker and Lewis 1973), Root Mean Square Error of Approximation (RMSEA; Steiger 1990) and Standardized Root Mean Square Residual (SRMR). In the tested models (see Fig. 9.3), all fit indices were acceptable (Byrne 1994; Hu and Bentler 1995).

The standardized regression coefficients (R^2) suggest that the PSCEFC Model contributes to explaining variance of FlowD1—Cognitive Absorption ($63< R^2 <69$) and of FlowD4—Autotelic Experience—Well-Being ($41< R^2 <43$) in an educational context.

Consistent with Heutte (2014) expectation, results cohere with the *Volitional Loop of Perceived Collective-Efficacy* (see in blue, Fig. 9.3). Standardized regression coefficients (R^2) are somewhat lower than expected in relation to the effect of

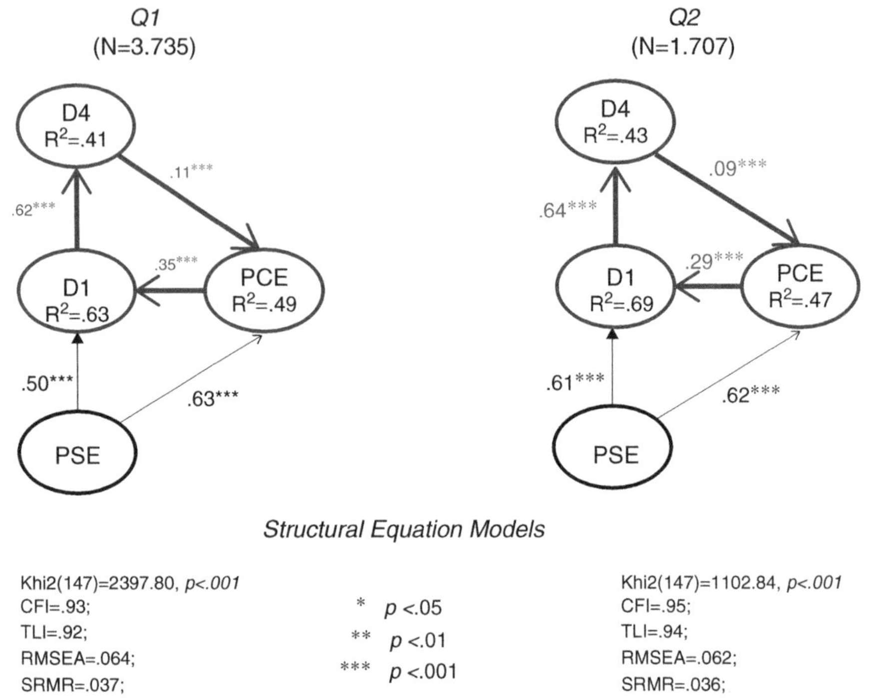

Fig. 9.3 The volitional loop of perceived collective-efficacy in Project Management MOOC, at start (*Q1*) and 6 weeks later (*Q2*). Note: *D1* FlowD1-cognitive absorption. *D4* FlowD4-autotelic experience—well-being. *PSE* perceived self-efficacy, *PCE* perceived collective-efficacy

Perceived Collective-Efficacy on FlowD1—Cognitive Absorption (0.29< R^2 <0.35) and FlowD4—Autotelic Experience—Well-Being on Perceived Collective-Efficacy (0.09< R^2 <0.11). This can perhaps be explained by student assignments being primarily individual rather than collective in the Project Management MOOC.

9.9 Conclusions and Prospects

This chapter has highlighted the relevance of using a flow in education model such as EduFlow to advance the study of optimal learning environments. Furthermore, the results from the research conducted with learners in the MOOC fit our extended conception of Cognitive Absorption. Cognitive Absorption emerges as a central characteristic in flow experiences within the context of learning (Heutte 2011, 2014). The model underpins the EduFlow Scale Construct. The EduFlow Scale has three advantages:

- It is suited to flow measurement in various educational contexts;
- It is short;
- It differentiates between four dimensions of flow that are related to cognitive process.

9.9.1 Further Exploration of the Social Conditions for Flow in Education

According to Fenouillet (2012), the explanatory level of group motivation is necessarily bound to the motivation of the individuals that compose it. Most theories refer to motivation and volition on the individual level. The challenge lies in applying these constructs to group processes. Heutte addresses the challenge using contributions from major theories of the self (Self-Determination, Self-Efficacy, and Autotelism-Flow). His proposal for a Heuristic Model of the *Individually Motivated Community*[2] (HMIMC, Heutte 2011, 2014) encompasses these three theories (see Fig. 9.4), although they do not share their views according to the Integrative Model of Motivation (Fenouillet 2012):

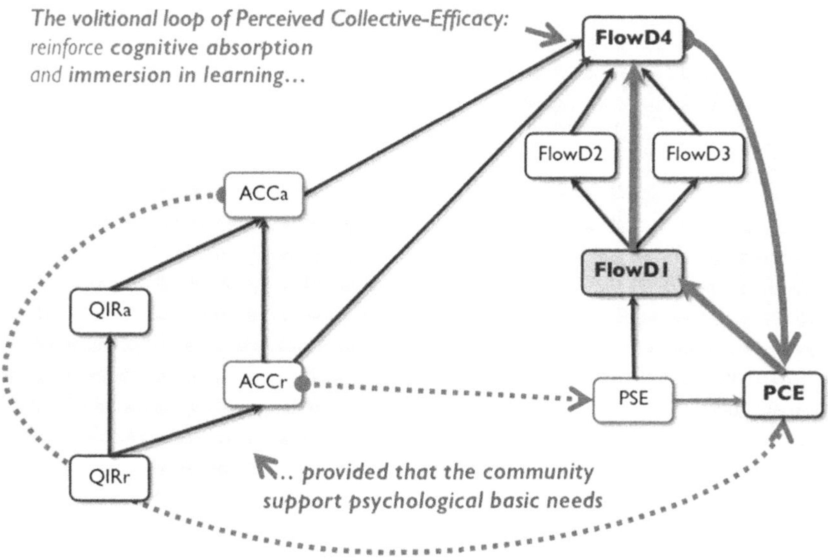

Fig. 9.4 Dynamic of the heuristic model of the individually motivated community (Heutte 2014)

[2] Modèle heuristique du *collectif individuellement motivé*, in French (MHCIM, Heutte 2011, 2014).

- Deci and Ryan (2000) consider the need for relatedness[3] to affect behavior orientation.
- Bandura (1997)) considers predictions of self -and collective-efficacy to affect engagement in tasks or activities.
- Csikszentmihalyi (1990) considers flow outcome to affect behavioral persistence in activities.

Well-being encompasses these three major theories (Heutte 2011).

QIRr:	Quality of interpersonal relationships with those who are responsible for the working or learning conditions (responsible)
QIRa:	Quality of interpersonal relationships between those who work or learn together (in activity)
ACCr:	Feelings of acceptance, and relatedness with those who are responsible for the working or learning conditions (responsible)
ACCa:	Feelings of acceptance, and relatedness between those who work or learn together (in activity)
PSE:	Perceived self-efficacy
PCE:	Perceived collective-efficacy
FlowD1:	Cognitive absorption
FlowD2:	Time transformation
FlowD3:	Loss of self-consciousness
FlowD4:	Autotelic experience—well-being

From a socio-cognitive standpoint, the environment composed of one's peers, needs to be accounted for. A learner will benefit from an upturned social climate through interactions with peers, which will support learner motivation and sustain volition. Flow and a sense of enjoyment provide for an optimal learning experience that in turn will contribute to the collective endeavor and will boost a sense of collective self-efficacy.

Being able to make choices is fundamental to autonomy—a basic psychological need. It affects well-being and contributes to self- and collective-efficacy. Feeling autonomous prepares the ground for engaging in an activity and supports persistence of effort to share, acquire, and construct knowledge.Directions for future exploration may include:

- Exploring cognitive absorption, autotelic activity and well-being in educational contexts.
- Carrying out comparative studies of mediating factors of flow that learners and instructors experience.
- Studying the ecological validity of the EduFlow Model as well as the heuristic model of the Individually Motivated Collective.

The EduFlow Model should prove useful to studies of cognitive activities in a variety of environments including learning within organizational contexts (Heutte

[3] In balance with two other basic psychological needs, *autonomy* and *competence*.

2014). Exploration on the personal, collective and institutional levels broadens our understanding by accounting for the intricate relations of factors within processes that are context bound, such as learning and knowledge creation.

References

Agarwal, R., & Karahanna, E. (2000). Time flies when you're having fun: Cognitive absorption and beliefs about information technology usage. *MIS Quarterly, 24*(4), 665–694.

Andersen, F. O. (2005). *International trends in primary school education: An overview based on case studies in Finland, Denmark & Japan*. Billund: Lego Learning Institute.

Bachelet R. (2014). *Data and success rates of MOOC GdP3*, website read 01/15/2015. http://goo.gl/StCLX9

Bakker, A. B. (2008). The work-related flow inventory: Construction and initial validation of the WOLF. *Journal of Vocational Behavior, 72*, 400–414.

Bandura, A. (1986). *Social foundations of thought and action: A social cognitive theory*. Englewood Cliffs: Prentice-Hall.

Bandura, A. (1997). *Self-efficacy: The exercise of control*. New York: Freeman.

Bentler, P. M. (1990). Comparative fit indexes in structural models. *Psychological Bulletin, 107*, 238–246.

Byrne, B. M. (1994). *Structural equation modeling with EQS and EQS/windows*. Thousand Oaks: Sage Publications.

Caron, P. A., Heutte, J., & Rosselle, M. (2014). *Présentation d'une méthode et d'outils pour évaluer les perceptions des apprenants dans un MOOC*., JOCAIR 2014, Paris, France, 27 juin.

Csikszentmihalyi, M. (1975). *Beyond boredom and anxiety: Experiencing flow in work and play*. San Francisco: Jossey-Bass.

Csikszentmihalyi, M. (1990). *Flow: The psychology of optimal experience*. New York: Harper and Row.

Csikszentmihalyi, M. (1993). *The evolving self. A psychology for the 3rd millennium*. New York: Harper Collins.

Csikszentmihalyi, M., & Larson, R. (1984). *Being adolescent*. New York: Basic Books.

Csikszentmihalyi, M., & LeFevre, J. (1989). Optimal experience in work and leisure. *Journal of Personality and Social Psychology, 56*(5), 815–822.

Deci, E. L., & Ryan, R. M. (2000). The "what" and "why" of goal pursuits: Human needs and the self-determination of behavior. *Psychological Inquiry, 11*, 227–268.

Deci, E. L., & Ryan, R. M. (2008). Facilitating optimal motivation and psychological well-being across life's domains. *Canadian Psychology, 49*, 14–23.

Delle Fave, A., & Massimini, F. (1992). The ESM and the measurement of clinical change: A case of anxiety disorder. *The experience of psychopathology: Investigating mental disorders in their natural settings*, 280.

Delle Fave, A., Massimini, F., & Bassi, M. (2011). *Psychological selection and optimal experience across cultures: Social empowerment through personal growth*. New York: Springer.

Engeser, S., & Schiepe-Tiska, A. (2012). Historical lines and overview of current research. In S. Engeser (Ed.), *Introduction to flow research*. New York: Springer.

Fenouillet, F. (2012). *Les théories de la motivation*. Paris: Dunod.

Fenouillet, F., Martin-Krumm, C., Heutte, J., & Besançon, M. (2014). *An urgent call for change: Flow, motivation and well-being in French School students*. 7th European Conference on Positive Psychology (ECPP), Amsterdam, The Netherlands.

Fu, F. L., Su, R. C., & Yu, S. C. (2009). Egameflow: A scale to measure learners' enjoyment of e-learning games. *Computers & Education, 52*(1), 101–112.

Gable, S. L., & Haidt, J. (2005). What (and why) is positive psychology? *Review of General Psychology, 9*(2), 103.

Heutte, J. (2011). La part du collectif dans la motivation et son impact sur le bien-être comme médiateur de la réussite des étudiants: Complémentarités et contributions entre l'autodétermination, l'auto-efficacité et l'autotélisme. (Unpublished Ph. D. thesis). Université Paris Ouest-Nanterre-La Défense (France).

Heutte, J. (2014) Persister dans la conception de son environnement personnel d'apprentissage: Contributions et complémentarités de trois théories du self. *STICEF, 21*, ISSN: 1764-7223

Heutte J.,Fenouillet F., Martin-Krumm C. (2013). Contribution de la psychologie positive au pilotage de l'innovation. *Congrès Francophone de Psychologie Positive*, Metz, France.

Heutte, J., Fenouillet, F., Boniwell, I., Martin-Krumm, C., & Csikszentmihalyi, M. (2014a). *Optimal learning experience in digital environments: Theoretical concepts, measure and modelisation, Symposium "Digital Learning in 21st Century Universities"*. Georgia Institute of Technology (Georgia Tech), Atlanta, GA.

Heutte, J., Galaup, M., Lelardeux, C., Lagarrigue, P., & Fenouillet, F. (2014b). Etude des déterminants psychologiques de la persistance dans l'usage d'un jeu sérieux: évaluation de l'environnement optimal d'apprentissage avec Mecagenius. *STICEF,* 21, ISSN: 1764–7223

Heutte, J., Kaplan, J., Fenouillet, F., Caron, P. A., & Rosselle, M. (2014c). MOOC user persistence—lessons from French educational policy adoption and deployment of a pilot course. In L. Uden, J. Sinclair, Y.-H. Tao, & D. Liberona (Ed.), *Learning technology for education in cloud. MOOC and Big Data (LTEC'14),* Communications in Computer and Information Science. 446: 13–24. Springer.

Hoffman, D. L., & Novak, T. P. (2009). Flow online: Lessons learned and future prospects. *Journal of Interactive Marketing, 23*(1), 23–34.

Hu, L. T., & Bentler, P. M. (1995). Evaluating model fit. In R. H. Hoyle (Ed.), *Structural equation modeling: Concepts, issues, and applications* (pp. 76–99). Thousand Oaks: Sage.

Jackson, S. A., & Eklund, R. C. (2002). Assessing flow in physical activity: The flow stateScale-2 and dispositional flow state scale-2. *Journal of Sport and Exercise Psychology, 24*, 133–115.

Jackson, S. A., & Eklund, R. C. (2004). *The flow scale manual*. Morgantown: Fitness Information Technology.

Jackson, S. A., & Marsh, H. W. (1996). Development and validation of a scale to measure optimal experience: The flow state scale. *Journal of Sport and Exercise Psychology, 18*, 17–35.

Jackson, S. A., Martin, A. J., & Eklund, R. C. (2008). Long and short measures of flow: The construct validity of the FSS-2, DFS-2, and new brief counterparts. *Journal of Sport and Exercise Psychology, 30*, 561–587.

Johnson, L. S. (2004). *Academic engagement from the perspective of flow theory: A comparative analysis of nontraditional and traditional schools*. Unpublished doctoral dissertation, Northern Illinois University, DeKalb.

Keller, J., & Landhäußer, A. (2012). The flow model revisited. In S. Engeser (Ed.), *Advances in flow research* (pp. 51–64). New York: Springer.

Maddux, J. E. (2002). *Self-efficacy: The power of believing you can. Handbook of positive psychology* (pp. 277–287). New York: Oxford University Press.

Mayers, P. (1978). Flow in adolescence and its relevation to school experience. Unpublished doctoral dissertation, University of Chicago. In C. R. Snyder, & S. J. Lopez (Eds.), *Handbook of positive psychology* (pp. 89–105). Oxford: University Press.

Mead, G.-H. (1934). *Mind, self, and society*. Chicago: University of Chicago Press.

Moneta, G. B. (2012). On the measurement and conceptualization of flow. In S. Engeser (Ed.), *Advances in. Flow research* (pp. 23–50). New York: Springer.

Nakamura, J., & Csikszentmihalyi, M. (2002). The concept of flow. In C. R. Snyder & S. J. Lopez (Eds.), *Handbook of positive psychology* (pp. 89–105). Oxford: Oxford University Press.

Nakamura, J., & Csikszentmihalyi, M. (2009). Flow theory and research. In S. J. Lopez & C. R. Snyder (Eds.), *Handbook of positive psychology* (pp. 195–206). New York: Oxford University Press.

Novak, T. P., Hoffman, D. L., & Yung, Y. (2000). Measuring the customer experience in online environments: A structural modeling approach. *Marketing Science, 19*(1), 22–42.

Parks, B. (1996). *Flow, boredom and anxiety in therapeutic work*. Unpublished doctoral dissertation, University of Chicago.

Procci, K., Singer, A. R., Levy, K. R., & Bowers, C. (2012). Measuring the flow experience of gamers: An evaluation of the DFS-2. *Computers in Human Behavior, 28*(6), 2306–2312.

Rathunde, K., & Csikszentmihalyi, M. (2005). Middle school students' motivation and quality of experience: A comparison of Montessori and traditional school environments. *American Journal of Education, 111*(3), 341–371.

Rheinberg, F. (2008). Intrinsic motivation and flow-experience. In H. Heckhausen & J. Heckhausen (Eds.), *Motivation and action* (pp. 323–348). Cambridge: Cambridge University Press.

Rheinberg, F., Vollmeyer, R., & Engeser, S. (2003). Die Erfassung des Flow-Erlebens. In J. Stiensmeier-Pelster & F. Rheinberg (Eds.), *Diagnostik von Motivation und Selbstkonzept* (pp. 261–279). Göttingen: Hogrefe.

Richer, S. F., & Vallerand, R. J. (1998). Construction et validation de l'échelle du sentiment d'appartenance sociale (ÉSAS). *European Review of Applied Psychology, 48*(2), 129–138.

Sawyer, R. K. (2007). *Group genius: The creative power of collaboration*. New York: Basic Books.

Schwarzer, R., & Jerusalem, M. (1995). Generalized self-efficacy scale. In J. Weinman, S. Wright, & M. Johnston (Eds.), *Measures in health psychology: A user's portfolio. Causal and control beliefs* (pp. 35–37). Windsor: NFER-NELSON.

Seligman, M. E. P., & Csikszentmihalyi, M. (2000). Positive psychology: An introduction. *American Psychologist, 55*(1), 5–14.

Shernoff, D. J., & Csikszentmihalyi, M. (2009). Flow in schools: Cultivating engaged learners and optimal learning environments. In R. C. Gilman, E. S. Heubner, & M. J. Furlong (Eds.), *Handbook of positive psychology in schools* (pp. 131–145). New York: Routledge.

Shernoff, D. J., Csikszentmihalyi, M., Schneider, B., & Shernoff, E. S. (2003). Student engagement in high school classrooms from the perspective of flow theory. *School Psychology Quarterly, 18*, 158–76.

Steiger, J. H. (1990). Structural model evaluation and modification: An interval estimation approach. *Multivariate Behavioural Research, 25*, 173–180.

Tucker, L. R., & Lewis, C. (1973). The reliability coefficient for maximum likelihood factor analysis. *Psychometrika, 38*, 1–10.

Vollmeyer, R., & Rheinberg, F. (2006). Motivational effects on self-regulated learning with different tasks. *Educational Psychology Review, 18*(3), 239–253.

Vygotsky, L. -S. (1962). *Thought and language*. MIT Press, Cambridge, Massachusetts.

Chapter 10
Using ESM to Study Flow in a STEM Project

Frans Ørsted Andersen

Abstract For decades, school students in the West have shown lower levels of interest in STEM subjects (science, technology, engineering and math) than in humanities, arts, finance or the media. But STEM competencies are increasingly in demand in modern societies. A Danish project, Future Learning Lab (FUF), conducted by two Danish ministries in concert with the Katafonden foundation and the Nynaturfag.dk project, aims to find ways to close this *STEM gap*. The goal is to create both (1) increased student motivation for STEM subjects and (2) better STEM teaching and learning. Recently a number of classes of Danish school students tested a new FUF learning lab designed to meet these goals. Researchers measured student flow during the test period, using ESM (Experience Sampling Method) in combination with observations and interviews. The research found high levels of student flow during the test period, and pointed to the following FUF characteristics as likely causes of the high flow levels detected in the experiment: (1) increased scope for hands-on activities, (2) increased use of open-ended experiments, (3) increased scope for working in groups, (4) increased scope for open internet search, and (5) increased scope for wild "myth buster" STEM activities engendering a (feeling of) lack of control.

10.1 Introduction

For decades in much of the Western world, school students have shown lower levels of interest in STEM subjects (science, technology, engineering and math) than in humanities, arts, finance, the media, sports, or social sciences. Yet STEM competencies are increasingly in demand in modern societies, so much so that STEM development and expansion are sometimes cited as the only solution to the crises of global warming, increasing social inequality, new diseases, and ever-scarcer resources (Thiel 2014).

Although there were subsequently minor improvements in the Danish and Norwegian PISA results of 2012, PISA 2006 (with science in focusu had revealed some very unfortunate attitudes toward science among Danish and Norwegian

F.Ø. Andersen (✉)
Department of Education, University of Aarhus, Aarhus, Denmark
e-mail: frans@edu.au.dk

L. Harmat et al. (eds.), *Flow Experience*, DOI 10.1007/978-3-319-28634-1_10

school students (Egelund 2010, 2013). Scandinavian school students generally did not value science very highly: e.g. only 40 % agreed with the statement: "Progress within science and technology normally leads to social progress as well" (Sølberg and Troelsen 2008).

Only 21 % of Scandinavian school students participating in the PISA 2006 study could see themselves in a future STEM career (Sølberg and Troelsen 2008). Another study of Scandinavian PISA science results looked further into the details of the students' low levels of interest in STEM (Schreiner 2006). This study pointed to non-engaging science teaching at primary and middle-school levels as a major reason for the low levels of STEM interest among high-school (higher secondary) students. A similar Scandinavian study showed that young Scandinavians see STEM subjects as irrelevant and meaningless to them (Schreiner and Sjøberg 2004). While initial STEM interest among Scandinavian (here: Danish and Norwegian) primary schoolchildren is high, it declines rapidly as early as fourth grade (Schreiner 2006). Consequently, a number of STEM-enhancing school projects have been launched in both Denmark and Norway. This chapter deals with one of these, the FUF project. ESM (Experience Sampling Method) flow measurements were part of the project's research design (see Chap. 9 by Heutte et al. in this volume). FUF stands for "Fremtidens Undervisnings Facilitet" or Future Learning Lab. FUF was initiated by the Danish ministry of education, the Danish ministry of science, technology and innovation, Sønderborg Municipality, and the Universefonden foundation (since 2015 called "Katafonden").

FUF aims to find ways to close this "STEM gap." FUF's objectives are to create:

1. Greater student motivation for and lifelong engagement in STEM subjects;
2. Better STEM teaching and deeper STEM learning; and
3. More constructive STEM teacher and student roles.

This chapter introduces the FUF concepts and lab, and outlines how the STEM labs were designed, constructed, and subsequently tested by schools. The FUF lab continues to this day to offer STEM education in its new experimental setting.

The project group that designed and ran (and still runs) the FUF facilities with its new STEM labs, drew on a wide range of existing research in the field of STEM teaching and learning (Merit and Nielsen 2006). Figure 10.1 below illustrates the process:

The design group established four physical zones in the STEM learning lab:

1. **The Workshop Zone** was a central feature of the concept. A well-functioning science learning environment has dedicated workshops that, while designed specifically for a science course, use normal workshop equipment that the students themselves can use freely, as well as a related stock of materials containing "useful junk."
2. **The Focus Zone** was equipped with tables and space for sitting and standing. Here the students could store their books and other equipment for preparation, as well as deciding on the distribution of roles for group work.

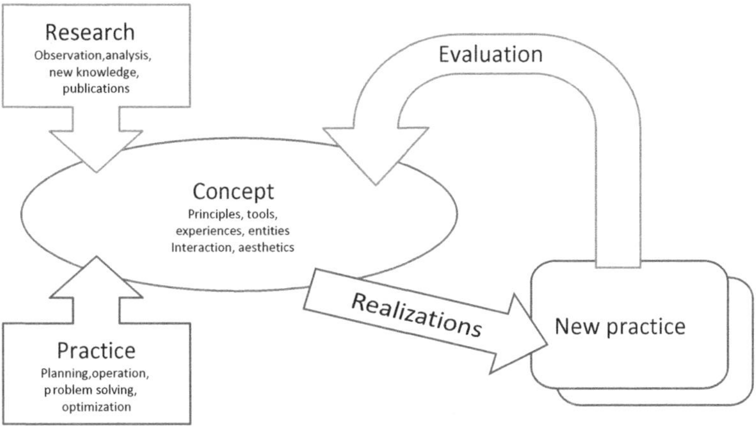

Fig. 10.1 FUF project process

3. **The Arena Zone** was a place for students to present their results. Here the teacher begins and ends the learning course, and here the students give their presentations to the rest of the class.
4. **The Model Zone** was a space for the student to get "into flow" by him- or herself, and to build models, create drafts, draw, or perform more focused activities. This zone can also function as a space for the "difficult" or "maladjusted" student.

You can see the design of the actual two-floor building constructed for FUF in Fig. 10.2.

10.2 Methods

The findings presented in this article are based on data collected over 10 days in the FUF labs. The labs opened in spring 2012 in the town of Nordborg, Southern Denmark, close to the science theme park Universe Parken. The test classes came from seven Danish public schools around the country. A total of eight classes participated in the study: seven classes in seventh grade, and one in eighth grade. The total number of students in the study was 187, of whom 107 were girls and 80 boys. The total number of teacher respondents was ten (Table 10.1).

The study measured student levels of both learning and flow. In the following, we will primarily focus on the flow measurements, which correspond to the learning measurements. It is documented that experiences of flow in connection with teaching can create sustained interest in the subject in question, which was precisely the overall objective of the FUF study (Csikszentmihalyi 1990). The study examined the following research question: how do the students experience the FUF labs, and to what extent do the students experience flow and the opportunity for learning in these labs?

The methods used were ESM, in combination with interviews with both students and teachers.

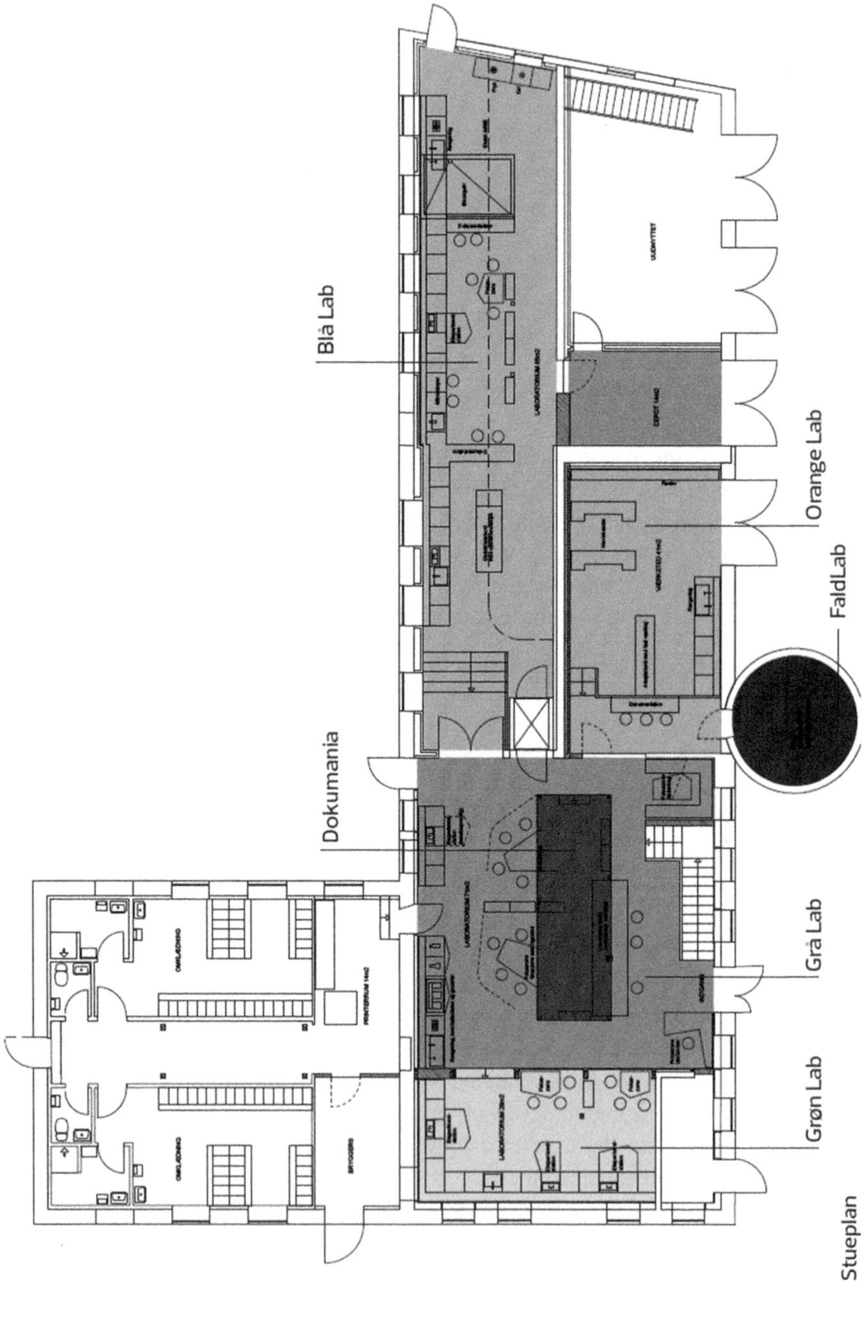
Blå Lab
Dokumania
Orange Lab
FaldLab
Grå Lab
Grøn Lab
Stueplan

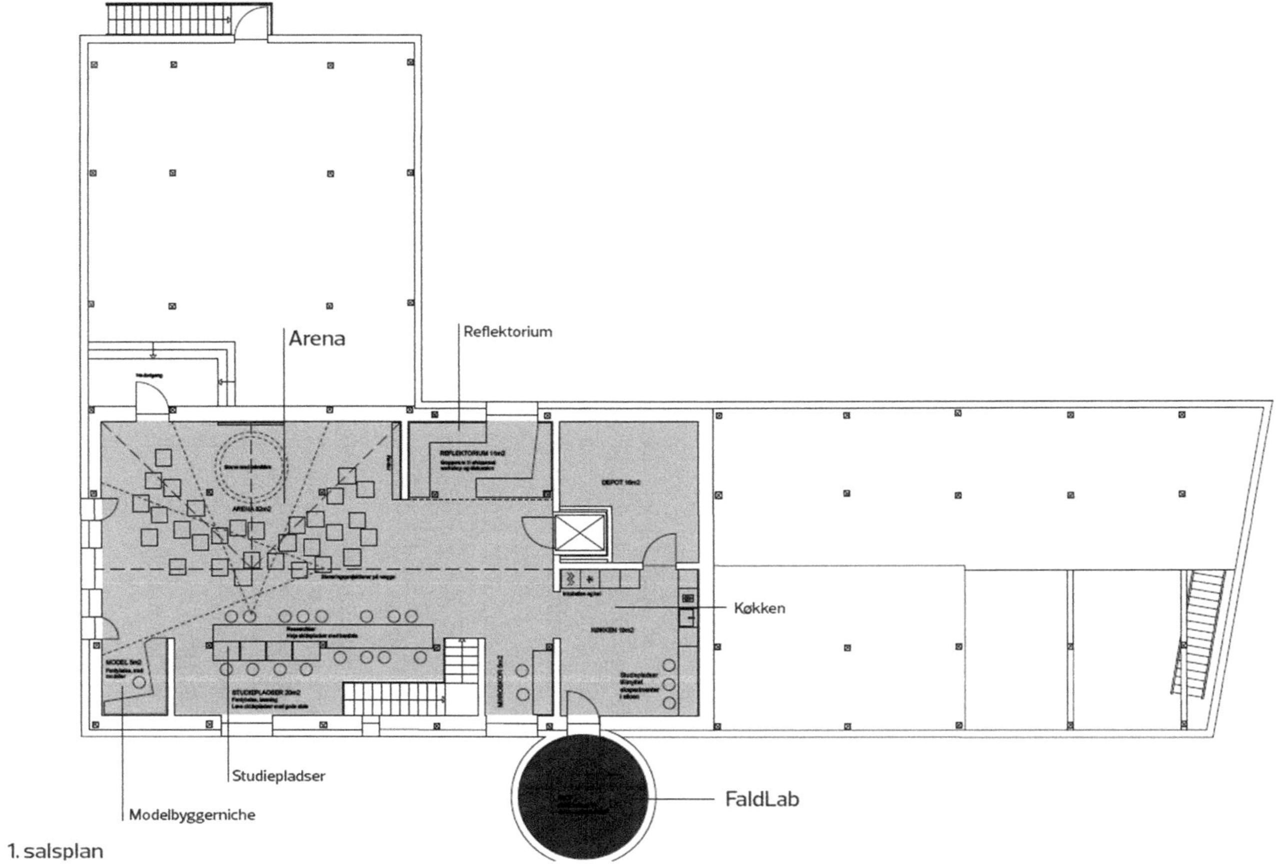

Fig. 10.2 Overview of the two-floor FUF labs. Key: Stueplan = Ground floor: Blå Lab = *Blue* lab, *Orange* Lab = *Orange* lab, Fald Lab = Drop lab, Grå Lab = *Gray* lab, Grøn Lab = *Green* lab, Dokumania = Documentary room *1*. Salsplan = first floor: Reflektorium = Reflection room, Arena = Arena, Køkken = Kitchen, Fald Lab = Drop lab, Studiepladser = Study tables, Modelbyggerniche = Modeling niche

Table 10.1 Overview of students and teachers (names changed) involved in the data-collecting period.

FUF	Date	Grades	Number of students	Girls	Boys	Teacher	Subject
1	17–04–12	7	11	4	7	Hans	Science
2	23–04–12	7	22	12	10	Ole	Science
3	25–04–12	7	19	14	5	Kenneth	Science
4	08–05–12	7	25	11	14	Jesper	Biology
5	09–05–12	7	22	12	10	Tom	Science
6	16–05–12	7	9	5	4	John	Science
7	25–05–12	7	21	10	11	Mads	Biology
8	29–05–12	7	11	5	6	Esben	Science
9	06–06–12	8	22	15	7	Trygve	Science
10	14–06–12	7	25	19	6	Erik	Science

10.2.1 ESM as Used in the Study

Studies of flow were implemented by use of ESM (Hektner et al. 2007). In the FUF experiment, all of the 187 participating students answered the same ESM questionnaire three times during each day-long teaching session. Concretely, the method consisted in the students receiving a bag containing three questionnaires and a pen at the beginning of the day. During the day, an alarm clock signaled three times for them immediately to fill in a questionnaire, which was then immediately collected. The actual ESM tool was developed from a current Danish translation of the German and English versions of Rheinberg's "Flow Kurz Skala" and "The Flow Short Scale" (Engeser and Rheinberg 2005, 2008). The following is the English version:

1. I feel just the right amount of challenge (skill – challenge balance)
2. My thoughts/activities run fluidly and smoothly (coherent, non-contradictory demands)
3. I do not notice time passing (time transformation)
4. I have no difficulty concentrating (centering of attention)
5. My mind is completely clear (centering of attention)
6. I am totally absorbed in what I am doing (merging of action and awareness)
7. The right thoughts/movements occur of their own accord (coherent, non-contradictory demands)
8. I know what I have to do each step of the way (coherent, non-contradictory demands)
9. I feel that I have everything under control (feeling of control)
10. I am completely lost in thought (loss of self-consciousness) (Rheinberg et al. 2003; Engeser 2012)

The Flow Short Scale (or Flow Kurz Skala) was originally developed by the German researcher Falko Rheinberg, who, together with colleagues, has used the scale not only in flow research projects (for example Rheinberg 2004), but also in projects studying flow in learning situations (Engeser and Rheinberg 2008). The Flow Short Scale is a scale consisting of the ten statements shown above. These statements are valid as defined by the criteria of flow experiences (Rheinberg et al. 2003). The scale is developed on the lines of a Likert scale, in which respondents indicate the degree of their agreement with each statement by ticking off a number between 1 (lowest degree of agreement) and 7 (highest degree of agreement) (Engeser and Rheinberg 2008). The ESM method has three basic characteristics:

In situ: Experiences are reported directly on the spot and in the actual environments in which they occur.

In real time: Experiences are reported just as they take place (or immediately thereafter).

On repeated time occasions: Experiences are reported repeatedly over time.

10.2.2 ESM Data Analysis

Data collected by ESM differs from many other kinds of dataset, because the respondents have answered the same questions several times. That makes it possible to take various different approaches to the analysis, the individual answers, and the individual respondents. Analyzing the individual answers provides brand new opportunities, because the answers represent different situations at different times. This gives access to an episodic representation of everyday life, something that is otherwise hard to quantify (Hektner et al. 2007).

10.2.3 The Experience Sampling Form

The Experience Sampling Form (ESF) constituted the study framework, while the questionnaire contained the ESM (see Fig. 10.3). Besides the ten statements listed above, the ESF contained a number of external questions related to the physical surroundings and concrete activities in progress at the moment the alarm went off. External questions were, for example: "What are you doing?" and "Where are you?" The former was an open question, while the latter was answered by marking an X on a map. As a quality control in ESM, the questionnaire also asks the respondents an open question, such as "What are you thinking about?" We did just that in our ESF study. The answer to this question is then compared to the answer to the question about what they are doing. If the subjects are thinking about the activity they are currently engaged in, the flow measurement is a meaningful expression of the purpose of FUF. Conversely, if subjects are thinking about something that has nothing to do with the STEM activity at the FUF labs, the flow measurement does not make sense (Hektner et al. 2007). "What are you thinking about?" was therefore added as an open question.

English translation of the Danish text in the form in Fig. 10.3.

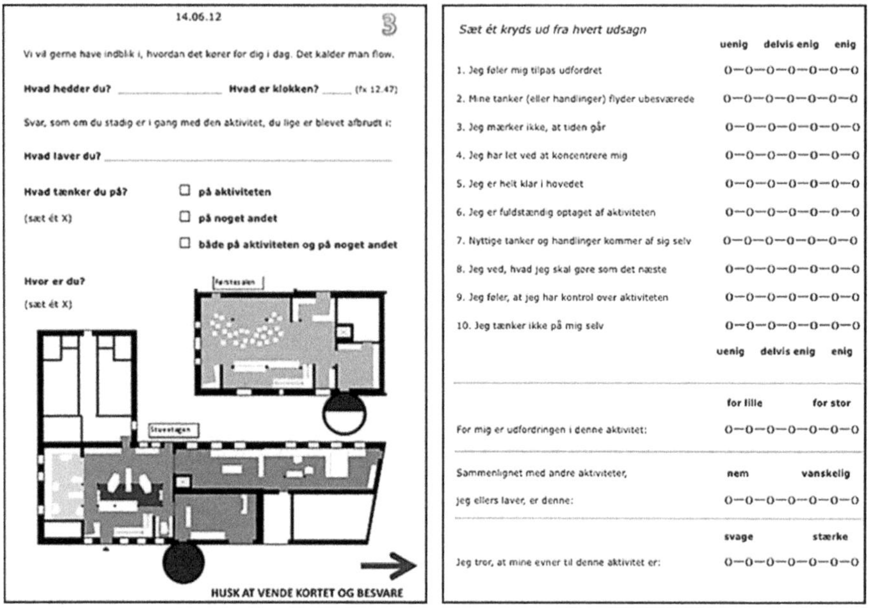

14.06.12

3

Vi vil gerne have indblik i, hvordan det kører for dig i dag. Det kalder man flow.

Hvad hedder du? ________ **Hvad er klokken?** ____ (fx 12.47)

Svar, som om du stadig er i gang med den aktivitet, du lige er blevet afbrudt i:

Hvad laver du? ________

Hvad tænker du på? (sæt ét X)

☐ **på aktiviteten**

☐ **på noget andet**

☐ **både på aktiviteten og på noget andet**

Hvor er du? (sæt ét X)

HUSK AT VENDE KORTET OG BESVARE

Sæt ét kryds ud fra hvert udsagn

	uenig	delvis enig	enig
1. Jeg føler mig tilpas udfordret	0—0—0—0—0—0—0		
2. Mine tanker (eller handlinger) flyder ubesværede	0—0—0—0—0—0—0		
3. Jeg mærker ikke, at tiden går	0—0—0—0—0—0—0		
4. Jeg har let ved at koncentrere mig	0—0—0—0—0—0—0		
5. Jeg er helt klar i hovedet	0—0—0—0—0—0—0		
6. Jeg er fuldstændig optaget af aktiviteten	0—0—0—0—0—0—0		
7. Nyttige tanker og handlinger kommer af sig selv	0—0—0—0—0—0—0		
8. Jeg ved, hvad jeg skal gøre som det næste	0—0—0—0—0—0—0		
9. Jeg føler, at jeg har kontrol over aktiviteten	0—0—0—0—0—0—0		
10. Jeg tænker ikke på mig selv	0—0—0—0—0—0—0		
	uenig	delvis enig	enig

	for lille	for stor
For mig er udfordringen i denne aktivitet:	0—0—0—0—0—0—0	

	nem	vanskelig
Sammenlignet med andre aktiviteter, jeg ellers laver, er denne:	0—0—0—0—0—0—0	

	svage	stærke
Jeg tror, at mine evner til denne aktivitet er:	0—0—0—0—0—0—0	

Fig. 10.3 The ESF/ESM form used in the study (in Danish)

14.06.12

We would like to know how it's going for you today. It's called flow

What's your name ?__________ **What's the time?** _______ (e.g. 12.47)

Answer as if you're still doing the activity that has just been interrupted:

What are you doing? ______________________

What are you thinking about? □ **the activity**

(mark with one X) □ **something else**

□ **the activity and something else**

Where are you?

(mark with one X)

→

PLEASE TURN OVER AND ANSWER

Make one mark for each statement

1. I feel just the right amount **disagree partly disagree**
agree
of challenge o—o—o—o—o—o—o

2. My thoughts(or activities) run **disagree partly disagree**
agree
fluidly and smoothly o—o—o—o—o—o—o

3. I do not notice time passing **disagree partly disagree**
agree
o—o—o—o—o—o—o

4. I have no difficulty concentrating **disagree partly disagree**
agree
o—o—o—o—o—o—o

5. My mind is completely clear **disagree partly disagree agree**
o—o—o—o—o—o—o

6. I am totally absorbed in what **disagree partly disagree agree**
I am doing o—o—o—o—o—o—o

7. The right thoughts/movements **disagree partly disagree**
agree
occur on their own record o—o—o—o—o—o—o

8. I know what I have to do each **disagree partly disagree**
agree
step of the way o—o—o—o—o—o—o

10.2.4 Data Collection and Analysis

The above ESF/ESM form was implemented as a paper/pen version in the study because of technical difficulties with the software that we were about to use (and had checked in small pilot studies). The form was collected manually, and answers were initially entered into Microsoft Access. The data was subsequently transferred to SPSS (Statistical Package for the Social Sciences) for statistical analysis. Data was drawn from answers rather than respondents, so that each ESF was registered individually. The respondent's ID number, name, date, and the time at which the alarm sounded together made up the identification of the individual ESF. Data was coded prior to the entries.

The open question "What are you doing?" was coded under the activity types "Nature sciences," "General science," and "Idle," and was included both as text and as number. The question "Where are you?" which the students answered by marking an X on the map of the FUF facilities, was coded to numbers twice: first to the specific place, categorized in 33 codes, and second, to the setting of the place, categorized in seven codes. Answers to the closed questions and the scaled statements were registered directly as numbers. Thereafter the data was cleaned and corrected for errors in the registration, definition of variables, values of variables, and relations between the values in the miscellaneous variable.

10.2.5 Total Amount of Flow Samplings

One hundred eighty-seven student experiences, reported three times per student, give an optimal total of 561 flow samplings. The present study, however, has a lower complete percentage of answers, as one respondent marked the line in between the value of gradation on all three of their ESFs, which therefore cannot be included in the total set of data. In addition, 19 samplings were excluded due to missing answers. The total data set was therefore 539 flow samplings (see Table 10.2).

10.2.6 Reliability

The ESF/ESM form was designed from student feedback in the pilot tests to ensure the best possible understanding of the questions and statements in the form. The Cronbach's Alpha pilot test was 0.91, and the table below shows Cronbach's Alpha for the revised, final scale. In the significantly larger set of data (57 in the pilot test, compared to 539 in the prototype study) reliability was expected to increase, but that did not happen. However, a Cronbach's Alpha of 0.846 still indicates good reliability (Tables 10.3 and 10.4).

Table 10.2 Total amount of flow samplings

Cases	N	%
Valid	53	96.6
	9	
Excluded	19	3.4
Total	558	100.0

Table 10.3 Reliability statistics

Cronbach's alpha	Cronbach's alpha based on standardized items	Number of items
0.846	0.848	10

Table 10.4 Item – total statistics and variable correlation

Flow scale statements	Corrected item – total correlation	C. Alpha if items 2 and 10 omitted
1. I feel just the right amount of challenge	0.440	0.841
2. My thoughts/activities run fluidly and smoothly	0.388	0.845
3. I do not notice time passing	0.502	0.836
4. I have no difficulty concentrating	0.724	0.815
5. My mind is completely clear	0.682	0.819
6. I am totally absorbed in what I am doing	0.703	0.817
7. The right thoughts/movements occur on their own record	0.614	0.827
8. I know what I have to do each step of the way	0.490	0.838
9. I feel that I have everything under control	0.602	0.827
10. I am completely lost in thought	0.341	0.850

10.2.7 Flow Rating

As usual in ESM, we employed a 7-point Likert scale with graduation:

disagree partly disagree agree

o — o — o — o — o — o — o

The mean number of the students' flow ratings is 4.6, which is above the middle value on a Likert scale (Table 10.5) The students' flow ratings are presented in mean numbers in Table 10.6 below. The middle value on a Likert scale is called "the scale's balance point," and it divides the scale between "negative rating" and "positive rating" of the value of statements (Rheinberg 2004). In this case, we see a positive rating of the total value of the scale.

Ratings from individual statements are shown in Table 10.6 below. Four statements are above the mean number, one statement is equal to the mean number, and five statements are below the mean number. Statement 3 ("I do not notice time passing") is the statement with the highest mean number.

Table 10.5 Total factor for flow rating mean and standard deviation

Mean	N	Standard deviation
4.5811	539	1.20095

Table 10.6 Item statistics with flow variables

Flow scale statements	Mean	Std. deviation	N
1. I feel just the right amount of challenge	4.36	1.869	539
2. My thoughts/activities run fluidly and smoothly	4.37	1.735	539
3. I do not notice time passing	5.02	1.984	539
4. I have no difficulty concentrating	4.80	1.861	539
5. My mind is completely clear	4.55	1.842	539
6. I am totally absorbed in what I am doing	4.26	1.875	539
7. The right thoughts/movements occur on their own record	4.65	1.639	539
8. I know what I have to do each step of the way	4.37	2.085	539
9. I feel that I have everything under control	4.85	1.748	539
10. I am completely lost in thought	4.58	1.865	539

10.2.8 Flow and Thoughts

According to Csikszentmihalyi, convergence between "experience of flow" and "thinking about the activity" can be used as an overall quality control of flow measurements using ESM (Hekter, Schmidt and Csikszentmihalyi 2007) (Fig. 10.4).

The responses in Table 10.7 show that the students who were thinking about the activity that they also indicate they were involved in were those with the highest flow rating (5.2), while the students who were thinking about something else have the lowest rating. Students who were thinking about both the activity and something else are located in between (but below the total average).

In terms of the overall purpose of the FUF study, namely seeking to boost interest in STEM subjects, there was an interesting correlation between the students' flow rating and the concrete activity they were engaged in at the moment when the ESM alarm went off. In the data processing, the answer to the question "What are you doing?" has been coded under three categories: "Nature sciences," "General sciences," and "Non-sciences."

The statistical results shown in Table 10.8 demonstrate that the students who reported a "nature sciences" activity were also the students with, in mean numbers, the highest flow rating (4.8, which is above the overall average at 4.6). Then there are "general sciences" and "non-sciences," both of which are placed below the total average. The rating in the "nature sciences" activity differs significantly from ratings in the two other activities, while the difference between "general sciences" and "non-sciences" is non-significant.

The external question "What are you doing?" documented the correlation between spatial location and concrete activity (Table 10.9).

What are you thinking of? ☐ **the activity**

(mark with one X) ☐ **something else**

☐ **the activity and something else**

Fig. 10.4 What are you thinking about?

Table 10.7 Descriptives: thoughts

Descriptives—thoughts	N	Mean	Std. deviation
Thinking about the activity	207	5.1831	0.93775
Thinking about something else	135	3.8533	1.27962
Thinking about both the activity and something else	188	4.3952	1.05203
Total	530	4.5649	1.19893

Table 10.8 Descriptives: activity, indicating flow rating and activity

Activity	N	Mean	Std. Deviation
Natural sciences	312	4.7728	1.14108
Non-sciences	76	4.1868	1.36776
General sciences	149	4.3772	1.16144
Total	537	4.5801	1.20195

Table 10.9 Descriptives: flow rating and setting

Setting	N	Mean	Std. deviation
General	209	4.4670	1.16681
Focus zone	90	4.3500	1.25977
Trial	161	4.7584	1.26726
Niche	23	4.8739	1.19477
Outside	15	5.0867	0.85178
Observer	3	5.6667	0.40415
Service	21	4.2619	0.66819
Total	522	4.5711	1.20477

10.3 Discussion

In a study like this, it is relevant to discuss the reactivity bias. The students knew that they were taking part in testing FUF, a program that was developed with the objective of providing better structures for STEM teaching. The very concept thus implicitly critiqued *the old format* that the students knew from their own school. The students' awareness that the project is seeking to provide a better structure may have affected their perception of the labs and the activities taking place there. Furthermore, the students knew that their behavior and actions were being observed, that their experience of flow was being measured, and that some of them would take part in group interviews after the trial. They also knew that their experience with FUF was important to the project.

One reactivity phenomenon of significance in this study might therefore be the so-called Hawthorne effect. The original Hawthorne study (reference) showed that no matter what you did to improve employees' physical working environments, any action at all had a positive effect. For instance, productivity increased when the premises got lighter, and it increased again when the premises were made darker. The conclusion was that productivity was not affected directly by the physical variable itself, but by the employees' knowledge that they were taking part in a study of the effects of improving the working environment. Csikszentmihalyi writes in his book *Good business*: *leadership, flow and the making of meaning* that the major consequence of the Hawthorne study is that physical environments have subsequently been seen as insignificant, the problem here being that the Hawthorne study measured only productivity, rather than employee well-being (Csikszentmihalyi 2003).

The FUF prototype learning lab was based on the hypothesis that the space in which we operate determines what we can do in it, and therefore also how we thrive in it. Consequently, the attempt was made to *embed* the conditions for creating flow *within the walls of the FUF labs*. In this context, it cannot be ruled out that the students' awareness of the aim of the project could have affected their flow ratings in a positive direction.

Another reactivity phenomenon of importance in this context could be the novelty effect (Kormi-Nouri et al. 2005). This has to do with the phenomenon that the presentation of something new sharpens the senses. The novelty effect describes the effect of the new, and one might say that the effect comes from the novelty itself (Kormi-Nouri et al. 2005). The novelty effect can thus be included as a bias in relation to increased achievement, not because respondents necessarily learned something new or developed their competencies in another way, but because they were interested by the new and their senses were therefore sharpened. At the opposite end of the spectrum, the novelty effect can also describe an increase in stress caused by the new, simply because it is new. Consequently, the novelty effect need not be a bias in the results only for the better; it can also have the opposite effect.

10.4 Conclusion

The research question was:

***How do the students experience the physical facilities, and to what extent do the students experience flow and the opportunity for learning in these labs*?**

Based on the ESM study and the associated interviews and classroom observations, we can conclude that the students at the FUF labs generally showed excite-

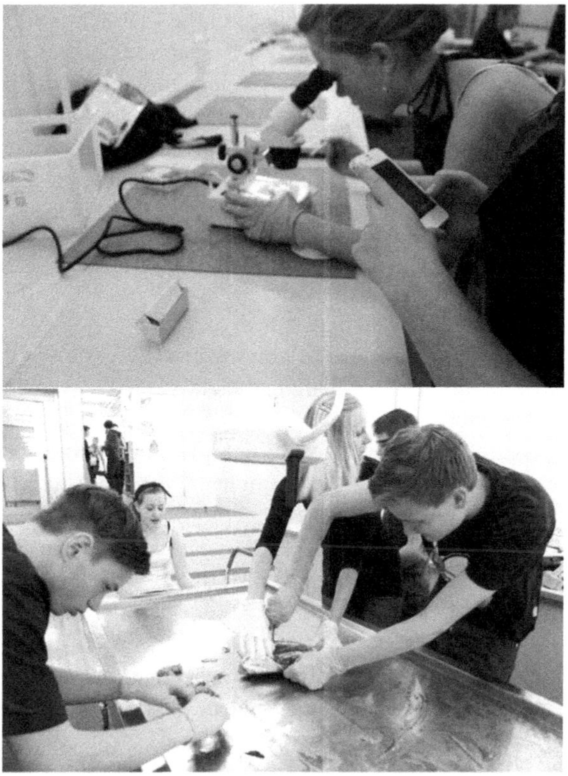

Fig. 10.5 FUF labs

ment at the new framework, the different approach to teaching, and the various different teacher and student roles. Our study showed that the students often forgot the time as they worked and studied in the FUF labs. Forgetting time and place is one of the most recognizable characteristics of flow experience. That the students forgot the time in the FUF labs may indicate that they were occupied by what they were doing.

A sense of control and the opportunity to concentrate are important additional aspects of flow experience. They are also important in order to improve the level of competency as challenges get harder. That the students experienced control and found it easy to concentrate is interpreted as a sign that they experienced good opportunities in the FUF labs both to reach flow and to learn (Fig. 10.5).

The study also shows that the new design, organization and decoration style of the FUF labs may beneficially affect social behavior within the rooms (teaching, learning, communication, etc.). The study indicates that the FUF labs (compared to normal teaching at the home school) gives good opportunities for:

- Varying approaches to teaching
- Different teacher roles
- Different student roles
- More frequent flow experiences
- Increased learning opportunities, i.e. both more numerous and in greater depth.

The teaching that takes place in the FUF labs still has to be well organized, the teachers still have to be well prepared and competent to make the teaching work, and the students still have to participate willingly and constructively. But by offering the new labs and by "turning the room around," new possibilities can be created for greater STEM engagement, motivation and learning.

Moreover, qualitative analysis of the complete data set (ESM, interviews and observations) points to the following elements in the STEM lab as likely to generate higher levels of flow:

1. More "hands-on" activities
2. More open-ended experiments
3. More opportunities for working and discussion in groups
4. More internet searching in the classroom
5. And more wild "myth buster" STEM activities in which a (feeling of) lack of control and security is present. (The FUF project aims to find ways to facilitate this without violating the students' sense of safety)

10.5 Perspectives

The science-teaching labs prototype that was tested as described here was not embedded in a school environment, and therefore was not tested as a part of the teachers' or students' everyday life. This means that a number of factors related to the informal context could have affected the results. In the trial, teaching the students meant a day trip out of their own school; in addition, the students had never been to the FUF labs before, and they knew that they were taking part in testing a whole new learning concept. This in itself could have affected their experience of both the labs and of the activities taking place there.

The results of the teaching trial therefore amount to hypotheses that require testing and appropriate organization in a new school environment. For the hypotheses to be confirmed or invalidated, additional research will be required, and this should also observe FUF's new decoration style in use in everyday life at the school for a longer period of time. Such a research program will render it possible continuously to review and evaluate the development of students' STEM interest, flow, and learning sciences—and to compare the results of the FUF concept with parallel studies of a control group in a "traditional" science room and "traditional" didactics in science.

References

Csikszentmihalyi, M. (1990). *Flow—the psychology of optimal experience*. New York: HarperCollins Publishers.

Csikszentmihalyi, M. (2003). *Good business—leadership, flow and the making of meaning*. New York: Hodder & Stoughton.
Egelund, N. (2010). *PISA 2009 undersøgelsen—en sammenfatning [PISA 2009—an abbreviation]*. Copenhagen: Danmarks Pædagogiske Universitetsforlag.
Egelund, N. (2013). *PISA 2012 undersøgelsen—en sammenfatning. [PISA 2012—an abbreviation]*. Copenhagen: KORA. Det Nationale Institut for Kommuners og Regioners Analyse og Forskning.
Engeser, S. (Ed.). (2012). *Advances in flow research*. New York: Springer.
Engeser, S., & Rheinberg, F. (2005). Motivation, Flow-Erleben und Lernleistung in universitären Lernsettings. *Zeitschrift für Pädagogische Psychologie/German Journal of Educational Psychology, 19*(3), 259–172.
Engeser, S., & Rheinberg, F. (2008). *Flow, performance and moderators of challenge-skill balance*. New York: Springer Science+Business Media.
Hektner, J. M., Schmidt, J. A., & Csikszentmihalyi, M. (2007). *Experience sampling method—measuring the quality of everyday life*. New York: Sage Publications.
Kormi-Nouri, R., Nilsson, L.-G., & Ohta, N. (2005). The novelty effect: Support for the novelty-encoding hypothesis. *Scandinavian Journal of Psychology, 46*, 133–143.
Merit, S., & Nielsen, T. (2006). *Vinderkoncepter. [Winner concepts]*. Copenhagen: Børsens Forlag.
Rheinberg, F. (2004). *Motivationsdiagnostik*. Göttingen: Hogrefe.
Rheinberg, F., Vollmeyer, R., & Engeser, S. (2003). Die Erfassung des Flow-Erlebens. In Stiensmeier-Pelster & Rheinberg (Eds.), *Diagnostik von Motivation und Selbstkonzept* (pp. 261–279). Göttingen: Hogrefe.
Schreiner, C. (2006). *Exploring a ROSE-garden; Norwegian youth's orientations towards science – seen as signs of late modern identities*. Doctoral thesis, University of Oslo, Faculty of Education, Olso.
Schreiner, C., & Sjøberg, S. (2004). Sowing the seeds of ROSE. *Acta Didactica*, no. 4. Oslo: University of Oslo.
Sølberg, J., & Troelsen, R. P. (2008). Et nuanceret billede af interesse for de naturvidenskabelige og teknologiske områder [A detailed picture of interest in scientific and technological fields]. In R.P. Troelsen, & J. Sølberg (Eds.), *Den danske ROSE-undersøgelse—en antologi [The Danish Rose-survey—an anthology*] (pp. 93–107). Aarhus University, Institut for Curriculumforskning, Danmarks Pædagogiske Universitetsskole.
Thiel, P. (2014). *Zero to one. Notes on startups, or how to build the future*. New York: Crown Business.

Chapter 11
Flow, Leisure, and Positive Youth Development

Teresa Freire, Dionísia Tavares, Eliana Silva, and Ana Teixeira

Abstract Leisure has been associated with several developmental opportunities that foster adolescents' optimal growth. Considering leisure as a context, activity or experience, researchers have focused on its role in the study of flow experience. Both leisure and flow experiences, and the way they interrelate, emerge as relevant to promoting positive youth development, daily and along life trajectories. This chapter aims to present and analyze conceptual and empirical evidence about the connection between positive youth development, leisure, and flow experience. Among the empirical evidence, we highlight studies from our Portuguese research team, the Research Group on Optimal Functioning – GIFOp, aimed at studying adolescents' optimal functioning. Specifically, we illustrate results according to different aims and methodologies. In this sense, we discuss adolescents' daily life perceptions of activities and quality of experiences, and future life goals, measured by retrospective self-report questionnaires; and flow, optimal experience and motivational aspects of subjective experience, by real-time measures, specifically the Experience Sampling Method (ESM). The conclusion sheds light on the importance of a psycho-social-ecological approach when studying adolescents' flow and leisure experiences and how these enhance positive youth development. Future research directions will consider the importance of merging school and leisure contexts, highlighting the role of leisure structured activities to promote flow and optimal experiences, when considered as different components of subjective experience. In addition, the use of different methodologies based on both retrospective and real-time measures, are addressed as being equally important and relevant to continue the main conceptual discussion around flow and optimal experiences in adolescence.

T. Freire (✉) • D. Tavares • E. Silva • A. Teixeira
School of Psychology, University of Minho, Braga, Portugal
e-mail: tfreire@psi.uminho.pt

L. Harmat et al. (eds.), *Flow Experience*, DOI 10.1007/978-3-319-28634-1_11

11.1 Introduction

Leisure is one of the most meaningful experiences that facilitate the construction of a positive, healthy and normative developmental life trajectory of adolescents. More than any other period of human development, in adolescence individuals seek for deep knowledge about themselves and their relation with others and the environment, making this period a pivotal opportunity for enhancing self-complexity.

From a conceptual point of view, leisure is a complex issue that can be analyzed within different frameworks and perspectives, making different kinds of definitions relevant. Following an integrative perspective headed by Caldwell and Faulk (2013), leisure can be studied threefold: as an experience, a context, or an activity. This highlights the ecological relevance that leisure experience has for adolescents' development and how it can facilitate the emergence and promotion of developmental assets. Leisure can be used as a conceptual filter to analyze and understand adolescents' psychosocial development making the concept of optimal leisure and positive development relevant (Freire 2013).

The main goal of this chapter is to show the conceptual relationship between *development*, *leisure* and *flow*, and its relevance for the study of adolescence. Specifically, we aim at understanding how these concepts integrate adolescents' actual lives and how they impact upon the construction of their future life trajectories. Our Portuguese research team (named Research Group on Optimal Functioning – GIFOp) focuses on the study of optimal functioning, integrating several research topics. Some of these are related to studies on flow/optimal experience and leisure experience and will be presented in this chapter.

So, flow, leisure, and positive youth development will define the contents of this chapter based on a structure organized along three specific but interrelated parts. In the first part, the introduction of the chapter, we briefly present the aims and main theoretical perspectives supporting the whole chapter. For this, two main subsections are structured. Firstly, adolescence issues, positive development and leisure are discussed as a general umbrella embracing main concepts for understanding leisure and positive development and their concomitant role in improving healthy and optimal growth in adolescence. Secondly, flow and leisure experiences are explored, by trying to understand how these two kinds of experiences potentiate positive trajectories in the present and for the future, mainly when co-occurring across daily activities and life contexts. These subsections are based on a review of the literature on those topics, trying to contribute to the state-of-the-art on the theme of the chapter.

In the second part, we present a series of studies about the quality of subjective experience of Portuguese adolescents, and the role of leisure and flow experiences in their daily lives and related trajectories. More than a collection of data we want to show how research has been designed and conducted according to conceptual approaches, what kind of methodologies have been used, and the main issues with respect to the results of the research about Portuguese adolescents.

Finally in the third part, we compile conclusions on Portuguese adolescents trying to integrate (and articulate) the conclusions in the actual empirical arena of this topic, shedding light on future research directions in the study of flow, leisure, and positive youth development.

11.1.1 Adolescents, Positive Development, and Leisure

Until the last decades, the scientific study of adolescence was characterized by a "deficit perspective", which conceptualized adolescence as a period of universal "storm and stress" (Hall 1904). Youth was seen as "problems to be managed" (Roth and Brooks-Gunn 2003), and if the term positive development was discussed, it was regarded to the absence or decrease of problems (Bowers et al. 2010). In the 1960s, researchers, practitioners, and policy makers began to question these assumptions, and later a new approach emerged for describing adolescence, designed as "positive youth development" (PYD, Damon 2004; Lerner 2005), which created a new milestone with significant impact in changing existent perspectives on adolescence. Following Lerner and Galambos (1998) definition, PYD is about the adolescents' engagement in pro-social behaviors and their avoidance of behaviors that can undermine or impair their health and their future (Freire and Soares 2000; Freire and Silva 2013; Silva and Freire 2014). Therefore, the exclusive focus on problems and corresponding resolution were replaced by an increased attention on the qualities, talents and strengths (Damon 2004; Lerner et al. 2005) and consequently, a (re) conceptualization of adolescents as "resources to be developed" (Roth and Brooks-Gunn 2003).

The PYD approach derived from the developmental systems theories (Damon 2004; Overton 2013) based in the plasticity of human development (Bowers et al. 2014; Lerner 2005). Derived from these theories, the "Five Cs" model of PYD (Bowers et al. 2010; Lerner et al. 2005) emerged as a more relevant proposal for the study of adolescents. This model defines positive development by Five Cs: *competence* (a positive view of one's actions in social, academic, cognitive, and vocational areas), *confidence* (overall positive self-worth and self-efficacy), *connection* (positive bonds with individuals and institutions), *character* (morality and integrity), and *caring* (empathy for other people). Youth who reveal these Five Cs are more likely to have a developmental trajectory with beneficial person-context relationships, developing an orientation to contribute to their community, which was characterized later on as the sixth "C" – *contribution* (Bowers et al. 2010).

This model also emphasizes that positive trajectories and youth thriving can be achieved through the mutually influential relations between the strengths of adolescents and their daily experiences and contexts (Bowers et al. 2010; Lerner et al. 2005). In this perspective, several studies have shown that leisure is an important daily context offering several developmental opportunities, such as identity and personal development, interpersonal relationships, initiative and teamwork, development of competence and academic achievement (Blomfield and Barber 2011;

Caldwell and Faulk 2013; Freire 2013; Trainor et al. 2010). Adolescents who engage in positive leisure activities are more susceptible to developmental experiences that foster a positive development (Blomfield and Barber 2011). Caldwell (2005) developed the Leisure Activity-Context-Experience (LACE) model in order to understand adolescents' development through the interaction of these three leisure components. This author considers that these three components are a key point because the way they combine may lead to positive or negative leisure experiences.

Following the LACE framework, and regarding leisure as an activity, recent studies have shown that the different types of leisure activities have different contributions regarding positive development of adolescents (Sarriera et al. 2014; Trainor et al. 2010; Weidman et al. 2012; Ward and Zabriskie 2011). For instance, participation in structured leisure activities (such as sports, volunteering, etc.) has been associated with high levels of well-being, self-esteem, self-concept, life satisfaction and psychological functioning (Blomfield and Barber 2011; Bradley and Inglis 2012; Sarriera et al. 2014; Trainor et al. 2010). On the other hand, participation in unstructured activities (such as watching television, using the computer and playing video games) has been negatively correlated with well-being, self-esteem, and life satisfaction levels, providing fewer developmental benefits (see Chap. 9 by Heutte et al. in this volume) (Bradley and Inglis 2012; Caldwell and Faulk 2013; Sarriera et al. 2014; Trainor et al. 2010). However, this structured and unstructured classification is not unique in the literature, and alternative classifications have been suggested (see for example Bradley and Inglis 2012).

As for leisure as a context, Caldwell and Faulk (2013) define context as "situational features surrounding the activity such as presence or absence of adults and opportunities for leadership" (p. 42). Depending on these features, leisure context can be considered a context for positive development, giving the opportunity for adolescents to develop leadership skills, self-determination, and competence; or considered a context for behavioral problems, such as delinquency, substance abuse, smoking and sexual risk behaviors (Caldwell and Smith 2006). Those contextual aspects of leisure that are considered to contribute to positive outcomes are adult supervision, adolescent opportunity to make decisions, to foster initiative, to develop new skills, to be valued and recognized, and to interact with peers (Caldwell and Faulk 2013).

Finally, leisure experience is about the way adolescents experience an activity. This emergent experience can be either positive or negative and is associated with personal dimensions, according to the type of leisure activity individuals are involved in and/or to the characteristics of the leisure context features and related impact (Caldwell and Smith 2006). For instance, engagement, interest, and motivation have been associated with positive outcomes such as initiative, self-efficacy, and competence, contributing to adolescent positive development. On the contrary, negative experiences (boredom, stress, and conflict) have been associated with negative outcomes, such as smoking, substance abuse, and delinquency (Caldwell and Faulk 2013; Caldwell and Smith 2006; Larson 2000). However, positivity or negativity associated with leisure is not a consensual issue within leisure studies, with some researchers in the field defending the unequivocal positivity of leisure experiences (cf. Freire 2013; Freire and Stebbins 2011).

Looking deeply into this experiential component, and following a developmental and ecological perspective, Freire (2013) focuses on leisure as subjective experience, understanding leisure as a set of opportunities for adolescents to be producers of their own development. The author distinguishes between leisure and free time, showing that "Adolescents can have different experiences during free time, but only some of them are related to leisure, and only some of these are considered optimal leisure experiences" (Freire 2013, p. 63–64). This optimal leisure concept demands a complex definition of leisure experience that integrates three different components: *personal leisure*, *social leisure* and *place or ecological leisure*. Together these components contribute to the adolescents' knowledge of themselves, others and the contexts. The personal leisure component refers to the individual and his/her personal characteristics (skills and resources) that can be developed through leisure activities and involvement in contexts. Social leisure refers to social interactions during leisure activities and contexts, contributing to the development of social competences and a sense of belonging. Finally, place or ecological leisure refers to the places where leisure activities happen, which has implications for the type of leisure activities and experiences that occur. For the author, the interaction among these three elements facilitates and promotes the development of adolescents' identity, one of the most complex and challenging tasks that adolescents have on their hands. In the same way, the author explored the concept of identity and dissected it into three types of identity, supported by psycho-social-environmental literature (for a more detailed description see Freire 2013): personal identity, social identity and place identity. These characteristics are directly associated with the three components of the leisure experience (personal leisure, social leisure and place leisure). It is the interaction between leisure experience and identity formation components that fosters optimal leisure and positive youth development (Freire 2013).

The emphasis on leisure daily subjective experience highlights the concept of flow and optimal experience as major topics in leisure studies. Leisure has been studied as an opportunity for inducing a flow state because it comprises high intrinsic motivation, concentration, and engagement, allowing the development of qualities and strengths, skills and competences, and meaningful relationships, which is about positive youth development (Larson 2000; Rich 2003). In the next topic of this chapter, we will discuss and deepen the knowledge on flow and leisure experiences.

11.1.2 Flow and Leisure Experience

Flow experience occurs when individuals are intensely involved in an activity, "making a voluntary effort to accomplish something difficult and worthwhile" (Csikszentmihalyi 1990, p. 3). Flow experience is characterized by the perception of a balance between high challenges and high skills, clear goals, immediate feedback, focused attention and high concentration, control of the situation and high intrinsic motivation (Csikszentmihalyi 1997). For this, some authors claim flow can be considered the most positive and complex experiential state that can occur in subjective experience of daily life (Nakamura and Csikszentmihalyi 2002).

Flow specific characteristics make this experience unique, different from other subjective experiences, connecting it in a perfect way to optimal growth and positive development. Being a rewarding experience, associated with positive affect, individuals seek to repeat it. As the challenges posed by an activity are overcome and in order to pursue personal goals and guarantee the similar level of enjoyment, the person looks for new and more complex challenges, giving rise to skill development and enhancing the complexity of the self (see Chap. 10 by Andersen in this volume) (Hunter and Csikszentmihalyi 2003; Massimini and Delle Fave 2000; Nakamura and Csikszentmihalyi 2002).

The connection between flow experience and leisure has been a central concern for many researchers. Perkins and Nakamura (2011) suggest that the goal of a positive leisure science should be "to understand the nature and conditions of optimal experience in leisure time/pursuits" (p. 141). The authors believe that the study of leisure can bring important contributions to flow theory but investigating the flow state can also inform the study of leisure. According to Elkington (2011), "flow and serious leisure are certainly not disparate frameworks, sharing much more than a simple theoretical kinship but are, in fact, mutually reinforcing" (p. 277). Albeit flow and leisure share specific features they are theoretically and empirically separate concepts (Freire 2006, 2011). Flow can be experienced in many contexts and activities other than leisure, and not all forms of leisure are conducive to flow experience. Despite the various conceptualizations of leisure, it is commonly accepted in scientific literature that leisure facilitates the entering into flow state and opens pathways to growth and development, especially when it provides structure and opportunities for action (Freire 2006; Perkins and Nakamura 2011). Although research linking flow and leisure is still scarce, particularly with adolescents, existing studies show important results on the topic.

Studies on adolescents' daily life showed that adolescents feel most intrinsically motivated, happy, alert, and active in leisure activities, especially in those that are highly structured like sports, arts and hobbies (Csikszentmihalyi and Larson 1986; Delle Fave and Bassi 2003). More than any other activity structured leisure activities offer the possibility of high engagement and intrinsic motivation, proving to be a source of well-being and optimal experience (Bassi and Delle Fave 2004; Delle Fave and Bassi 2000; Mesurado 2009). This happens because adolescents are working toward their own chosen goals, which gives them a sense of freedom from adult control (Csikszentmihalyi and Larson 1986; Perkins and Nakamura 2011). Due to its central features (clear goals, immediate feedback, group identification, individual differentiation, engagement in progressively more complex challenges), structured leisure creates a unique experiential profile fertile to the occurrence of flow (Delle Fave and Bassi 2003; Freire 2006). Still there are some other activities that being associated with positive leisure experiences have rarely been associated with optimal experience, as it is the case of relaxed leisure usually characterized by low mood and low engagement (Delle Fave and Bassi 2003). Similarly, Stebbins (1997) states that casual leisure fails to produce a sense of optimal experience for its participants, which tend to occur mainly in serious leisure activities. Yet, the author points out that serious leisure and flow experience are not synonymous (Stebbins 2010).

More recently, in the last 5 years, the few studies investigating the relationship between flow and leisure in adolescents were focused on the quality of experience (including flow) in general or in a specific leisure activity (e.g., sports, arts or games) and, on trying to identify some predictors of motivation and flow (Cassidy and Paisley 2013; Coterón et al. 2013; Lee and Choe 2011; Moreno et al. 2010; Sinnamon et al. 2012; Steca et al. 2011; Trayes et al. 2012; Zhao et al. 2011).

In general, studies that investigated adolescents' daily experience showed that the majority of adolescents experienced flow during leisure activities. Results confirm the high and positive quality of experience associated with the performance of structured leisure activities and the occurrence of flow during these activities (Cassidy and Paisley 2013; Lee and Choe 2011; Sinnamon et al. 2012; Trayes et al. 2012). For example, when involved in a music-game or music activity and a performing arts competition, adolescents generally reported high levels of flow (Lee and Choe 2011; Sinnamon et al. 2012), although some differences were identified in flow dimensions between amateur or elite practitioners: amateurs scored lower in challenge-skill balance and clear goals dimensions, but scored higher on loss of self-consciousness than elite students (Sinnamon et al. 2012). Despite experiencing flow during leisure activities, adolescents also experienced flow in productive activities, while experiencing less flow in maintenance activities (Lee and Choe 2011). Positive emotions, togetherness, integrity, excitement, enthusiasm, pride, feeling relaxed yet excited, happy, alert, and active were the main characteristics experienced during the performance of the leisure activity, besides flow features (Cassidy and Paisley 2013; Lee and Choe 2011; Sinnamon et al. 2012; Trayes et al. 2012). One of the studies also showed that frustration was a negative predictor while boredom and nervousness were not predictors of the desire to repeat the experience in female adolescents (Trayes et al. 2012).

Steca et al. (2011) also analyzed adolescents' daily experience in different contexts, including leisure, comparing adolescents with high and low parents' perceived parental self-efficacy (PSE). The group of adolescents with low parents' PSE reported experiencing leisure more frequently but, simultaneously, reported a significantly lower percentage of optimal experiences than adolescents with parents with high PSE. The latter group reported more challenging activities in daily life in which to invest personal skills and attention. Results showed that both groups had optimal experiences in different kind of activities: productive activities, leisure, interactions, and maintenance (Steca et al. 2011).

Other studies tried to report predictors of flow experience, showing that basic psychological needs (competence, autonomy, and relatedness) predict the occurrence of flow experience in sports (Coterón et al. 2013; Moreno et al. 2010) and in Internet use (Zhao et al. 2011). In particular, the authors found that satisfaction of competence need was a significant predictor of dispositional flow (i.e. the typical frequency in which an individual experiences flow states in a particular activity) and, as the relatedness dimension, had a significant effect on motivation to do the activity (curiosity and enjoyment), while autonomy (support from teacher) only affected curiosity (Coterón et al. 2013; Zhao et al. 2011). Task and ego orientations and self-determined motivation were also found to predict dispositional flow, although task dimensions showed more prediction power than the ego dimensions (Moreno et al. 2010).

Fewer studies in flow and leisure research directly investigated the relationship between flow and any dimension of leisure. In this domain, Lee et al. (2011) found that flow experience had a significant effect on the establishment of sport values and positive leisure attitude among adolescents who participated in marine-leisure sport (windsurfing, water-skiing, and wakeboarding).

The above-mentioned empirical studies represent the actual state-of-the-art in the field of flow and leisure in adolescence. In sum, serious or structured leisure activities seem to be the ideal context for the occurrence of flow experience in adolescents, being associated with a high and positive quality of subjective experience. Nevertheless, individual (e.g., motivational aspects) and familiar factors seem to predict more or less the occurrence of flow in this type of activities. Despite these important findings, research in this area should be extended, including other individual and contextual variables and by using a diverse range of adolescent samples. In the last years, our Portuguese research team has developed some studies that address these concerns, using both retrospective and real-time measures. The Portuguese results on flow and leisure constructs are presented in the next sections.

11.2 Studies on the Quality of Subjective Experience in the Daily Life of Portuguese Adolescents: What About Flow and Leisure?

In this section, we will illustrate some of the Portuguese studies that contribute to understanding flow and leisure in adolescents' lives. Our purpose is to show the main research features of these studies, in terms of their main conceptual aims and addressed issues, design and methodologies, and finally results and discussions. These Portuguese studies will be organized in two main sections, according to the study design and methodologies: a section comprising studies that used self-report questionnaires for assessing information on the quality of subjective experience in daily life of adolescents on a retrospective basis, titled "Daily Life Perceptions on Activities and Quality of Experience, and Future Life Goals"; and another section devoted to studies using real-time measures, concretely the Experience Sampling Method (ESM), titled "Optimal Experience and the Motivational Dimension of the Subjective Experience: from Individual Characteristics to Social Contexts".

Participants in all these studies were adolescents, including boys and girls aged from 14 to 19 years old, and they were all students in high schools in 10th, 11th and 12th grades.

11.2.1 Daily Life Perceptions on Activities and Quality of Experiences, and Future Life Goals

For the purpose of this section, we analyzed the quality of subjective experience in daily life of Portuguese adolescents, in order to know if they could find flow in their daily activities and in which kind of activities; what their main challenging activities were in the present moment and what their future goals were. Data presented in this section integrate a total of 138 adolescents (61 % girls) and were collected by means of the *Flow Questionnaire* (FQ, Csikszentmihalyi 1975; Csikszentmihalyi and Csikszentmihalyi 1988; Delle Fave and Massimini 1988, Portuguese version) to assess the optimal experience or flow, and the *Life Theme Questionnaire* (LT, Delle Fave 2004, Portuguese version) for the assessment of individuals' life themes. We used the Flow Questionnaire (FQ) to assess flow activities, wished activities and related constraints; and the Life Theme Questionnaire (LT) to assess the present challenges and future life goals of adolescents. For both, data were collected through open answers that were then coded using a coding system defined in previous studies (international and national), with high results in inter-rater reliability measures (e.g., Cohen's kappa).

Overall, results on general daily life showed that among all activities associated with optimal experience about 55 % were related to leisure, contrasting with the second most reported category of activities, studying (about 15 %). This means that when adolescents were remembering in what kind of activities a flow experience occurred (as described in FQ), they reported leisure activities as a main source of flow experience. The quality of experience reported from activities associated with flow experience was evaluated significantly higher than those associated with studying experience, showing high values of involvement, intrinsic motivation, no boredom, no attention effort, and enjoyment. Studying experience was associated with lower levels of intrinsic motivation and with higher levels of boredom and attention effort. Perception of skills was mainly reported in the activities associated with studying. To be with family was associated with average quality of experience' values when comparing to studying or flow/leisure experiences, and thereby highlighting the importance of the school and leisure contexts in adolescents' lifetime.

Nevertheless, a deeper focus on adolescents' perceptions of wished or preferred activities, highlights new insights about the way they think about their present and future lives. These adolescents reported different perceptions about activities if they were considering the present moment of their lives or something about future life goals. When considering the present moment, leisure activities were the most frequent reported category in terms of wished activities (35 % of the total of reported activities). However, when considering future goals, the frequency of the category associated with the activity of study led the reported categories. It seems that despite leisure being considered the preferred activity in the present moment of their lives, it does not have the same importance when adolescents are considering their future life goals. In the same way, when considering the most challenging activities in the present moment, it is "study" again that has the higher frequency, with the leisure category having the lower frequency. As for constraints associated with wished activities, leisure was never considered a constraint or obstacle to the achievement of wished activities, contrary to other types of activities that can be simultaneously considered as wished activities, but also as constraints to the achievement of other activities. For example, the family category integrates several wished activities (e.g., "to travel with my parents"), but at the same time it appears as constraints (e.g., "not to have the permission from my parents to go to a party").

These results make the type of leisure activities adolescents are involved in relevant. It seems that Portuguese adolescents are mainly involved in passive and non-structured leisure, which contrasts with the formal school structure that they perceived as less pleasurable. To complement these results, the next section focuses on experiences captured in real-time that highlight momentary processes that regulate flow and leisure during the day.

11.2.2 Flow, Optimal Experience and Motivational Aspects of Subjective Experience: From Individual Characteristics to Social Contexts

Motivational aspects have emerged as one of the main ingredients of flow and optimal experience and also of leisure experience, mainly if distinguishing between short-term desirability and long-term meaning. Following this, we were interested to know how motivation is influenced by both individual characteristics and life contexts, analyzing these variables according to momentary information on daily experience.

For this we studied a total of 158 adolescents (39 % boys and 61 % girls), using the Experience Sampling Method (ESM – Csikszentmihalyi et al. 1977) to assess daily contexts and associated momentary subjective experiences in real life. ESM provides repeated real-time information based on the daily life of participants, considering internal (quality of subjective experience) and external (activities, social context and location) variables of the daily life of participants (see Chap. 9 by Heutte et al. in this volume). Following general procedures defined for this methodology (cf. Hektner et al. 2007) and according to previous Portuguese studies (Freire et al. 2007), our participants received a booklet of ESM reports and an electronic device programmed to emit 8 beeps at random moments each day, between 8 a.m. and 10 p.m., completing ESM questionnaires for seven consecutive days (1 week).

After each beep, participants completed open questions and Likert scales ranging from 0 "not at all" to 12 "extremely", concerning current contexts (activity, company, location) and affective, cognitive, and motivational components of momentary subjective experience. At the present, we use electronic devices specifically built for the purposes of ESM in Portuguese studies, within a multidisciplinary team integrating engineers and our own team's expertise on ESM procedures (Psychobeeper, Machado et al. 2009).

According to the aims of this study, we focused on some of the questions of the ESM, using both subject level and beep level for analysis. For individual characteristics, we defined autotelic and non-autotelic participants; and for life contexts, we distinguished between school and leisure. Motivation related to daily activities was analyzed, as short-term desirability (e.g., wanting to do the activity at the moment) and long-term meaning (e.g., importance of the activity to future goals). According to the literature, autotelic subjects tend to have high frequency of optimal experiences during a week (cf. Asakawa 2010). Therefore, we calculated the percentage of optimal experiences, identifying autotelic and non-autotelic adolescents (respectively above cut point group mean and follow P75; and below cut point and follow P25). The final number of participants (total of 78 adolescents) corresponded to a balanced distribution in terms of autotelic personality (39 autotelic adolescents and 39 non-autotelic, both with a majority of girls: 59.7 % autotelic and 61.8 % non-autotelic). This experimental design showed that short-term motivation was more associated with the context than to the personality. There were no differences between autotelic and non-autotelic groups, but a statistically significant difference existed in terms of short-term motivation by context (school vs. leisure): when in school both groups wished to be doing something else showing lower short-term desirability in school than in leisure; and while in leisure, they wished to be doing the present activity, showing higher short-term desirability in leisure than in school (F (1,76) = 77.69, $p < .001$). The same pattern of results was obtained in terms of the importance of the activity to future life goals. Long-term motivation appeared to be different by context (school vs. leisure) for both groups of adolescents: when in school they reported the activity as being important to future goals (more than in leisure); and when in leisure they reported the activity as less important to future goals (F (1,76) = 59.14, $p < .001$). Nevertheless, in both contexts the autotelic adolescents reported higher values of importance to future goals.

These results highlight the role of life contexts and the impact that activities have in experiential dimensions such as motivation. The different patterns obtained on short-term desirability and long-term meaning across the two contexts make some questions relevant in the role of the socialization process and associated meanings. Looking in terms of contexts, it seems school has a negative side for adolescents: it is synonymous of obligation, and it is associated with positive experience deprivation. It seems that the consciousness of its importance for future goals does not influence their present motivation for engagement in this kind of activity. On the contrary, leisure seems to be more positively evaluated: it is about non-obligation and thus about pleasure; but the consciousness of a higher short-term desirability does not influence future motivation in terms of its role in future goals. Finally, results also showed that having frequent optimal experiences during the course of daily life (autotelic adolescents) does not change this motivational pattern associated with contexts, yet, those who had frequent optimal experiences (autotelic) achieved higher levels of short and long-term motivation.

11.3 Conclusions and Future Research Directions

Leisure became a major concept when considering adolescents' development along their life trajectories. By considering leisure as an activity, an experience or a life context, leisure serves several developmental functions and facilitates positive personal and social achievements highlighting the concept of *optimal leisure* (Freire 2013). Therefore, leisure is also about developmental assets, which are intrinsically associated with adolescence.

Our concept of leisure experience based on a psycho-social-ecological perspective matches the concept of flow experience and emphasizes the importance of subjective experiences across daily life. This match is important when considering positive development and the enhancement of personal skills and resources that make possible to overcome with success developmental tasks.

As illustrated in this chapter, the study of leisure and flow experiences illustrates how socio-cognitive processes and behaviors of adolescents are associated with the type of activity involvement. According to Portuguese results, a mix of social and individual meanings tends to emerge from these involvements building a constellation of motives and goals that shape individual experiences in the present moment and the way they will be integrated in their future life. Concretely, Portuguese adolescents seem to appreciate leisure in their present lives, enjoy it and understand it as a positive and grateful experience, but at the same time they do not consider it an important and relevant issue in terms of their future projects. This has been a frequent result in our studies that deserves particular attention in terms of leisure education that aims to promote individuals' consciousness about the benefits of leisure and its contribution to the enhancement of the quality of life (Freire 2006).

These individual and social processes impact individuals' choices about what to do, how to do it and for what reason. The gap between the way adolescents think about the present moment and about future life needs to be explored in order to know if this is just a question of age or a developmental stage, or a regular pattern associated with a specific person-contextual interaction. Intervention aimed at promoting adolescents' positive development needs to analyze individual characteristics as well as contextual opportunities and related facilities for involvement and engagement that promote their self-complexity.

Following our previous studies and empirical literature highlighted in this chapter, several main issues can be addressed in future research and empirical studies. From a contextual perspective, to merge leisure and school contexts and related experiences can benefit the development of adolescents, with parents or other significant adults/educators intentionally mediating and supervising this process. Each context demands for different skills, social interactions, and specific environmental involvements. These two specific contexts are, not only, the contexts where adolescents spend most of their time, but also the contexts where demanding skills can be developed and transferred from one to the other through the involvement in activities.

This is especially relevant for leisure activities that are structured and supervised, include social interactions, and provide opportunities for the development of skills, competences, and initiative. Engagement in these kinds of leisure activities can be an adaptive alternative to the engagement in risky behaviors and delinquency or to avoid boredom and apathy. Flow activities have been reported as relevant for inducing a positive mood and positive affect that, in turn, will motivate adolescents for action and proactivity. Flow experience can be induced and promoted by leisure experience generating a *continuum* of growth, self-awareness, and self-complexity, crossing internal and external dimensions. In line of the search for the differences between flow and optimal experience (as previously considered by Freire 2011), this chapter contributes to the discussion on this topic, reinforcing a possible conceptual difference between flow and optimal experience, when considering proximal/future conceptualizations of adolescents and retrospective/real-time measures of their subjective leisure experience.

Our research group envisages the relationship between flow and leisure as one of the most relevant future research areas in the study of adolescence. Leisure constitutes a major opportunity for the study of flow experience and the main conditions for its emergence, maintenance, and incorporation in the self. For this, methodological tools need to integrate both retrospective and real-time measures following an intra-individual and longitudinal level of analysis in order to overcome stated limitations associated with a unique form of methodology. Integration of different data offers unique lenses for understanding adolescence and associated psycho-social-ecological issues. From this perspective, understanding adolescents' quality of leisure experience can bring new insights to normative developmental processes and to the onset of psychopathology or disorders, shedding light on new clues to appropriate interventions across different life contexts.

Acknowledgements and Funding This study was conducted at Psychology Research Centre, University of Minho, and supported by the Portuguese Foundation for Science and Technology and the Portuguese Ministery of Education and Science through national funds and when applicable co-financed by FEDER under the PT2020 Partnership Agreement (UID/PSI/01662/2013).

References

Asakawa, K. (2010). Flow experience, culture, and well-being: How do autotelic Japanese college students feel, behave, and think in their daily lives? *Journal of Happiness Studies, 11*(2), 205–223. doi:10.1007/s10902-008-9132-3.

Bassi, M., & Delle Fave, A. (2004). Adolescence and the changing context of optimal experience in Time: Italy 1986–2000. *Journal of Happiness Studies, 5*(2), 155–179. doi:10.1023/B:JOHS.0000035914.66037.b5.

Blomfield, C. J., & Barber, B. L. (2011). Developmental experiences during extracurricular activities and Australian adolescents' self-concept: Particularly important for youth from disadvantaged schools. *Journal of Youth and Adolescence, 40*(5), 582–594. doi:10.1007/s10964-010-9563-0.

Bowers, E. P., Li, Y., Kiely, M. K., Brittian, A., Lerner, J. V., & Lerner, R. M. (2010). The five Cs model of positive youth development: A longitudinal analysis of confirmatory factor structure and measurement invariance. *Journal of Youth and Adolescence, 39*(7), 720–735. doi:10.1007/s10964-010-9530-9.

Bowers, E. P., Johnson, S. K., Buckingham, M. H., Gasca, S., Warren, D. J. A., Lerner, J. V., et al. (2014). Important non-parental adults and positive youth development across mid- to late-adolescence: The moderating effect of parenting profiles. *Journal of Youth and Adolescence, 43*(6), 897–918. doi:10.1007/s10964-014-0095-x.

Bradley, G. L., & Inglis, B. C. (2012). Adolescent leisure dimensions, psychosocial adjustment, and gender effects. *Journal of Adolescence, 35*(5), 1167–1176. doi:10.1016/j.adolescence.2012.03.006.

Caldwell, L. L. (2005). Recreation and youth development. In P. A. Witt & L. L. Caldwell (Eds.), *Recreation and youth development* (pp. 169–189). State College: Venture Publishing.

Caldwell, L. L., & Faulk, M. (2013). Adolescent leisure from a developmental and prevention perspective. In T. Freire (Ed.), *Positive leisure science* (pp. 41–60). Dordrecht: Springer Netherlands.

Caldwell, L. L., & Smith, E. A. (2006). Leisure as a context for youth development and delinquency prevention. *Australian & New Zealand Journal of Criminology, 39*(3), 398–418. doi:10.1375/acri.39.3.398.

Cassidy, G. G., & Paisley, A. M. J. M. (2013). Music-games: A case study of their impact. *Research Studies in Music Education, 35*(1), 119–138. doi:10.1177/1321103x13488032.

Coterón, J., Sampedro, J., Franco, E., Pérez-Tejero, J., & Refoyo, I. (2013). The role of basic psychological needs in predicting dispositional flow of basketball players in training. Differences by sex. *Revista de Psicología del Deporte, 22*(1), 187–190.

Csikszentmihalyi, M. (1975). *Beyond boredom and anxiety: Experiencing flow in work and play*. San Francisco: Jossey-Bass Publishers.

Csikszentmihalyi, M. (1990). *Flow: The psychology of optimal experience*. New York: Harper & Row.

Csikszentmihalyi, M. (1997). *Finding flow: The psychology of engagement with everyday life*. New York: Basic Books.

Csikszentmihalyi, M., & Csikszentmihalyi, I. S. (1988). *Optimal experience: Psychological studies of flow in consciousness*. Cambridge: Cambridge University Press.

Csikszentmihalyi, M., & Larson, R. (1986). *Being adolescent: Conflict and growth in the teenage years*. New York: Basic Books.

Csikszentmihalyi, M., Larson, R., & Prescott, S. (1977). The ecology of adolescent activity and experience. *Journal of Youth and Adolescence, 6*(3), 281–294. doi:10.1007/bf02138940.

Damon, W. (2004). What is positive youth development? *The Annals of the American Academy of Political and Social Science, 591*(1), 13–24. doi:10.1177/0002716203260092.

Delle Fave, A. (2004). Editorial: Positive psychology and the pursuit of complexity. *Ricerche di Psicologia, 27*(1), 7–12.

Delle Fave, A., & Bassi, M. (2000). The quality of experience in adolescents' daily lives: Developmental perspectives. *Genetic, Social, and General Psychology Monographs, 126*(3), 347–367.

Delle Fave, A., & Bassi, M. (2003). Italian adolescents and leisure: The role of engagement and optimal experience. *New Directions for Child and Adolescent Development, 2003*(99), 79–94. doi:10.1002/cd.68.

Delle Fave, A., & Massimini, F. (1988). Modernization and the changing contexts of flow in work and leisure. In M. Csikszentmihalyi & I. S. Csikszentmihalyi (Eds.), *Optimal experience: Psychological studies of flow in consciousness*. Cambridge: Cambridge University Press.
Elkington, S. (2011). What it is to take the flow of leisure seriously. *Leisure/Loisir, 35*(3), 253–282. doi:10.1080/14927713.2011.614838.
Freire, T. (2006). Experiências óptimas e lazer: sobre a qualidade da experiência subjectiva na vida diária. *Psicologia: Teoria, Investigação e Prática, 11*(2), 243–258.
Freire, T. (2011). From flow to optimal experience: (Re)searching the quality of subjective experience throughout daily life. In I. Brdar (Ed.), *The human pursuit of well-being* (pp. 55–63). Dordrecht: Springer Netherlands.
Freire, T. (2013). Leisure experience and positive identity development in adolescents. In T. Freire (Ed.), *Positive leisure science* (pp. 61–79). Dordrecht: Springer Netherlands.
Freire, T., & Silva, E. (2013). Adolescentes e desenvolvimento positivo: para uma abordagem inovadora da adolescência. In T. Medeiros (Ed.), *Adolescência: desafios e riscos* (pp. 47–70). Ponta Delgada: Letras Lavadas Edições.
Freire, T., & Soares, I. (2000). A intervenção na adolescência através do lazer e a promoção do desenvolvimento positivo. *Psicologia, Educação e Cultura, IV*(2), 329–343.
Freire, T., & Stebbins, R. A. (2011). Activités de loisir optimales et développement positif des adolescents: un rapprochement entre les perspectives psychologiques et sociologiques. In C. Martin-Krumm & C. Tarquinio (Eds.), *Traité de psychologie positive: fondements théoriques et implications pratiques* (pp. 557–576). Brussels: De Boeck.
Freire, T., Fonte, C., & Lima, I. (2007). As experiências óptimas na vida diária de adolescentes: Implicações para um desenvolvimento positivo. *Revista de Psicologia, Educação e Cultura, XI*(2), 223–242.
Hall, G. S. (1904). *Adolescence: Its psychology and its relations to physiology, anthropology, sociology, sex, crime, religion and education*. New York: Appleton.
Hektner, J. M., Schmidt, J. A., & Csikszentmihalyi, M. (2007). *Experience sampling method: Measuring the quality of everyday life*. Thousand Oaks: SAGE Publications.
Hunter, J. P., & Csikszentmihalyi, M. (2003). The positive psychology of interested adolescents. *Journal of Youth and Adolescence, 32*(1), 27–35. doi:10.1023/A:1021028306392.
Larson, R. W. (2000). Toward a psychology of positive youth development. *American Psychologist, 55*(1), 170–183. doi:10.1037/0003-066X.55.1.170.
Lee, H.-J., & Choe, I.-S. (2011). A study for quality of life in musically talented students using experience sampling method. *Journal of Gifted/Talented Education, 21*(1), 57–81. doi:10.9722/JGTE.2011.21.1.057.
Lee, K. Y., Yoon, Y. S., & Kim, H. T. (2011). The effects of flow experience of marine-leisure sport on sport values and leisure attitude among middle school students. *Journal of Leisure & Recreation Studies, 35*(4), 99–111.
Lerner, R. M. (2005). *Promoting positive youth development: Theoretical and empirical bases [white paper]*. Washington, DC: National Academies of Science.
Lerner, R. M., & Galambos, N. L. (1998). Adolescent development: Challenges and opportunities for research, programs, and policies. *Annual Review of Psychology, 49*(1), 413–446. doi:10.1146/annurev.psych.49.1.413.
Lerner, R. M., Almerigi, J. B., Theokas, C., & Lerner, J. V. (2005). Positive youth development: A view of the issues. *The Journal of Early Adolescence, 25*(1), 10–16. doi:10.1177/0272431604273211.
Machado, C., Gomes, J., & Freire, T. (2009). *The psycho beeper* [Electronic beeper software]. (0.9 ed.). Braga: University of Minho.
Massimini, F., & Delle Fave, A. (2000). Individual development in a bio-cultural perspective. *American Psychologist, 55*(1), 24–33. doi:10.1037/0003-066X.55.1.24.
Mesurado, B. (2009). Actividad estructurada vs actividad desestructurada, realizadas en solitario vs en compañía de otros y la experiencia óptima. *Anales de Psicología, 25*(2), 308–315.
Moreno, J. A., Gimeno, E. C., & Gonzále-Cutre, D. (2010). The achievement goal and self-determination theories as predictors of dispositional flow in young athletes. *Anales de Psicología, 26*(2), 390–399.

Nakamura, J., & Csikszentmihalyi, M. (2002). The concept of flow. In C. R. Snyder & S. Lopez (Eds.), *Handbook of positive psychology* (pp. 89–105). New York: Oxford University Press.

Overton, W. F. (2013). Relationism and relational developmental systems: A paradigm for developmental science in the post-Cartesian era. In R. M. Lerner, & J. B. Benson (Eds.), *Advances in child development and behavior: Embodiment and epigenesis: Theoretical and methodological issues in understanding the role of biology within the relational developmental system* (2013/07/10 ed., Vol. 44, pp. 21–64). London: Elsevier.

Perkins, K., & Nakamura, J. (2011). Flow and leisure. In T. Freire (Ed.), *Positive leisure science* (pp. 141–157). Dordrecht: Springer Netherlands.

Rich, G. J. (2003). The positive psychology of youth and adolescence. *Journal of Youth and Adolescence, 32*(1), 1–3. doi:10.1023/A:1021017421413.

Roth, J. L., & Brooks-Gunn, J. (2003). What exactly is a youth development program? Answers from research and practice. *Applied Developmental Science, 7*(2), 94–111. doi:10.1207/S1532480XADS0702_6.

Sarriera, J. C., Casas, F., Bedin, L., Paradiso, Â. C., Abs, D., & González, M. (2014). Aspects of leisure on adolescent's well-being in two countries. *Child Indicators Research, 7*(2), 245–265. doi:10.1007/s12187-013-9220-8.

Silva, E., & Freire, T. (2014). Programas de mentoria e promoção do desenvolvimento positivo de adolescentes. *Revista Portuguesa de Educação, 27*(1), 157–176.

Sinnamon, S., Moran, A., & O'Connell, M. (2012). Flow among musicians: Measuring peak experiences of student performers. *Journal of Research in Music Education, 60*(1), 6–25. doi:10.1177/0022429411434931.

Stebbins, R. A. (1997). Casual leisure: A conceptual statement. *Leisure Studies, 16*(1), 17–25. doi:10.1080/026143697375485.

Stebbins, R. A. (2010). Flow in serious leisure: Nature and prevalence. *Leisure Studies Association Newsletter, 87*, 21–23.

Steca, P., Bassi, M., Caprara, G. V., & Fave, A. D. (2011). Parents' self-efficacy beliefs and their children's psychosocial adaptation during adolescence. *Journal of Youth and Adolescence, 40*(3), 320–331. doi:10.1007/s10964-010-9514-9.

Trainor, S., Delfabbro, P., Anderson, S., & Winefield, A. (2010). Leisure activities and adolescent psychological well-being. *Journal of Adolescence, 33*(1), 173–186. doi:10.1016/j.adolescence.2009.03.013.

Trayes, J., Harré, N., & Overall, N. C. (2012). A youth performing arts experience: Psychological experiences, recollection, and the desire to do it again. *Journal of Adolescent Research, 27*(2), 155–182. doi:10.1177/0743558411417867.

Ward, P. J., & Zabriskie, R. B. (2011). Positive youth development within a family leisure context: Youth perspectives of family outcomes. *New Directions for Youth Development, 2011*(130), 29–42. doi:10.1002/yd.395.

Weidman, A. C., Fernandez, K. C., Levinson, C. A., Augustine, A. A., Larsen, R. J., & Rodebaugh, T. L. (2012). Compensatory internet use among individuals higher in social anxiety and its implications for well-being. *Personality and Individual Differences, 53*(3), 191–195. doi:10.1016/j.paid.2012.03.003.

Zhao, L., Lu, Y., Wang, B., & Huang, W. (2011). What makes them happy and curious online? An empirical study on high school students' Internet use from a self-determination theory perspective. *Computers & Education, 56*(2), 346–356. doi:10.1016/j.compedu.2010.08.006.

Part V
Flow in Every Day Experiences

Chapter 12
Flow in the Context of Daily Experience Fluctuation

Marta Bassi and Antonella Delle Fave

Abstract Flow is just one of the various experiences that occur in daily life. Research has shown that different experiential profiles can be identified based on the subjective perception of environmental opportunities for action (challenges) and of the personal capabilities possessed to cope with them (skills). The different patterns of relationship between these two variables were operationalized through the Experience Fluctuation Model, leading to the identification of eight different experiences: arousal, flow, control, relaxation, boredom, apathy, worry, and anxiety. Besides allowing researchers to identify qualitative fluctuations of daily experience, the model provides information on how each specific experience can change quantitatively, as levels of challenges and skills increase or decrease. In this chapter, we will first present the Experience Sampling Method (ESM), a procedure that allows the gathering of real-time repeated samplings of individuals' experience as daily situations and events unfold. Starting from ESM assessments, we will then illustrate the Experience Fluctuation Model, and we will provide empirical support to the eight experiential profiles identified by the model. We will finally present findings from groups of participants differing in age and culture, highlighting the potential of flow to promote growth in complexity and well-being.

12.1 Introduction

From a common-sense perspective, conscious experience is defined as those states of sentience or awareness that typically begin when we wake from a dreamless sleep and continue through the day until we fall asleep again (Searle 1998; Tononi and Edelman 1998). At the phenomenical level, it consists of a continuous stream

M. Bassi (✉)
Department of Biomedical and Clinical Sciences "Luigi Sacco", University of Milan, Milan, Italy
e-mail: marta.bassi@unimi.it

A. Delle Fave
Department of Pathophysiology and Transplantation, University of Milano, Milano, Italy
e-mail: antonella.dellefave@unimi.it

L. Harmat et al. (eds.), *Flow Experience*, DOI 10.1007/978-3-319-28634-1_12

of thoughts, images, sensations, memories, emotions, motivations, goals, that is cognitive, affective, motivational and volitional components which uniquely combine to make up the complex experiential configurations all individuals report in their daily life (Hilgard 1980). The essential characteristic of consciousness is unified qualitative subjectivity (Searle 1998). Conscious states are subjective by definition, as they imply a subject who experiences a certain condition in a given moment. The content of consciousness is thus original and primarily accessible only to the person who experiences it. Each conscious experience also has a specific qualitative feel to it; tasting wine is very different from hearing a sonata, and both are yet qualitatively different from smelling a flower or seeing a sunset (Searle 1998). Finally, consciousness represents a unified field in which single components are not perceived in isolation but as global configurations. As such, conscious experience represents one of the most intriguing characteristics of human beings, having far-reaching implications in shaping individuals' life trajectories and in influencing the long-term development of the human species (Delle Fave et al. 2011; see Chap. 1 in this volume). An increasing number of studies have stressed its role in directing human behavior, giving individuals the ability to self-regulate and monitor current actions, plan long-term objectives, and anticipate future outcomes and emotional reactions (for a review see Baumeister et al. 2011). In this chapter, we will delve deep into individuals' quality of subjective experience and, in particular, into the potentials of flow in promoting growth in complexity and well-being. In the first part, we will introduce the role of perceived opportunities for action (challenges) and personal capabilities (skills) in shaping individuals' quality of experience. We will then present the Experience Sampling Method (Hektner et al. 2007) a procedure developed to collect real-time repeated samplings of everyday situations and associated experience. Consequently, we will describe the Experience Fluctuation Model, allowing researchers to represent real-time data based on the subjective perception of challenges and skills (Massimini and Carli 1988; Massimini et al. 1987). Drawing from our research work, the second part of this chapter will be devoted to presenting empirical findings supporting the model, and providing insight into individuals' experience fluctuation in various contexts and life situations, including pregnancy and family building, risky sports, and learning activities. The chapter will conclude with future research suggestions, which could advance our knowledge on the phenomenology of conscious experience.

12.2 Challenges, Skills and the Quality of Experience

Subjective experience ultimately represents the moment-by-moment conscious processing of information coming from the external environment and the inner world of a person (Csikszentmihalyi 1982). The content of consciousness is thus perennially changing, giving rise to a stream of unique unrepeatable experiences (James 1890).

In the history of psychology, a large number of scholars have stressed that the quality of experience changes based on individuals' perception of the opportunities for action retrieved in the environment (challenges) and of the personal capabilities possessed to face them (skills; for a review, Delle Fave 2013). Among them, Lazarus (1966) formulated the well-known cognitive transactional theory of stress, according to which individuals judge a current situation based on the demands it entails (primary appraisal) and on the resources and options available to cope with the demands (secondary appraisal). When demands are perceived as threatening vis-à-vis low available resources, the situation is evaluated as stressful. Similarly, Bandura (1997) focused on self-efficacy beliefs as individuals' perceived capabilities to exercise control over environmental demands. Such beliefs influence the ongoing subjective experience, aspirations and goal pursuit, level of motivation and perseverance in the face of difficulties, as well as causal attribution for success and failure.

The relationship between perceived challenges and skills is also central to the concept of flow (Csikszentmihalyi; 1990; Csikszentmihalyi and Csikszentmihalyi 1988). In Csikszentmihalyi's book *Beyond Boredom and Anxiety* (1975/2000), different combinations of perceived challenges and skills are described, giving rise to at least three qualitatively different experiential states. When individuals perceive low challenges in the face of high skills in a given situation, the experience of boredom is reported. Conversely, when challenges are perceived as exceeding personal skills, anxiety ensues. Flow is conceptualized as a positive and complex experience stemming from the balance between high environmental challenges and high personal skills. In more recent theoretical formulations, a fourth experiential profile was identified as being the opposite of flow. This condition, characterized by a balance between low challenges and low skills, was labelled as apathy (Massimini and Carli 1988). A large number of subsequent studies substantially confirmed the challenge-skill match as an important antecedent of optimal experience, using both correlational research (Delle Fave and Massimini 2005; Delle Fave et al. 2011; Inkinen et al. 2014; Moneta and Csikszentmihalyi 1996; Schiefele 2013) and experimental designs (Keller and Bless 2008; Keller and Blomann 2008). In addition, it is to the perceived match between high challenges and skills that flow owes its dynamic characteristic (Csikszentmihalyi 1975/2000; Delle Fave and Bassi 2000). As flow is a highly positive and rewarding experience associated with stimulating activities and situations in which individuals can mobilize their personal resources, such activities are likely to be replicated and cultivated over time. This leads to a progressive increase in personal competence and to the consequent search for higher challenges in order to match augmented skill levels, to avoid a state of boredom, and to continue experiencing the deep engagement, concentration and involvement which characterize flow. This dynamic process gives rise to a virtuous circle fostering individual development, through both the acquisition of increasingly complex information and competence enhancement (Massimini and Delle Fave 2000; see Chap. 1 in this volume).

12.3 Experience Sampling Method

The best way to investigate individuals' content of consciousness and its daily fluctuations is to adopt ecological momentary assessment tools (EMA; Trull and Ebner-Priemer 2009). These tools allow researchers to gather ecologically valid real-time data on the stream of experience as daily events and situations unfold. Compared to single-administration questionnaires, the immediacy and contingency of individuals' response reduce distortions due to retrospective memory biases, according to which individuals are more likely to recall experiences and events that stand out as significant or unusual (salience effect), that occurred more recently (recency effect), or that are congruent with their present mood (mood-congruent memory effect).

Among EMA tools, Experience Sampling Method (ESM) is a widely used procedure developed by Csikszentmihalyi et al. (1977) to collect repeated samples of individuals' daily time-budget and experience fluctuation over time. Its psychometric properties, reliability, validity, as well as participants' compliance and technical characteristics are thoroughly described in the literature (Hektner et al. 2007). Individuals are usually provided with an electronic device (be it an electronic agenda, a palmtop computer or a mobile phone), which sends random acoustic signals (beeps) during waking hours. While length of study, number and time distribution of beeps depend on the investigator's research aims, studies have generally shown that sending six to eight random signals a day (usually from 8.00 am to 10.00 pm) for 1 week can provide a representative sample of individuals' daily experiences and activities (Hektner et al. 2007). When participants are beeped, they are asked to fill in one questionnaire sheet (Experience Sampling Form; ESF), comprising a series of open-ended questions, which investigate the participant's ongoing activity ("what was the main activity you were doing?"), social context ("who were you with?"), and location ("where were you?"). In ESF, participants are also asked to rate how they felt when they were beeped on a list of 20 adjectives (e.g., happy, strong, sociable, active, involved, free), and with queries measuring concentration ("How well were you concentrating?"), ease of concentration ("Was it hard to concentrate?", reverse scored), control ("Were you in control of the situation?"), unselfconsciousness ("How self-conscious were you?", reverse scored), satisfaction ("Did you feel satisfied with yourself?"), wish to perform the activity ("Did you wish you had been doing something else?" reverse scored), stakes ("Was there anything at stake for you in the activity?") and goals ("Was the activity you were doing important for some overall life goal?"). In addition, participants are asked about their time perception (from slowly to fast) in the ongoing situation, as well as their levels of challenges and skills (A sample ESF is reported in Delle Fave et al. 2011).

Once information is gathered, answers to open-ended questions are coded by researchers using extant manuals, and then grouped into content categories according to functional criteria based on the aims of the study (Csikszentmihalyi 1997a; Delle Fave and Bassi 2000; Delle Fave et al. 2011; Hektner et al. 2007). For example, activities can be grouped into broad domains – like productive tasks, maintenance and free time – or into more specific categories, e.g. free time can be broken down into hobbies, sports, media use, and so forth. Concerning scaled items, data are usually standardized for each individual based on their global weekly mean for each item (*z*-scores; Hekner et al. 2007; Larson and Delespaul 1992). Standardization presents two advantages. On the one hand, the individual's weekly average score of an item provides a within-person cut-off point representing the reference to which to compare daily moment-by-moment scores for that item. On the other hand, at the inter-individual level, standardization of individuals' experience ratings provides a common metric to compare experience across participants.

12.4 The Experience Fluctuation Model

Starting from ESM repeated on-line assessments of individuals' daily experience, an original Quadrant Model was built based on the subjective perception of challenges and skills (Csikszentmihalyi and LeFevre 1989). Values of these variables are standardized for each individual over the mean of the sampling period (usually a week). The Cartesian plane is divided into four quadrants, each representing a specific ratio interval of skills on the x-axis and challenges on the y-axis: high challenges and high skills, low challenges and high skills, low challenges and low skills, and high challenges and low skills. This original broad division of the challenge-skill space proved to offer a rather rough picture of the world of experience (Moneta 2012; Inkinen et al. 2014; Lambert et al. 2013).

Consequently, the Experience Fluctuation Model (EFM) was built providing a more fine-grained partition of the Cartesian plane into eight channels – that is arc sectors of 45° – and of the associated experience (Delle Fave and Bassi 2000; Delle Fave et al. 2011; Massimini and Carli 1988; Massimini et al. 1987). Because values of challenges and skills are standardized for each individual, the center of the model corresponds to zero (subjective mean; SM). As shown in Fig. 12.1, channels 1, 3, 5 and 7 are centered upon the two main axes, starting from 90° and proceeding clockwise; the others are positioned on the bisectors of the four right angles.

According to theoretical expectations, when both challenges and skills are above subjective mean (channel 2), optimal experience is likely to be reported, whereas apathy is associated with below-average challenges and skills (channel 6). When challenges are below and skills are above subjective mean (channel 4), an experience of relaxation arises; and when challenges are higher and skills lower than subjective mean (channel 8), an individual is more likely to report a state of anxiety. The remaining challenges/skills ratios are defined transition channels as they are expected to be associated with experiential profiles presenting hybrid features from their neighboring channels: arousal (channel 1), control (channel 3), boredom (channel 5), and worry (channel 7; Csikszentmihalyi 1997b; Delle Fave et al. 2011).

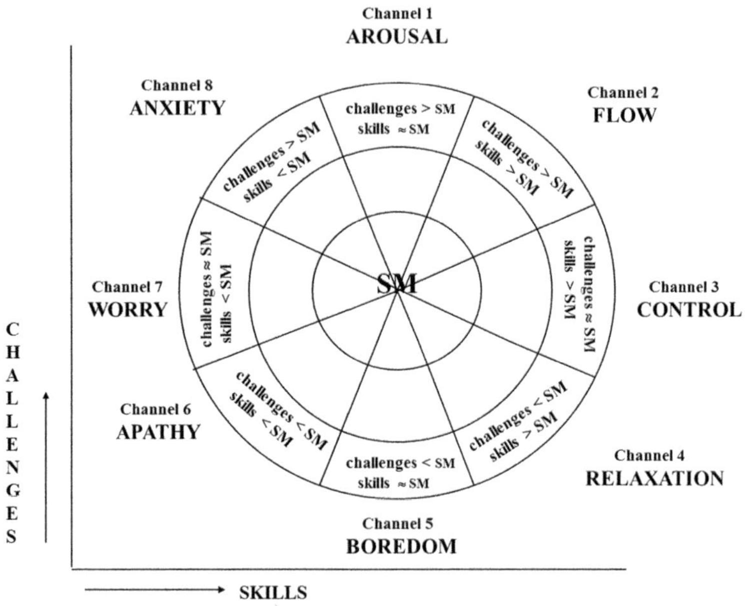

Fig. 12.1 The Experience Fluctuation Model (*SM* subjective mean; from Delle Fave et al. 2011, p. 73)

Across samples (Csikszentmihalyi 1990; Delle Fave and Massimini 2005; Delle Fave et al. 2011), theoretical expectations were met, and a recurrent association emerged between channels and specific experiential profiles. To illustrate this association, in Fig. 12.2 we report the quality of experience of a sample of Italian adolescents across channels (Delle Fave et al. 2011). Analysis focused on the variables concentration, ease of concentration, control, involvement, wish to do the activity, happiness, time perception and goals.

Findings highlighted that channel 2 is associated with high and effortless concentration, involvement, control of the situation, clear goals, wish to do the activity, positive affect, and perception of time passing faster than usual. All these characteristics are central features of optimal experience (Csikszentmihalyi 1975/2000; Csikszentmihalyi and Csikszentmihalyi 1988). As for channel 6, apathy was characterized by a globally negative profile with low values of all the cognitive, emotional, motivational and volitional components of experience. In channel 4, relaxation was not only characterized by positive affect and a wish to do the activity, but also by low cognitive investment and below-average importance in relation to life goals. In channel 8, individuals in the condition of anxiety did not feel in control of the situation: They reported high involvement and cognitive investment, but also negative affect and low intrinsic motivation.

Like the four major channels, the transition ones – though less extensively studied – show recurrent experiential profiles across samples. Arousal in channel 1

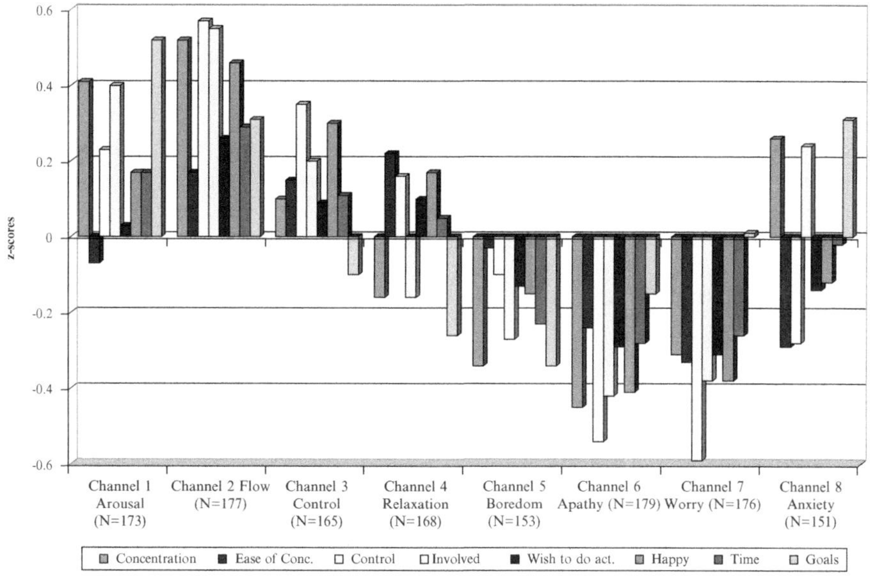

Fig. 12.2 Quality of experience in the EFM channels (*N* number of participants; *N* self-reports = 7,616; from Delle Fave et al. 2011, p. 74)

is primarily characterized by above-average concentration, involvement and goals; on the contrary, control in channel 3 is described as a substantially passive experience in which the person perceives below-average goals, does not need to invest her/his cognitive resources, but exerts control over the situation and is happy about it. Compared to relaxation, boredom associated to channel 5 presents substantially negative features in terms of below-average cognitive investment, involvement, affect and goals. Finally, also the experience of worry in channel 7 is mostly negative in all its dimensions, with prevailing low levels of control of the situation.

Besides allowing researchers to identify how experience fluctuates qualitatively across the channels based on challenges/skills combinations, the EFM provides information on how experience can change quantitatively as levels of challenges and skills decrease or increase within a given channel. As shown in Fig. 12.1, in each channel three concentric areas or rings are depicted. They represent the ranges of standardized values of challenges and skills, increasingly differing from average (zero, the center of the model; Delle Fave and Bassi 2000). Ring 1 ranges between 0 and 0.90 standard deviations from the center, ring 2 from 0.90 to 1.8, and ring 3 from 1.8 to 2.7. Research has shown that as the values of challenges and skills increase – either below or above the subjective mean – moving from ring 1 to ring 3, the experiential profile associated with each channel undergoes quantitative changes, becoming more intense and clear cut (Delle Fave and Bassi 2000; Delle Fave et al. 2011). In channel 2, the positive and complex features of flow become intensified, as individuals perceive increasing opportunities for action matched by increasing abilities in facing them. This may also be related to the distinction between "deep-flow" and "micro-flow" originally proposed by Csikszentmihalyi (1975/2000). In channel 6, apathy becomes more pronounced as challenges and skills plummet below the center of the model. In channel 4, higher positive affect and lower cognitive investment become distinguishing marks of relaxation, and in channel 8 higher cognitive investment and lower positive affect are enhanced in anxiety.

12.5 Capturing Flow with the Experience Fluctuation Model

The main assumptions on which the EFM was based are: (1) the quality of subjective experience is related to perceived challenges and perceived skills in a given situation; (2) different experiential profiles can be identified based on the relationship between perceived challenges and skills. While the available studies concerning experience fluctuations empirically supported these assumptions (Delle Fave et al. 2011; Inkinen et al. 2014), criticism has primarily focused on the ability of the model to capture flow. Particularly, researchers focusing solely on optimal experience have questioned the way the EFM operationalizes the high challenges and skills balance (considered as the primary flow antecedent; see Sect. 12.2), and the standardization procedure adopted to identify channels, particularly channel 2.

Concerning the challenges/skills balance, Keller and Landhäußer (2012) have argued that perceived task demands and required skills are not independent constructs, as the evaluation of demands necessarily involves reference to one's skills. Accordingly, they proposed that the perceived fit between these variables be measured with a unidimensional construct rating the degree to which the demands of the task fit with the skills in the task. While this solution can be profitable in measuring flow vs non-flow conditions, it fails to detect the variety of experiential profiles that can fall under the non-flow condition (e.g. anxiety, boredom). In addition, Moneta and Csikszentmihalyi (1996, 1999) showed that challenges and skills could both have independent and interaction effects on different experiential dimensions. Indeed, in our ESM studies, correlations between challenges and skills were quite low, amounting to $r=.18$, $p<.001$ among rock climbers (Bassi and Delle Fave 2010; Delle Fave et al. 2003), $r=.21$, $p<.001$ among adolescents (Bassi et al. 2007), and $r=.32$, $p<.001$ among pregnant women at 22 weeks of gestation (Pozzo 2015). Modelling challenges/skills balance as (a) challenge by skill cross-product, (b) absolute difference between challenges and skills, and (c) quadratic terms of challenges and skills following axis rotation (similarly to EFM), Moneta and Csikszentmihalyi (1999) concluded that both the rotated and the absolute difference models were to be preferred in predicting the experiential component of concentration, a central feature of flow.

Concerning standardization of challenges and skills for the identification of the EFM channels, some flow researchers questioned whether it is meaningful to compute average levels of perceived challenges and skills across the various activities an individual is engaged in. They claim that this would – unlikely – imply that individuals have an absolute standard in mind against which to compare perceived challenges and skills (Keller and Landhäußer 2012; Moneta 2012). Standardization was introduced in the EFM for both conceptual and empirical reasons (Massimini and Carli 1988): While Csikszentmihalyi (1975/2000; Csikszentmihalyi and Csikszentmihalyi 1988) originally maintained that flow is experienced when people perceive a balance between challenges and skills, later empirical studies showed that in such a condition individuals did not necessarily feel better than in other conditions. There were instances in which the balance between challenges and skills was indeed associated with low scores of all the components of experience, which could not be explained by theoretical assumptions. Massimini and his colleagues thus posited that perceived challenges and skills should be evaluated against an individual's cut-off point (Massimini and Carli 1988). Particularly, they proposed that optimal experience would be likely to arise only when challenges and skills were in balance above a certain level. By standardizing challenges and skills ratings, the zero – which corresponds to the individual's mean for challenges and skills over the tested period – becomes the starting point above which optimal experience is likely to be reported. When both challenges and skills are balanced, but their scores are below the person's average (that is, below zero), a person would report a different negative experience, which was labeled apathy in the EFM model. Empirical findings supported this interpretation, as shown in Sect. 12.4.

The methodological issue about standardization essentially revolves around researchers' ability to capture optimal experience indirectly, by assessing the relationship between perceived challenges and skills (Schmidt et al. 2007). This issue substantially concerns all measurement instruments – including ESM – and experimental designs, which rely on challenges/skills balance as primary antecendent of flow. To a certain extent, it also concerns single-administration scales – such as those developed by Jackson and Eklund (2002, 2004) – which measure flow as a continuous construct characterized by various experiential components (concentration, control, merging of action and awareness, autotelic experience, unselfconsciousness, time transformation, goals, clear feedback from the activity and challenge/skill balance) without specific validated criteria for cut-off scores of flow dimensions (Delle Fave et al. 2011; Moneta 2012).

To the best of our knowledge, to date no alternative solution to the standardization procedure has been brought forward in relation to the real-time measurement of flow within the broad spectrum of conscious experiences (i.e. different relationships between challenges and skills), as proposed by EFM. Like any other model in science, EFM represents a schematic description, a simplification of relevant aspects of the real world needed to systematically study and make sense of them. Even though EFM classification of experiences remains probabilistic in nature, it allowed us to gather precious information on (a) flow phenomenology, (b) the pattern of experience fluctuation in various situations and life contexts, and (c) the implications of the experiential profiles in terms of personal growth and well-being. In the following section, we will summarize some relevant findings we have gathered in our research work on the quality of subjective experience using the EFM (for a review, Delle Fave et al. 2011).

12.6 From Theory to Everyday Life

As reported in Sect. 12.4, ESM data analysis through the EFM allowed us to describe in detail the quality of experience associated with channel 2, namely the match between above-average challenges and above-average skills that is likely to be related to optimal experience. In all the studies across samples varying in cultural background, age, profession, and educational level (Delle Fave et al. 2011), channel 2 was associated with a positive and gratifying state of consciousness presenting central characteristics of optimal experience in terms of effortless and focused concentration, deep involvement, sense of control over the situation, positive affect, transformation of time, clear long-term goals, and intrinsic motivation as measured through the item "wish to do the activity" (Fig. 12.2). Contrary to theoretical expectations, participants reported being more self-conscious than usual. Mixed findings about the unselfconscious aspect of optimal experience were also obtained through single-administration questionnaires using multiple items (Hektner et al. 2007; Jackson and Eklund 2002), possibly hinting at participants' difficulty in understanding and answering the related question, or in consciously observing oneself during engagement in a task (Keller and Blomann 2008).

In-depth analyses further showed that the quality of experience in channel 2 presents some stable characteristics as well as variable features depending on the kind of activity performed (Delle Fave and Massimini 2005). Particularly, a stable cognitive core was detected including high concentration and control of the situation, while affective, volitional and motivational variables fluctuated across activities. During productive tasks like work and study, for instance, participants reported below-average values of positive affect and wish to do the activity as well as above-average goals. By contrast, during structured leisure like sports and hobbies, participants reported above-average positive affect and wish to do the activity, along with below-average goals. As shown in Delle Fave (2007), these experiential patterns were replicated in cross-cultural studies through the administration of Flow Questionnaire, a direct self-report measure of optimal experience (Delle Fave and Massimini 1988; Delle Fave et al. 2011; see Chap. 19 by Riva, Freire and Bassi in this volume). In addition, adopting a Self-Determination Theory approach to motivation (Deci and Ryan 2000), further investigation of productive tasks under the high challenges and high skills condition (channel 2) showed that these activities can be associated not only with intrinsic motivation, but also – and actually, more frequently – with extrinsic motivation and internalized extrinsic motivation (Bassi and Delle Fave 2012a, b). As expected, compared to extrinsic motivation, intrinsic motivation had a positive impact on most cognitive, affective and motivational components of experience. At the same time, however, no differences in terms of quality of experience were observed between intrinsic motivation and internalized extrinsic motivation during productive activities in channel 2.

Our findings point to flow as a positive experiential configuration mostly characterized by absorption and concentration, and dynamically changing in its motivational, volitional and affective components according to activity typology.

Flow, however, is just one of the various experiences that occur in everyday life. Based on the EFM, evidence was gathered on a variety of experiential profiles, as shown in Fig. 12.2, and on the pattern of experience fluctuation among the different daily situations and events. First of all, compared to the other experiential profiles, experience in channel 2 can be defined as optimal, not because all its components are most intense or "peaking", but because they are both positive and balanced. In addition, flow is not the only positive experience per se. In arousal, for instance, individuals experience high cognitive investment and involvement, and perceive long-term goals; in control, and to a certain extent relaxation, individuals perceive high levels of positive affect and intrinsic motivation (Inkinen et al. 2014; Lambert et al. 2013). Even anxiety, though associated with below-average control and average positive affect, is characterized by above-average concentration, long-term goals and involvement (Delle Fave et al. 2003; Delle Fave and Massimini 2005). When the discrepancy between perceived high challenges and low skills is not too wide, anxiety can represent a stimulating experience for the individual; on the contrary, when the gap widens (moving from ring 1 to 3; Fig. 12.1), the associated experience becomes extremely negative at the motivational and affective levels.

These experiential configurations are all common ingredients of everyday life: For example, findings showed that relaxation is mostly related to maintenance activities and watching TV, which represent typical opportunities for energy restoration and rest in Western societies (Bassi and Delle Fave 2004; Delle Fave et al. 2011). By contrast, boredom, apathy and worry represent negative experiential profiles, possibily associated with stagnation and psychic disorganization when they become pervasive in one's life. In particular, high frequencies of apathy were detected in a case study with an agoraphobic patient at the beginning of psychotherapy (Delle Fave and Massimini 1992). High frequencies of boredom, apathy and worry were also found in relation to activities such as personal care (including eating and physical exercise) among obese women (Preziosa et al. 2008), and unstructured activities (vs rehabilitation activities) among psychiatric patients attending a Psychiatric Rehabilitation Center (Bassi et al. 2012) and patients undergoing hospital rehabilitation (Sartori et al. 2014).

Overall, findings from different samples showed that individuals' quality of experience fluctuates according to life priorities, areas of investment, and ultimately meaning, as posited by the theory of psychological selection (Massimini and Delle Fave 2000; see Chap. 1 in this volume). To investigate the relationship between quality of experience and parenthood, for example, we carried out a study among five couples expecting their first child (Delle Fave and Massimini 2004). Women and their husbands were monitored longitudinally for four ESM sessions during pregnancy (10th, 20th, 30th and 35th week of gestation), as well as four sessions after child birth (3rd and 7th week, 3rd and 6th month). In each couple, the husband and wife received synchronized beeps. As expected, findings showed that becoming a parent requires reorganization of daily activities and priorities, especially for women who cut down both on work activities as well as leisure time. Interestingly, parents' quality of experience associated with childcare was substantially similar: It was characterized by the perception of high challenges, engagement, positive affect and intrinsic motivation. In addition, the majority of ESM self-reports referring to parenting (71.8 %) were associated with channels in which challenges were perceived as above average: channels 8, 1 and 2. Becoming parents for the first time was clearly reflected in the high levels of anxiety (channel 8; 25.9 %) and also arousal (channel 1; 24.9 %) associated with childcare, compared to low-challenging experiences such as relaxation. At the same time, around 21 % of the self-reports dealing with parenting was associated with optimal experience (channel 2). This is an important finding in light of mothers' and fathers' long-term commitment to childcare, making it an opportunity for enjoyable resource investment, quality time and personal fulfilment in the face of risks of depression and disengagement that can potentially undermine the post-partum period (Delle Fave et al. 2013; Pozzo 2015).

Similarly, leisure time can become an important area of long-term personal investment. This was shown in studies involving six climbers monitored with ESM for one and a half months during an expedition on Thalay Sagar (6,904 m) in the Himalayas, and for 1 month during their daily life in Italy (Bassi and Delle Fave 2010; Delle Fave et al. 2003; Delle Fave et al. 2011). Participants were not professional sportsmen, but skilled amateurs who usually devoted time to climbing when they were off work. Inspection of the self-reports distribution in the eight channels of the EFM showed that during the expedition climbers mostly retrieved occasions for optimal experience (21.2 %), mainly followed by relaxation (19.4 %), apathy (19.2 %) and arousal (15.5 %). In particular, while flow was primarily associated with camp and climbing activities (respectively, 34.8 % and 52.2 %), relaxation and apathy were primarily linked to maintenance tasks such as eating and resting, which were necessary for keeping in good health (respectively, 23.9 % and 28.2 %). Paradoxically, few self-reports were associated with anxiety (7.5 %), in spite of the structural components of real or perceived danger characterizing rock climbing (Ewert and Hollenhorst 1997). By contrast, participants at home experienced twice as much anxiety (16.8 %), and also fewer occasions for flow (12.8 %). Such data suggest a preferential long-term investment in climbing activities to such an extent that participants felt more comfortable and competent under the seemingly risky and uncertain conditions in the mountains than in their cozy and safe living environment at home.

Besides crucial life transitions such as parenthood and extreme sport conditions, our ESM studies also targeted more general phenomena like learning (Bassi and Delle Fave 2004; Bassi et al. 2007; Delle Fave and Bassi 2000; Delle Fave and Massimini 2005). In Western countries, studying represents a pervasive task from childhood until at least adolescence, providing learners necessary knowledge to integrate in their communities as active members. Our research among various samples of adolescents from North and Central Italy globally showed that participants describe studying as a compulsory activity associated with low levels of happiness, but also as a potential opportunity for cognitive investment in relation to long-term goals. However, essential differences in experience fluctuation were detected across type of activity (Bassi and Delle Fave 2004). Homework was more frequently associated with optimal experience (21.4 %) compared to apathy (16.4 %): Students perceived control in the learning process while at home, and felt autonomous to decide how and when to invest their time in learning according to their own pace. By contrast, schoolwork was more frequently associated with apathy (17.8 %) than flow (13.2 %). Formal education basically consisted of activities, such as listening to lectures and taking notes that were primarily directed by teachers, and were perceived as passive and low challenging by students. Interestingly, such experiential differences between types of activity were not detected among students from Asian countries such as Nepal (Lombardi 2003), where formal education is strongly considered as a crucial opportunity for personal development and professional future. For Nepalese teenagers schoolwork and homework were predominantly associated with optimal experience (respectively, 24.5 % and 22.4 %) compared to apathy (6.7 % and 13.4 %). Nonetheless, for all students, experiencing flow in learning activities was associated with both short and long-term benefits. In the short-term, students derived enjoyment, gratification and sense of mastery from the learning tasks (Delle Fave and Bassi 2000). In the long-term, those who found flow in academic activities also perceived higher academic self-efficacy, placed more importance on academic attainments and aspired to higher educational levels (Bassi et al. 2007).

12.7 Back to Base for Future Research Directions

After this quick journey into the individuals' worlds of conscious experience, it is now time to go back to base for some considerations. As illustrated in this chapter, it is not easy to capture subjective experience and its fluctuations in the stream of daily life. Conscious experience ultimately represents a private complex phenomenon that researchers try to access through available real-time instruments such as the ESM, breaking it down into its cognitive, affective, motivational and volitional components as daily events and situations unfold. In this respect, EFM proved to offer a theory-led model to make sense of the myriad of empirical data collected with the ESM, highlighting complex experiential patterns with different meaning and impact on individuals' lives.

However, much still needs to be done to advance our knowledge on the phenomenology of conscious experience. On the one hand, the combined use of real-time measures, single-administration questionnaires and participants' interviews may contribute to unravel the experiential characteristics of flow, which are still a matter of dispute among researchers after 40 years from Csikszentmihalyi's first publication (1975/2000). Besides the proximal role of challenges and skills, top on researchers' agenda is the identification of the distal antecedents of flow, including individual characteristics like gender and age, health conditions, personality, meaning-making and goal-setting, as well as cultural and contextual features, such as family and community life (Bassi et al. 2014; Delle Fave et al. 2011; Engeser 2012). On the other hand, studies using EFM as a framework for data analysis have mostly focused on the main experiences of flow, relaxation, apathy, and anxiety. More information should be gathered on the other experiential profiles (arousal, control, boredom, and worry), and particularly on the combined role of all the eight profiles in individuals' optimal daily functioning. In this respect, it is not clear yet whether there exists a "healthy" combination of all the experiential configurations such that, for example, high frequencies of flow and relaxation in daily life may compensate for frequent occasions of apathy or anxiety. It is also not yet clear how individuals move from one experience to the other, whether there are predictable patterns of experience fluctuation, and whether there may be a "critical value" beyond which quality of experience inevitably changes, as shown in preliminary studies using nonlinear dynamical system models (Ceja and Navarro 2011, 2012).

With such challenging objectives in mind, we are ready to go back to everyday life with new research directions guiding our next journey into the intricacies of human conscious experience.

References

Bandura, A. (1997). *Self-efficacy: The exercise of control*. New York: Freeman.

Bassi, M., & Delle Fave, A. (2004). Adolescence and the changing context of optimal experience in time: Italy 1986–2000. *Journal of Happiness Studies, 5*, 155–179.

Bassi, M., & Delle Fave, A. (2010). Impact of extreme weather conditions on high-altitude climbers' goals and quality of experience. *Journal of Leisure Research, 3*, 469–488.

Bassi, M., & Delle Fave, A. (2012a). Optimal experience and self-determination at school: Joining perspectives. *Motivation and Emotion, 36*, 425–438.

Bassi, M., & Delle Fave, A. (2012b). Optimal experience among teachers: New insights into the work paradox. *Journal of Psychology, 146*, 533–557.

Bassi, M., Steca, P., Delle Fave, A., & Caprara, G. V. (2007). Academic self-efficacy beliefs and quality of experience in learning. *Journal of Youth and Adolescence, 36*, 301–312.

Bassi, M., Ferrario, N., Ba, G., Delle Fave, A., & Viganò, C. (2012). Quality of experience during psychosocial rehabilitation: A real-time investigation with experience sampling method. *Psychiatric Rehabilitation Journal, 35*, 447–453.

Bassi, M., Steca, P., Monzani, D., Greco, A., & Delle Fave, A. (2014). Personality and optimal experience in adolescence: Implications for well-being and development. *Journal of Happiness Studies, 15*, 829–843.

Baumeister, R. F., Masicampo, E. J., & Vohs, K. D. (2011). Do conscious thoughts cause behavior? *Annual Review of Psychology, 62*, 331–361.

Ceja, L., & Navarro, J. (2011). Dynamic patterns of flow in the workplace: Characterizing within-individual variability using a complexity science approach. *Journal of Organizational Behavior, 32*, 627–651.

Ceja, L., & Navarro, J. (2012). 'Suddenly I get into the zone': Examining discontinuities and nonlinear changes in flow experiences at work. *Human Relations, 65*, 1101–1127.

Csikszentmihalyi, M. (1975/2000). *Beyond boredom and anxiety*. San Francisco: Jossey Bass.

Csikszentmihalyi, M. (1982). Toward a psychology of optimal experience. In L. Wheeler (Ed.), *Review of personality and social psychology* (Vol. 3, pp. 13–36). Sage: Beverly Hills.

Csikszentmihalyi, M. (1990). *Flow. The psychology of optimal experience*. New York: Harper & Row.

Csikszentmihalyi, M. (1997a). Activity, experience and personal growth. In J. Curtis & S. Russell (Eds.), *Physical activity in human experience: Interdisciplinary perspectives* (pp. 59–88). Champaign: Human Kinetics.

Csikszentmihalyi, M. (1997b). *Finding flow. The psychology of engagement with everyday life*. New York: Basic Books.

Csikszentmihalyi, M., & Csikszentmihalyi, I. (Eds.). (1988). *Optimal experience. Psychological studies of flow in consciousness*. New York: Cambridge University Press.

Csikszentmihalyi, M., & Lefevre, J. (1989). Optimal experience in work and leisure. *Journal of Personality and Social Psychology, 56*, 815–822.

Csikszentmihalyi, M., Larson, R. W., & Prescott, S. (1977). The ecology of adolescent activity and experience. *Journal of Youth and Adolescence, 6*, 281–294.

Deci, E. L., & Ryan, R. M. (2000). The "what" and "why" of goal pursuits: Human needs and the self-determination of behavior. *Psychological Inquiry, 11*, 227–268.

Delle Fave, A. (2007). Individual development and community empowerment: Suggestions from studies on optimal experience. In J. Haworth & G. Hart (Eds.), *Well-being: Individual, community, and societal perspectives* (pp. 41–56). London: Palgrave McMillan.

Delle Fave, A. (2013). Past, present, and future of flow. In S. A. David, I. Boniwell, & A. Conley Ayers (Eds.), *The Oxford handbook of happiness* (pp. 60–72). Oxford: Oxford University Press.

Delle Fave, A., & Bassi, M. (2000). The quality of experience in adolescents' daily life: Developmental perspectives. *Genetic, Social, and General Psychology Monographs, 126*, 347–367.

Delle Fave, A., & Massimini, F. (1988). Modernization and the changing contexts of flow in work and leisure. In M. Csikszentmihalyi & I. Csikszentmihalyi (Eds.), *Optimal experience. Psychological studies of flow in consciousness* (pp. 193–213). New York: Cambridge University Press.

Delle Fave, A., & Massimini, F. (1992). The ESM and the measurement of clinical change: A case of anxiety disorder. In M. W. deVries (Ed.), *The experience of psychopathology: Investigating mental disorders in their natural settings* (pp. 280–289). New York: Cambridge.

Delle Fave, A., & Massimini, F. (2004). Parenthood and the quality of experience in daily life: A longitudinal study. *Social Indicators Research, 67*, 75–106.

Delle Fave, A., & Massimini, F. (2005). The investigation of optimal experience and apathy: Developmental and psychosocial implications. *European Psychologist, 10*, 264–274.

Delle Fave, A., Bassi, M., & Massimini, F. (2003). Quality of experience and risk perception in high-altitude rock climbing. *Journal of Applied Sport Psychology, 15*, 82–99.

Delle Fave, A., Massimini, F., & Bassi, M. (2011). *Psychological selection and optimal experience across cultures: Social empowerment through personal growth*. Dordrecht: Springer.

Delle Fave, A., Pozzo, M., Bassi, M., & Cetin, I. (2013). A longitudinal study on motherhood and well-being: Developmental and clinical implications. *Terapia Psicologica, 31*, 21–33.

Engeser, S. (Ed.). (2012). *Advances in flow research*. Dordrecht: Springer.

Ewert, A. W., & Hollenhorst, S. J. (1997). Adventure recreation and its implications for wilderness. *International Journal of Wilderness, 3*, 21–26.

Hektner, J. M., Schmidt, J., & Csikszentmihalyi, M. (2007). *Experience sampling method. Measuring the quality of everyday life*. Thousand Oaks: Sage.

Hilgard, E. R. (1980). The Trilogy of the mind: Cognition, affection, and conation. *Journal of the History of Behavioral Sciences, 16*, 107–117.

Inkinen, M., Lonka, K., Hakkarainen, K., Muukkonen, H., Litmanen, T., & Salmela-Aro, K. (2014). The interface between core affects and the challenge-skill relationship. *Journal of Happiness Studies, 15*, 891–913.

Jackson, S. A., & Eklund, R. C. (2002). Assessing flow in physical activity: The flow state scale-2 and dispositional flow scale-2. *Journal of Sport and Exercise Psychology, 24*, 133–150.

Jackson, S. A., & Eklund, R. C. (2004). *The flow scale manual*. Morgantown: Fitness Information Technology.

James, W. (1890). *The principles of psychology*. New York: Holt.

Keller, J., & Bless, H. (2008). Flow and regulatory compatibility: An experimental approach to the flow model of intrinsic motivation. *Personality and Social Psychology Bulletin, 34*, 196–209.

Keller, J., & Blomann, F. (2008). Locus of control and the flow experience: An experimental analysis. *European Journal of Personality, 22*, 1–19.

Keller, J., & Landhäußer. (2012). The flow model revisited. In S. Engeser (Ed.), *Advances in flow research* (pp. 51–64). Dordrecht: Springer.

Lambert, J., Chapman, J., & Lurie, D. (2013). Challenges to teh four-channel model of flow: Primary assumption of flow support the moderate challenging control channel. *Journal of Positive Psychology, 8*, 395–403.

Larson, R. W., & Delespaul, P. A. E. G. (1992). Analyzing experience sampling data: A guidebook for the perplexed. In M. deVries (Ed.), *The experience of psychopathology – Investigating mental disorders in their natural settings* (pp. 58–78). Cambridge: Cambridge University Press.

Lazarus, R. (1966). *Psychological stress and the coping process*. New York: McGraw-Hill.

Lombardi, M. (2003). *La qualità dell'esperienza di un gruppo di adolescenti nepalesi: applicazione transculturale di experience sampling method* [The quality of experience in a group of Nepalese adolescents: A cross-cultural application of ESM]. Doctoral dissertation at Università degli Studi di Milano, Italy.

Massimini, F., & Carli, M. (1988). The systematic assessment of flow in daily experience. In M. Csikszentmihalyi & I. Csikszentmihalyi (Eds.), *Optimal experience. Psychological studies of flow in consciousness* (pp. 266–287). New York: Cambridge University Press.

Massimini, F., & Delle Fave, A. (2000). Individual development in a bio-cultural perspective. *American Psychologist, 55*, 24–33.

Massimini, F., Csikszentmihalyi, M., & Carli, M. (1987). Optimal experience: A tool for psychiatric rehabilitation. *Journal of Nervous and Mental Disease, 175*, 545–549.

Moneta, G. B. (2012). On the measurement and conceptualization of flow. In S. Engeser (Ed.), *Advances in flow research* (pp. 23–50). Dordrecht: Springer.

Moneta, G. B., & Csikszentmihalyi, M. (1996). The effect of perceived challenges and skills on the quality of subjective experience. *Journal of Personality, 64*, 275–310.

Moneta, G. B., & Csikszentmihalyi, M. (1999). Models of concentration in natural environments: A comparative approach based on streams of experiential data. *Social Behavior and Personality, 27*, 603–638.

Pozzo, M. (2015). *Psychosocial resources and risk factors before and after childbirth: a longitudinal study among second time mothers*. Unpublished doctoral dissertation, University of Milano, Milano, Italy.

Preziosa, A., Riva, G., & Delle Fave, A. (2008). L'esperienza soggettiva dell'obesità: Implicazioni diagnostico- terapeutiche [The subjective experience of obesity: Diagnostic-therapeutic implications]. *Psicologia della Salute, 1*, 39–55.

Sartori, R. D. G., Marelli, M., Garavaglia, P., Castelli, L., Busin, S., & Delle Fave, A. (2014). The assessment of patients' daily qualità of experience: Autonomy level and perceived challenges. *Rehabilitation Psychology, 59*, 267–277.

Schiefele, U. (2013). Response to Engeser (2012): On the nature of flow experience. *Psychological Reports, 112*, 529–532.

Schmidt, J., Shernoff, D., & Csikszentmihalyi, M. (2007). Individual and situational factors related to the experience of flow in adolescence: A multilevel approach. In A. D. Ong & M. van Dulmen (Eds.), *The handbook of methods in positive psychology* (pp. 542–558). Oxford: Oxford University Press.

Searle, J. R. (1998). How to study consciousness scientifically. *Philosophical Transactions of the Royal Society of London, Series B, 353*, 1935–1942.

Tononi, G., & Edelman, G. M. (1998). Consciousness and complexity. *Science, 282*, 1846–1851.

Trull, T. J., & Ebner-Priemer, U. W. (2009). Using Experience Sampling Methods/Ecological Momentary Assessment (ESM/EMA) in clinical assessment and clinical research: Introduction to the special section. *Psychological Assessment, 21*, 457–462.

Chapter 13
Flow Within Everyday Emotions and Motivations: A Reversal Theory Perspective

Jon Wright

Abstract This chapter introduces reversal theory in relation to flow theory and explains why it could be helpful in exploring flow within everyday emotions and motivations. Reversal theory itself is described and the methods by which people are thought to move between metamotivational states are explained. It is argued that flow and reversal theory have similarities, but differ in how they propose people enter and leave optimal states and in the number and type of optimal state that are thought to be part of human experience. Reversal theory's emphasis on the dynamic nature of people's emotions and motivations, combined with the suggestion that there are eight different types of optimal state, appear compatible with findings from phenomenological research that explored the flow process. The rationale for undertaking phenomenological research exploring the flow process will be provided. The methodology of phenomenology will be justified and explored and clarification given to the method used within these phenomenological studies.

13.1 Introduction

It might appear odd to write about flow within everyday emotions and motivations, when flow has been considered to be *an experience that is not accessible in "everyday life"* (Csikszentmihalyi 1975, p. 132). Equally, it could appear strange that in a chapter discussing empirical data, the focus will be on phenomenological research that utilizes lived experiences, rather than quantitative approaches using experiments and statistics. However, it will be argued that the topic and focus of the chapter are not odd, but legitimate for two reasons. First, because flow has been found to be a common occurrence (Donner and Csikszentmihalyi 1992; Kennedy and Vectis 2004). Second, because Csikszentmihalyi (2002) has argued that phenomenology is, *the clearest way to examine the main facets of what happens in the mind, in a way that can be useful in the actual practice of everyday life* (p. 25).

J. Wright, Ph.D. (✉)
School of Health Sciences, University of Brighton, Eastbourne, East Sussex, UK
e-mail: j.wright@brighton.ac.uk

L. Harmat et al. (eds.), *Flow Experience*, DOI 10.1007/978-3-319-28634-1_13

13.2 The Problem of Definition

The complexity of defining flow has been explored in earlier chapters, but it is important to return to this thorny issue to explain how a reversal theory perspective could contribute to our understanding. It could be argued that a reason why flow experiences have been difficult to define is that they have not been precisely differentiated from more everyday emotions, experiences and states. For example, the characteristics of flow that are commonly used when defining flow have been described as including intense concentration (Csikszentmihalyi 2002) but does these mean that a person will necessarily experience flow if s/he is able to concentrate intensely? Or putting it another way is it possible for people to experience other states in moments when they are intensely concentrating? If you believe the answer to this question is that it would be possible to experience states other than flow, you would probably agree that precision in definition is important. Milne (2007) certainly thought so. Milne (2007) argued that when we are making empirical definitions we needed to use the criteria that had been laid down in the Concise Oxford English Dictionary (COED 2004), which includes the need for precision. In order to be fulfill the criteria for precision:

> *A definition needs to state the precise, essential meaning of a word or a concept that makes it distinct.* (Milne 2007, p. 438)

Thus, in order to define flow by the intensity of concentration, one would need to be precise about how intense concentration during flow is distinct from intense concentration within other psychological states that occur in everyday life. Establishing distinct differences between intense concentration during flow and other states has so far proved elusive. It could be helpful to explore and understand our everyday emotions and motivations in order to help us define flow precisely and understand the nature of optimal experiences. A reversal theory perspective could be useful in helping us to understand flow within everyday emotions, because it includes the range of human emotions and motivations, rather than just optimal experience (Apter 2007).

It could be argued that it is not only how flow has been defined that has been problematic for researchers, but occasionally Csikszentmihalyi's assertions as to what flow is, has also led to a degree of confusion. For example, Csikszentmihalyi (1993, p. 176) provided the following quotation to illustrate a mother's flow experience:

> Oh yes, when I'm working with my daughter; when she's discovering something new. A new cookie recipe that she has accomplished, that she had made herself, an artistic work that she had done that she's proud of. Her reading is one thing that she is really into and we read together. She reads to me and I read to her, and that's a time when I sort of lose touch with the rest of the world, I'm totally absorbed in what I'm doing.

Although it would appear that this mother was enjoying being absorbed in reading with her daughter, the extent to which all the characteristics of flow were present is unclear, for example, whether listening to her daughter read was particularly challenging. Additionally, although Csikszentmihalyi has stated that *almost every activity has the potential to produce flow* (p. 189), it could be argued that listening to one's daughter read would be a different type of experience than might be experienced when rock climbing (rock climbers being a group that Csikszentmihalyi (1975) has also studied). It has remained unclear if flow should be conceptualised as being on a continuum of experiences, as originally suggested by Csikszentmihalyi, or if there are different types of optimal experience, each on a continuum of experience, that could be explained from a reversal theory perspective (Wright et al. 2014a).

13.3 Introduction to Reversal Theory

Reversal theory has been defined as, *a structural-phenomenological theory of motivation, emotion, and personality* in everyday life (Apter 2007, p. 3). Richard Mallows (2013, p.668) when President of the British Psychological Society described reversal theory as, *an intriguing general approach to psychology, once referred to by Sternberg as psychology's best-kept secret... The theory emphasises the variability, inconsistency and even self-contradictions that occur in human personality, and the motivational and emotional patterns that underlie these.*

Reversal theory has rarely been referred to in connection to flow. This might be considered surprising if Rea (1993, p. 76) was correct in his assertion that the many similarities between flow theory and reversal theory could, *provide a common ground for comparison and integration.* Rea perceived them both to be psychological theories, which aimed to describe human motivation and were concerned with phenomenological experience and how motivation was structured psychologically. He saw flow and reversal theory as, *non-homeostatic theories which define motivation as a harmonic process of dynamic equilibrium* and that, *given this theoretical compatibility, these two theories can provide a mutually enriching perspective on optimal experience* (p. 76). Since Rea introduced this possibility, only the work of Wright et al. (2014a, b) has focused on the relationship between flow and reversal theory. Apter, one of the originators of reversal theory has, however, continued to occasionally refer to flow theory in his writing (Apter 2006; Apter and Heskin 2001).

Flow and optimal experiences within reversal theory may have received modest consideration in theoretical and research literature because reversal theory encompasses all of everyday human experience. Researchers exploring reversal theory have consequently been able to explore a wide assortment of issues other than optimal experience. In the area of sport and exercise reversal theory research has focused on issues related to participating in physical activity in middle-aged women (Sit et al. 2008), high-risk sports (Florenthal and Shoham 2001; Kerr et al. 2004; Kerr and Vlaminkx 1997), baseball (Fujiyama et al. 2005), rugby (Wilson and Kerr 1999), women's field hockey (Kerr et al. 2005a), lacrosse (Kerr and Males 2010, 2011), athletics (Grange and Kerr 2011), javelin throwers (Legrand and LeScanff 2003), aerobics, circuit training and Tai Chi (Frith et al. 2011), high and low-frequency exercisers (Segatto and Lafreniere 2013), football fans' responses to their teams winning and losing (Kerr et al. 2005b) and the motivational orientations of participants in sport (Lindner and Kerr 2000, 2001; Kerr et al. 2006b; Sit and Lindner 2005). People who had eating disorders and who were considered to be exercise dependent, regularly participating in highly active amateur sport have also been investigated (Blaydon et al. 2004).

Outside the sporting arena reversal theory research has been conducted into a variety of areas, such as smoking cessation (Burris and O'Connell 2003; Lee et al. 2012), stress (Lafreniere 1997; Martin and Svebak 1997, 2001), adventure activities (Houge Mackenzie et al. 2011, 2013; Houge Mackenzie and Kerr 2012), toy design (Gielen et al. 2011), disaffection with school mathematics (Lewis 2013), academic performance of secondary school students (Sit et al. 2013), humor (Apter and Desselles 2012), addictions (Brown 2001), health promoting behaviour (Apter and Spirn 1997; O'Connell and Brooks 1997; Svebak and Martin 1997), modern dance (Kerr et al. 2000, 2006a), music and rebelliousness (Carpentier et al. 2003), rebelliousness (Boddington and McDermott 2012; Lafreniere et al. 2013; McDermott 2001); street robbery offenders (Piotrowski 2011); watching natural disasters and watching violence on television (Portrell and Mullet 2014) and intelligence (Giraudeau et al. 2007). Interest has also explored reversal theory in organisations (Apter and Carter 2001; Fontana and Valente 1997), stress at work (Houge Mackenzie and Kerr 2013), risk taking (Apter and Batler 1997; Gerkovitch 2001; Howard et al. 2002; O'Neil and Lafreniere 2014; Skakoon-Sparling and Cramer 2014; Trimpop et al. 1999), espionage (Wilson 2012) and measurement of aspects of reversal theory including motivational states (Apter et al. 1998; Desselles et al. 2014; Gotts et al. 2000; Lafreniere and Cramer 2006; O'Connell and Calhoun 2001).

13.4 The Background to My Research of the Flow Process

My interest in flow and reversal theory began through my professional background as an occupational therapist and a personal curiosity about the relationship between what people do in their everyday lives, or their occupations and their health and well-being. I came across flow indirectly through reading a book by Oliver James (1998) who was more interested in why people were unhappier in the UK at the end of the twentieth century, than they had been 50 years before, despite being relatively more affluent. Specifically, James cited research that demonstrated that levels of depression, violence and compulsive behaviour had all increased significantly since 1950. He argued that the British people's comparatively unhealthy state could largely be accounted for by social comparison. Although James made his case well, I wondered if these apparent changes in the health and well-being of the British people could also been influenced by changes in the way people lived their lives. I discussed this idea with my colleague Gaynor Sadlo, who encouraged me to read the work of Csikszentmihalyi. Through my reading it became clear that a possible avenue for exploring the relationship between our everyday occupations and our health was through flow. Initially I hoped that investigating flow could help to reveal the therapeutic potential of occupation and contribute to the evidence base for my profession. Initially I wanted to conduct applied research that would have clear implications for occupational therapy practice. Specifically, I wanted to develop a method of measuring flow that had clinical utility and could be used as an outcome measure to judge the effectiveness of intervention. I also wanted to examine the relationship between flow and schizophrenia, as there was conflicting evidence as to whether a person with schizophrenia could experience flow or not (Csikszentmihalyi 2002; Emerson et al. 1998; Gerhardsson and Jonsson 1996) and I was aware that occupational therapists within mental health services were tending to work predominately with people who had enduring mental health problems, such as schizophrenia. However, the more I read the more *puzzling* flow became. Before conducting applied flow research I decided that I needed to have a greater understanding about flow process i.e. what happened before, during and after a flow experience, and the nature of flow itself. The overall aims of my research were therefore to understand the flow process and what flow is. My research questions addressed these aims by asking what the processes of flow were in the context of human experience and asking the same question of people who performed an activity with different levels of skill. The focus on human experience led me to phenomenology, a methodology that will be introduced in the next section.

13.5 Phenomenological Exploration of Flow

Both Csikszentmihalyi (2002) and Apter (2007) have recognised the importance of phenomenology in developing flow and reversal theory. Although more recently phenomenology has been considered to be a research methodology, originally it was a philosophy (Giorgi 2000; Moran 2000). Moran described phenomenology as, *a radical way of doing philosophy, a practice rather than a system. Phenomenology is best understood as radical, anti-traditional style of philosophising, which emphasises the attempt to get to the truth of matters, to describe phenomena, in the broadest sense as whatever appears in the manner in which it appears, that is as it manifests itself to consciousness, to the experiencer* (p. 4).

- Various authors have defined phenomenology, for example, Van Manen (1990, p. 10) stated that, *phenomenology asks for the very nature of a phenomenon, for that which makes a some-'thing' what it is-and without which it could not be what it is.* What Van Manen appeared to suggest was that phenomenology offers the possibility of understanding what makes an optimal experience distinct from other types of experience. Becker (1992, p. 39) defined phenomenology as the study of situations, *in the everyday world from the viewpoint of the experiencing person.* The implication of how Becker viewed phenomenology is that in order to explore flow process, in-depth interviews needed to take place with people who have had *direct* experience of the phenomenon under study, or what is termed *lived experience*. Van Manen described phenomenology in the following way:

- *Phenomenology aims at gaining a deeper understanding of the nature or meaning of our everyday experiences... Anything that presents itself to consciousness is potentially of interest to phenomenology, whether the object is real or imagined, empirically measurable or subjectively felt. Consciousness is the only access human beings have to the world. Or rather, it is by virtue of being conscious that we are already related to the world. Thus all we can ever know must present itself to consciousness. Whatever falls out of consciousness therefore falls outside the bounds of possible lived experience... A person cannot reflect on lived experience while living through the experience. For example, if one tries to reflect on one's anger while being angry, one finds that the anger has already changed or dissipated. Thus, phenomenological reflection is not* ***introspective*** *but* ***retrospective****. Reflection on lived experience is always recollective; it is reflection on experience that it is already passed or lived through* (p. 9–10).

Van Manen's description of the retrospective nature of phenomenological reflections is very apt in the exploration of flow, as any reflection upon a flow experience could only be achieved once flow had ended. Thus, it has to be acknowledged that a phenomenological exploration of flow, similar to other research methods, such as flow questionnaires and the ESM, inevitably means that participants are asked remember their lived experiences of flow after they have happened. It could be argued that methods of exploring flow that rely on participants' interpretations and recollections of human consciousness, such as occurs in phenomenological research, has its limitations. However, until flow can be studied rigorously in 'real time' they remain the most appropriate tools to use within flow research.

13.6 Phenomenological Method

- The choice of phenomenological method is not an easy one, for reasons Giorgi (2000, p. 11) has explained:
  - The amorphousness of phenomenology is both a boon and a bane. It is the former because it offers possibilities for resolving all kinds of issues in human affairs within its broad, inviting context; it is the latter because precise guidelines are lacking as to which level of phenomenological praxis to adopt and precisely what to do once the phenomenological invitation has been taken up.
- In order to examine the flow process, Becker's (1992) empirical phenomenological method was chosen because it offered reasonable, if not comprehensive, guidelines on what to do. Researchers using the empirical phenomenological method, *ask people to describe life events and then use these descriptions to understand the general structure* (or essence) *or nature of a phenomenon* (p. 32). Becker's method is based on her adaptation of the approach and procedures that were used by Giorgi, which emphasise the importance of researchers bracketing their preconceptions and being rigorous in focusing on the phenomenon. By such

methods Giorgi could be described as attempting to implement Husserl's phenomenology. In adopting this descriptive phenomenological method it is however acknowledged that some interpretation is inevitable by both participant and researcher as knowers, perceivers and believers. For a full description of the research method used within the research, readers are advised to read the published articles that explore the flow process (Wright et al. 2006, 2007, 2014b).
- From Becker's (1992) perspective, researchers orientated in phenomenology *design empirical studies that highlight phenomena as they are experienced by people. They study everyday events from the inside, from within the world of the person experiencing them. In doing so, they strive to understand what phenomena* ***are*** *for the experiencing person* (p. 33). Becker stated that phenomenologist's assume that *experience is a valid source of knowledge* and *people's everyday experiences contain rich insights into phenomena* (p. 34). Becker suggested that it is because scientific truths arise from and return to the everyday world that phenomenologist's need to *get back to the things themselves* (p. 34). In this instance, I wanted to return to the essence of flow process, exploring what happens before, during and after flow experiences. In order to achieve this aim I chose to utilise a phenomenological method that involved interviewing people who reported having flow experiences. By interviewing participants I also returned to the method that Csikszentmihalyi (1975) himself first used when trying to understand what 'autotelic experiences' are.

13.7 A Reversal Theory Perspective of Flow Experiences in Everyday Life

To date my research exploring the flow process has consisted of three studies (Wright et al. 2006, 2007, 2014b). In the first two studies the participants' descriptions of optimal experiences indicated that there might be various psychological states in which a person may be absorbed in an enjoyable occupation to the extent that they lose track of time and forget everything else apart from what they are focusing on at that particular moment. After the interviews in the third study had begun it became clear that as had happened previously, participants were involved in a complex process describing **different** experiences when describing flow. Although reversal theory had received little attention in flow literature, after careful consideration it was incorporated into the structural analysis of the third study. The rationale being that reversal theory appeared to be consistent with the findings from all three studies that suggested that there is more than one type of optimal experience and that people regularly move between different states of consciousness. The advantages of using reversal theory to examine flow experiences were that it provided a framework to understand how a person entered and left optimal states, and gave possible explanations for the variety of participants' experiences. The results of the phenomenological studies suggested that different optimal states had similar characteristics including a balance between the challenges and skills of an activity.

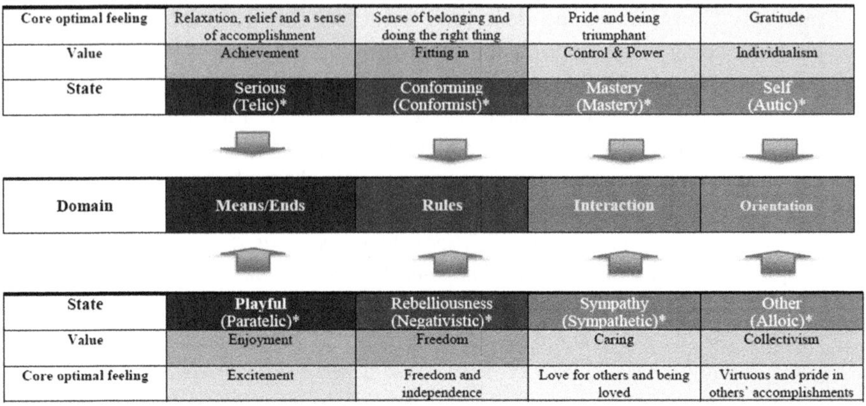

Fig. 13.1 Optimal feelings from 'Eight Ways of Being' (Apter International Limited 2003)

It should be clarified at this point that it is the phenomenological and psychological *concomitants* of flow experiences that were examined. It is not the intention to make any definitive claims about the causal significance of reversal theory states as determinants of flow experience, even though this is possibly the case.

Reversal theory states that what people experience and how they react in their everyday lives will be shaped by which metamotivational state they are in at a particular moment (Apter 2007). Apter (2007) has found four domains of being: means/end, rules, interaction and orientation. Each domain has a pair of opposite metamotivational states that are termed: telic/paratelic, conformist/negativistic, mastery/sympathetic and autic/alloic states (see Fig. 13.1). Reversal theory states that people will 'reverse', or switch between these opposite states during their everyday lives. Perhaps most importantly in relation to flow, reversal theory posits that each of the eight metamotivational states has at its core a feeling that a person will seek to optimise. Hence, from a reversal theory perspective there are eight different types of optimal experience, which will now be introduced.

Within the *telic/paratelic domain* it is proposed that in our everyday lives people are normally doing things that are either 'serious', aimed at working towards or achieving a particular goal, or 'playful' when doing something purely for enjoyment and its own sake (Apter International 2003). In this domain either people are concerned with how they can enjoy themselves (the 'means') or achieving a goal (the 'ends'). Optimal emotions within the telic state include relaxation, relief and a sense of accomplishment; negative emotions include anxiety and feelings of being overwhelmed. In the paratelic state optimal emotions include excitement and feeling that one has high energy levels; negative emotions include boredom. In reversal theory the telic/paratelic states are classified as somatic states (Apter 2007) i.e. the emotion felt is dependent on the level of arousal a person is experiencing at that particular time. For example, the lower a person's level of arousal in the telic state, the more relaxed s/he would be. The higher the arousal felt in the paratelic state the more excitement would be felt. Therefore, the level of arousal that a person feels when in an optimal telic or paratelic state is therefore important in determining how 'optimal' a person perceives an experience to be.

The *conformist/negativistic domain* is concerned with the 'rules' that are apparent in the social groups that occur in our everyday lives. When the conformist state is the focus of attention "our motivation is based on knowing the rules and keeping to them. The rules may be explicit or implicit, commands or conventions, moral or practical, light-hearted or gravely important" (Apter International 2003, p. 6). Optimal emotions associated with the conformist state "include a sense of belonging to a group and the comfort of knowing one is doing the right thing"; negative emotions include feelings of embarrassment and guilt if individuals consider they have failed to live up to expectations (p. 6). Apter (2007) proposed that in the negativistic, or rebelliousness state, rules are perceived as restricting and confining. People in a negativistic state will want to break free and might be seen as being defiant, eccentric or unconventional. Optimal emotions in the negativistic state include feelings of freedom and independence. When the negativistic state is at the forefront of people's attention and their occupations are being restricted by rules, they are likely to become frustrated and angry. In reversal theory conformist/negativistic states are also classified as somatic states (Apter 2007). Therefore, a person's level of arousal would determine the extent to which an experience was perceived as being 'optimal'.

The *mastery and sympathy domain* is concerned with our 'interactions' with others, for example, people, animals and plants, or situations or tasks we might face everyday (Apter International 2003). According to Apter (2007) in the mastery state people are concerned with a struggle for power and control and the extent to which people perceive that they are winning or losing. When the mastery state is the focus of attention, people will try to control objects, dominate others and solve problems. Optimal emotions include feelings of pride and being triumphant. When people in the mastery state think that they have lost, they might feel humiliated. When the sympathetic state is at the forefront of attention, building and maintaining relationships, giving and receiving affection, and caring will be of importance. Optimal emotions include both feeling love for others and being loved. Negative emotions associated with the sympathy state include feelings of being unloved and rejected. In reversal theory mastery and sympathy states are classified as transactional states (Apter 2007) i.e. what a person feels is partly dependent upon what has been termed the *felt transactional outcome*. Felt transactional outcome varies between high loss and high gain, for example, winning or losing, doing well or doing badly and succeeding and failing. Therefore, in the mastery state the more a person perceives him or herself to have triumphed the more 'optimal' the experience would be. Similarly, in the sympathetic state the more a person feels that he or she is loved the more 'optimal' the experience.

In the *autic and alloic domain* ('orientation') the motivational focus is either on self or others. In the autic state people are trying to do "the best one can for oneself"; people strive for personal satisfaction and judge situations primarily by assessing how they have been affected personally (Apter International 2003, p. 10). Optimal emotions in the autic state include feelings of gratitude and the satisfaction from doing a job well. In the alloic state "people do the best that they can for others and will judge situations primarily in terms of how they affect other people" (p. 11). Commonly, people may identify with someone, or something other than themselves, such as a football team or the community in which they live. Optimal emotions might include feeling "virtuous from helping others or feeling pride in the accomplishments of others" (p. 11). Negative emotions in the alloic state include guilt if people believe that they have not helped others enough. In reversal theory autic and alloic states are classified as transactional metamotivational states (Apter 2007). Therefore, how 'optimal experience will be perceived will vary depending, for example, on how much a person feels they have to be grateful for (in the autic state) or how much pride he or she feels for someone (in the alloic state).

Within flow theory, it is posited that people enter flow when they perceive a balance between the challenges of an occupation and the skills that they have. An imbalance between challenge and skills would theoretically prevent a flow experience, or lead to a flow experience ending (Csikszentmihalyi 2002). Alternatively, from a reversal theory perspective, moving between different psychological states, including optimal states, occurs by various means. Reversal theory proposes that people "spend their lives moving between the motivational states – experiencing an ever-changing kaleidoscope of combinations" (Apter International 2003, p. 13). Despite regularly moving between states, people will only experience one state within each domain at any one time e.g. either the telic state or the paratelic state (Apter 2007). Furthermore, normally only one or two states, from no more than two domains, will be at the focus of a person's attention. According to Apter two kinds of movement are possible in order for people to satisfy optimal feelings in all of the states, reversal within a pair of metamotivational states and a change of focus across the different domains. The different mechanisms by which movement is possible will now be explained.

13.8 The Role of Protective Frames in Optimal Experiences Within the Paratelic State

In order for people to move from the telic to the paratelic state and to attain an optimal feeling in the paratelic state, they need to perceive that protective frames are in place (Apter 2007). Apter believed that there are three types of protective frame: confidence, safety-zone and detachment. In the *confidence frame* "the individual faces up to real problems and dangers but feels such confidence in facing them that they do not seem like genuine threats" (p. 51). For example, dangerous sports enthusiasts might feel excited rather than anxious because they have confidence in their ability and/or the safety of their equipment and/or the other people who are sharing the risk with them.

Apter (2007) proposed that in the *safety-zone frame* the individual is "ensconced within a zone which is removed from risk and threat and where one becomes so enthralled and absorbed in what one is doing that one becomes totally unaware of a world outside" (p. 51). The safety-zone would seem to echo what might be thought to occur during a flow experience in which a person would be absorbed in an enjoyable activity and would forget his or her worries (Csikszentmihalyi 2002). Apter provided examples from sport to clarify how a safety-zone frame might work. In sports and games there are specially demarcated areas, such as a football pitch, in which normally no one apart from the players and officials can enter once the game has begun. Systems of rules can also help to provide a safety-zone during sporting competitions by providing a psychological space where players know in advance what can happen and that a referee or umpire will uphold the rules. Within a sporting safety-zone problems of the real world may arise when someone gets injured, or from understanding the implications of winning or losing a game, but generally, especially for amateurs, sport seems to be a good means of providing a protective safety-zone frame.

The *detachment frame* has been considered to be different from the other two protective frames, because in the detachment zone "one always feels oneself to be experiencing the world from the vantage point of complete safety" (Apter 2006, p. 65). In the detachment frame "the individual participates in what is going on, but only as an observer and is consequently detached from the action" (Apter 2007, p. 51). Apter proposed that when a person is in a detachment frame they have no goal to achieve or danger to avoid and are protected from the need to do anything. However, by observing other people trying to obtain goals and avoid danger through a combination of empathy, identification, arousal and protective frames a person can experience enjoyment in the paratelic state. Apter stated that various occupations could be undertaken within a detachment frame, for example, slowing down on the motorway to see the results of an accident, daydreaming, or by identifying with people portrayed in books, films, plays or television. What seems to occur in such instances is that people perform a self-substitution, when in order to become aroused they identify with one or other of the central characters and the emotions they might feel (Apter 2006). However, because of the detachment frame people can experience not only high arousal emotions such as excitement, but also all high arousal emotions even if the feelings would be likely to feel unpleasant outside of the detachment frame. For example, when watching a film it is quite possible to feel a variety of emotions including anger, horror, and grief that would normally be unpleasant, but when in the detachment frame could be enjoyed. Apter (2007, p. 53) termed these feelings "parapathic emotions". One circumstance it might be useful to acknowledge the influence of parapathic emotions is reading. Csikszentmihalyi (2002) has stated that people can obtain flow states from activities such as reading, but has never fully explained why reading could be so enjoyable. For those who are sufficiently literate the challenge-skills balance would not appear to easily fit with reading a book. The detachment frame and the ability to experience arousal through parapathic emotions that would be enjoyed in the paratelic state provide an alternative theoretical possibility.

13.9 Reversals Between Metamotivational States

Reversals between metamotivational states are termed *contingent*, *frustration* and *satiation* (Apter 2007). These reversals happen instantaneously and involuntarily (Apter International 2003). *Contingent reversals* for instance occur when a situation changes, for example, one could be absorbed in playing the piano in the paratelic state when your telephone rings and you switch to a telic state to answer in a formal manner (Apter 2007). *Frustration* in one state may lead to reversal into another. For example, a golfer who initially played in a paratelic state might reverse into a telic state after becoming frustrated at his failure to hole a putt. *Satiated reversals* occur when people have been in a state long enough to naturally reverse into another state. The time it takes to become satiated varies between seconds to hours and changes constantly for each person (Apter International 2003). Although Apter has stated that people are unable to change metamotivational states at will, it is thought possible to reverse between states indirectly by changing our situations or the way we perceive them.

13.10 Conclusion

Reversal theory provides a potentially important role in our understanding of flow within our lives, as it is a theory that encompasses all of our everyday emotions, motivations, including optimal states (Apter 2007). Reversal theory could be particularly helpful in enabling us to define flow more precisely by clearly differentiating between our normal, everyday emotions and motivations within the different motivational states and the associated optimal core feelings. Csikszentmihalyi (1993) has stated that he believes that almost all activities in our everyday lives could produce a flow experience. Three phenomenological studies that explored the process of flow in a variety of activities found that participants reported experiencing different types of flow whilst performing the same activities, as well as between different activities (Wright et al. 2006, 2007, 2014b). Flow theory did not provide an adequate explanation for these findings. However, reversal theory's identification of eight different metamotivational states, each with an associated core feeling that could be optimized, provided a theoretical framework to explain the participants' phenomenological accounts. Reversal theory might have an important role in future research into optimal experiences, as it could help researchers to qualify the type of flow experience under examination.

References

Apter, M. (2006). *Danger: Our quest for excitement*. Oxford: Oneworld Publications.
Apter, M. (2007). *Reversal theory: The dynamics of motivation, emotion and personality* (2nd ed.). Oxford: Oneworld Publications.

Apter International. (2003). *Eight ways of being: Insights from the Apter motivational style profile*. Loughborough: Apter International Ltd.
Apter, M. J., & Batler, R. (1997). Gratuitous risk: A study of parachuting. In S. Svebak & M. J. Apter (Eds.), *Stress and health: A reversal theory perspective* (pp. 119–130). Washington, DC: Taylor and Francis.
Apter, M. J., & Carter, C. (2001). Management in organisations. In M. J. Apter (Ed.), *Motivational styles in everyday life: A guide to reversal theory* (pp. 251–262). Washington, DC: American Psychological Association.
Apter, M. J., & Desselles, M. (2012). Disclosure humor and distortion humor: A reversal theory analysis. *Humor, 25*(4), 417–435.
Apter, M. J., & Heskin, K. (2001). Basic research on reversal theory. In M. J. Apter (Ed.), *Motivational styles in everyday life: A guide to reversal theory* (pp. 77–96). Washington, DC: American Psychological Association.
Apter, M. J., & Spirn, N. (1997). Motives for donating blood. In S. Svebak & M. J. Apter (Eds.), *Stress and health: A reversal theory perspective* (pp. 145–156). Washington, DC: Taylor and Francis.
Apter, M. J., Mallows, R., & Williams, S. (1998). The development of the motivational style profile. *Personality and Individual Differences, 24*, 7–18.
Becker, C. (1992). *Living & relating: An introduction to phenomenology*. Newbury Park: Sage.
Blaydon, M. J., Linder, K. J., & Kerr, J. H. (2004). Metamotivational characteristics of exercise dependence and eating disorders in highly active amateur sport participants. *Personality and Individual Differences, 36*, 1419–1432.
Boddington, E. L., & McDermott, M. R. (2012). Predicting resistance to health education messages for cannabis use: The role of rebelliousness, autic mastery, health value and ethnicity. *Journal of Health Psychology, 18*(2), 157–166. doi:10.1177/1359105312438111.
Brown, R. A. F. (2001). Addictions. In M. J. Apter (Ed.), *Motivational styles in everyday life: A guide to reversal theory* (pp. 155–166). Washington, DC: American Psychological Association.
Burris, R. F., & O'Connell, K. A. (2003). Reversal theory states and cigarette availability predict lapses during smoking cessation among adolescents. *Research in Nursing & Health, 26*, 263–272.
Carpentier, F. D., Knobloch, S., & Zillmann, D. (2003). Rock, rap and rebellion: Comparisons of traits predicting selective exposure to defiant music. *Personality and Individual Differences, 35*, 1643–1655.
Concise Oxford English Dictionary. (11th ed.). (2004). New York: Oxford University Press.
Csikszentmihalyi, M. (1975). *Beyond boredom and anxiety: The experience of play of play in work and games*. San Francisco: Jossey-Bass.
Csikszentmihalyi, M. (1993). Evolution and flow. In M. Csikszentmihalyi (Ed.), *The evolving self* (pp. 175–205). New York: Harper Collins.
Csikszentmihalyi, M. (2002). *Flow: The classic work on how to achieve happiness*. London: Rider.
Desselles, M. L., Murphy, S. L., & Theys, E. (2014). The development of the reversal theory state measure. *Journal of Motivation, Emotion, and Personality, 2*(1), 10–21.
Donner, E. J., & Csikszentmihalyi, M. (1992). Transforming stress to flow. *Executive Excellence, 9*(2), 16–17.
Emerson, H., Cook, J., Polatajko, H., & Segal, R. (1998). Enjoyment experiences as described by persons with schizophrenia. *Canadian Journal of Occupational Therapy, 65*(1), 183–192.
Florenthal, B., & Shoham, A. (2001). The impact of persuasive information on changes in attitude and behavioural intentions towards risky sports for arousal-seeking versus arousal-avoidance individuals. *Sport Marketing Quarterly, 10*(2), 83–95.
Fontana, D., & Valente, L. (1997). Stress in the workplace: Causes and treatments. In S. Svebak & M. J. Apter (Eds.), *Stress and health: A reversal theory perspective* (pp. 199–208). Washington, DC: Taylor and Francis.

Frith, J. J., Kerr, J. H., & Wilson, G. V. (2011). Immediate improvements in emotions and stress following participation in aerobics, circuit training and Tai Chi. *International Journal of Sport Psychology, 4*, 1–18.

Fujiyama, H., Wilson, G. V., & Kerr, J. H. (2005). Motivational state and emotional tone in baseball: The reciprocity between reversal theory and field research. *Revue Européenne de Psychologie Appliquée, 55*, 71–83.

Gerhardsson, C., & Jonsson, H. (1996). Experience of therapeutic occupations in schizophrenic subjects: Clinical observations organized in terms of the flow theory. *Scandinavian Journal of Occupational Therapy, 3*, 149–155.

Gerkovitch, M. M. (2001). Risk-taking. In M. J. Apter (Ed.), *Motivational styles in everyday life: A guide to reversal theory* (pp. 215–228). Washington, DC: American Psychological Association.

Gielen, M., Van Leeuwen, L., & Westwood, D. (2011). Designing for the real child: Toy designers and psychologists in dialogue on reversal theory. In N. F. M. Roozenburg, L. L. Chen, P. J. Stappers (Eds.), Proceedings of the fourth world conference on design research. TUDelft.

Giorgi, A. (2000). Concerning the application of phenomenology to caring research. *Scandinavian Journal of Caring Sciences, 14*, 11–15.

Giraudeau, C., Chasseigne, G., Apter, M. J., & Mullet, E. (2007). Adults' lay views about intelligence: A reversal theory approach. *Personality and Individual Differences, 42*, 169–179.

Gotts, G. H., Kerr, J. H., & Wangeman, J. F. (2000). Towards an international scale of telic-paratelic dominance. *Personality and Individual Differences, 28*, 217–227.

Grange, P., & Kerr, J. H. (2011). Do athletes renowned for their aggressive play transfer aggression to non-sport settings? An exploratory qualitative study. *Journal of Aggression, Maltreatment and Trauma, 20*, 359–375.

Houge Mackenzie, S., & Kerr, J. H. (2012). A (mis)guided adventure tourism experience: An autoethnographic analysis of mountaineering in Bolivia. *Journal of Sport and Tourism, 17*, 125–144.

Houge Mackenzie, S., & Kerr, J. H. (2013). Stress and emotions at work: An adventure tour guide's experiences. *Tourism Management, 36*, 3–14.

Houge Mackenzie, S., Hodge, K., & Boyes, M. (2011). Expanding the flow model in adventure activities: A reversal theory perspective. *Journal of Leisure Research, 43*(4), 519–544.

Houge Mackenzie, S., Hodge, K., & Boyes, M. (2013). The multi-phasic and dynamic nature of flow in adventure experiences. *Journal of Leisure Research, 45*(2), 214–232.

Howard, R., Yan, T. S., Ling, L. H., & Min, T. S. (2002). Risk taking and metamotivational state. *Personality and Individual Differences, 32*, 155–165.

James, O. (1998). *Britain on the couch: Treating a low serotonin society*. London: Arrow Books.

Kennedy, B. L., & Vectis, R. N. (2004). Contexts of the flow experience of women with HIV/AIDS. *OTJR: Occupation, Participation and Health, 24*(3), 83–91.

Kerr, J. H., & Males, J. R. (2010). The experience of losing: Qualitative study of elite lacrosse athletes and team performance at a world championship. *Psychology of Sport and Exercise, 11*, 394–401.

Kerr, J. H., & Males, J. R. (2011). Experiencing aggression in sport: Insights from a lacrosse world championship tournament. *Sport and Exercise Psychology Review, 7*, 26–33.

Kerr, J. H., & Vlaminkx, J. (1997). Gender differences in the experience of risk. *Personality and Individual Differences, 22*(2), 293–295.

Kerr, J. H., Kawaguchi, C., Oiwa, M., Terayama, Y., & Zukawa, A. (2000). Stress, anxiety and other emotions in Japanese modern dance performance. *Pacific Journal of Psychology, 11*(1), 16–33.

Kerr, J. H., Au, C. K. F., & Lindner, K. J. (2004). Motivation and level of risk in female and male recreational sport participation. *Personality and Individual Differences, 37*, 1245–1253.

Kerr, J. H., Wilson, G. V., Bowling, A., & Sheahan, J. P. (2005a). Game outcome and elite Japanese women's field hockey player's experience of emotions and stress. *Psychology of Sport and Exercise, 6*, 251–263.

Kerr, J. H., Wilson, G. V., Nakamura, I., & Sudo, Y. (2005b). Emotional dynamics of soccer fans at winning and losing games. *Personality and Individual Differences, 38*, 1855–1866.
Kerr, J. H., Fujiyama, H., Wilson, G. V., & Nakamori, K. (2006a). The experience of a modern dance group: Arousal, motivation and self-rated performance. *Research in Dance Education, 7*(2), 125–140.
Kerr, J. H., Wilson, G. V., Svebak, S., & Kirkaldy, B. D. (2006b). Matches and mismatches between telic dominance and type of sport: Changes in emotions and stress pre to post performance. *Personality and Individual Differences, 40*, 1557–1567.
Lafreniere, K. D. (1997). Paratelic dominance and the appraisal of stressful events. In S. Svebak & M. J. Apter (Eds.), *Stress and health: A reversal theory perspective* (pp. 35–43). Washington, DC: Taylor and Francis.
Lafreniere, K. D., & Cramer, K. M. (2006). Examining reversal theory measures in relation to NEO personality dimensions and consideration of future consequences. *Personality and Individual Differences, 40*, 1387–1397.
Lafreniere, K. D., Menna, R., & Cramer, K. M. (2013). Rebelliousness, effortful control, and risky behavior: Metamotivational and temperamental predictors of risk-taking in older adolescents. *Journal of Motivation, Emotion, and Personality, 1*, 17–26.
Lee, J. T., Smith, D. W., & Colwell, B. (2012). An exploration of transactional states and cessation-related social variables within adolescent smokers. *Tobacco Induced Diseases, 10*, 20.
Legrand, F., & LeScanff, C. (2003). Tension-stress, effort-stress and mood profiling with an elite javelin performer. *Psychology of Sport and Exercise, 4*, 429–436.
Lewis, G. (2013). A portrait of disaffection with school mathematics: The case of Anna. *Journal of Motivation, Emotion, and Personality, 1*, 36–43.
Lindner, K. J., & Kerr, J. H. (2000). Metamotivational orientations in sport participants and non-participants. *Psychology of Sport and Exercise, 1*, 7–25.
Lindner, K. J., & Kerr, J. H. (2001). Predictability of sport participation motivation from metamotivational dominances and orientations. *Personality and Individual Differences, 30*, 759–773.
Mallows, R. (2013). President's column. *Psychologist, 26*, 668.
Martin, R. A., & Svebak, S. (1997). The psychobiology of telic dominance and stress. In S. Svebak & M. J. Apter (Eds.), *Stress and health: A reversal theory perspective* (pp. 69–80). Washington, DC: Taylor and Francis.
Martin, R. A., & Svebak, S. (2001). Stress. In M. Apter (Ed.), *Motivational styles in everyday life: A guide to reversal theory* (pp. 119–138). Washington, DC: American Psychological Association.
McDermott, M. R. (2001). Rebelliousness. In M. Apter (Ed.), *Motivational styles in everyday life: A guide to reversal theory* (pp. 167–186). Washington, DC: American Psychological Association.
Milne, D. (2007). An empirical definition of clinical supervision. *British Journal of Clinical Psychology, 46*(4), 437–447.
Moran, D. (2000). *Introduction to phenomenology*. Oxon: Routledge.
O'Connell, K. A., & Brooks, E. (1997). Resisting urges and adopting new behaviours. In S. Svebak & M. J. Apter (Eds.), *Stress and health: A reversal theory perspective* (pp. 157–171). Washington, DC: Taylor and Francis.
O'Connell, K. A., & Calhoun, J. E. (2001). The telic/paratelic instrument (T/PSI): Validating a reversal theory measure. *Personality and Individual Differences, 30*, 193–204.
O'Neil, A. I., & Lafreniere, K. D. (2014). Metamotivational tendencies, sociocultural attitudes, and risky eating behaviors. *Journal of Motivation, Emotion, and Personality, 2*(1), 50–57.
Piotrowski, P. (2011). Street robbery offenders: Shades of rationality and reversal theory perspective. *Rationality and Society, 23*(4), 427–451. doi:10.1177/1043463111414125.
Portrell, M., & Mullet, E. (2014). Why do people enjoy watching natural disasters and human violence on television? A reversal theory perspective. *Journal of Motivation, Emotion, and Personality, 2*(1), 38–49.

Rea, D. W. (1993). Reversal theory explanations of optimal experience. In M. J. Apter, D. Fontana, & S. Murgatroyd (Eds.), *Advances in reversal theory* (pp. 75–88). Amsterdam: Swets and Zeitlinger.

Segatto, B. L., & Lafreniere, K. D. (2013). Motivational and personality predictors of body esteem in high-and low-frequency exercisers. *Journal of Motivation, Emotion, and Personality, 1*, 27–35.

Sit, C. H. P., & Lindner, K. J. (2005). Motivational orientations in youth sport participation: Using achievement goal theory and reversal theory. *Personality and Individual Differences, 38*, 605–618.

Sit, C. H. P., Kerr, J. H., & Wong, I. T. F. (2008). Motives for and barriers to physical activity participation in middle-aged Chinese women. *Psychology of Sport and Exercise, 9*, 266–283.

Sit, C. H. P., Braman, O. R., Kerr, J. H., & Lindner, K. J. (2013). Motivational style and actual and perceived academic performance of secondary school students in Hong Kong. *School Psychology International, 34*, 17–32.

Skakoon-Sparling, S., & Cramer, K. (2014). Paratelic/telic state, sexual arousal, and sexual risk-taking in university students. *Journal of Motivation, Emotion, and Personality, 2*(1), 32–37.

Svebak, S., & Martin, R. A. (1997). Humour as a form of coping. In S. Svebak & M. J. Apter (Eds.), *Stress and health: A reversal theory perspective* (pp. 173–184). Washington, DC: Taylor and Francis.

Trimpop, R. M., Kerr, J. H., & Kirkcaldy, B. (1999). Comparing personality constructs of risk taking behaviour. *Personality and Individual Differences, 26*, 237–254.

Van Manen, M. (1990). *Researching lived experience: Human science for an action sensitive pedagogy*. New York: State University of New York Press.

Wilson, L. R. (2012). Reversal theory: Understanding the motivational styles of espionage. *International Journal of Intelligence Ethics, 3*(1), 76–100.

Wilson, G. V., & Kerr, J. H. (1999). Affective responses to success and failure: A study of winning and losing in competitive rugby. *Personality and Individual Differences, 27*, 85–99.

Wright, J. J., Sadlo, G., & Stew, G. (2006). Challenge-skills and mindfulness: An exploration of the conundrum of flow process. *OTJR: Occupation, Participation and Health, 26*(1), 25–32.

Wright, J. J., Sadlo, G., & Stew, G. (2007). Further explorations of the conundrum of flow process. *Journal of Occupational Science, 14*(3), 136–144.

Wright, J. J., Wright, S., Sadlo, G., & Stew, G. (2014a). Exploring optimal experiences: A reversal theory perspective of flow and occupational science. *Journal of Occupational Science, 21*(2), 188–201. doi:10.1080/14427591.2012.713312.

Wright, J. J., Wright, S., Sadlo, G., & Stew, G. (2014b). A reversal theory exploration of flow process and the flow channel. *Journal of Occupational Science, 21*(2), 173–187. doi:10.1080/14427591.2012.713313.

Part VI
The Social Flow

Chapter 14
Social Psychology of Flow: A Situated Framework for Optimal Experience

Marco Boffi, Eleonora Riva, Nicola Rainisio, and Paolo Inghilleri

Abstract Flow research is traditionally focused on subjective experience and well-being, with less concern for the impact of these aspects on the broader social context. This chapter, introducing a situated framework of research, assigns instead a central role to flow in generating social change. We highlight how social and physical environments are continuously modeled through optimal experience and its social dissemination. Whilst some models drive their attention to flow in groups as a facilitator of performance, our approach focuses on the study of the link between flow and socio-cultural experience. This link between the person and the external context regards both the intrapsychic relationship that individuals build with cultural artifacts and the influence of affective relations and participation in groups. This perspective is supported through new research data from three different areas of study.

14.1 Introduction: Flow of Consciousness as a Link Between Individual and Socio-Cultural Context

Flow research is traditionally focused on subjective experience and well-being, with less concern for the impact of these aspects on the broader social context. Indeed, optimal experience is one of the main mediators of the relationship between the individual and the cultural system, as a trigger of the psychological selection (Inghilleri 1999). Hence, some artifacts of our culture are selected according to their ability to generate flow whereas others are set aside (Csikszentmihalyi and Massimini 1985). Also our socio-physical environment may be considered as an artifact, since both physical spaces and social organizations are basically produced by human culture (Rainisio and Inghilleri 2013). The link between flow and socio-cultural experience regards both the intrapsychic relationship that individuals build with cultural artifacts and the influence of affective relations and participation in groups. Social and physical environments are continuously modeled through

M. Boffi (✉) • E. Riva • N. Rainisio • P. Inghilleri
Department of Cultural Heritage and Environment, University of Milan, Milan, Italy
e-mail: marco.boffi@unimi.it

L. Harmat et al. (eds.), *Flow Experience*, DOI 10.1007/978-3-319-28634-1_14

optimal experience and its social dissemination (Inghilleri 2014). Modern society offers, day after day, challenges of increasing complexity. The global citizen is constantly stimulated by demands from the world of work, family and the social environment. Simultaneously people realize how necessary it is, in a busy and hectic life, to find some time for themselves, to cultivate their own physical and mental health, and to carve out spaces for leisure, hobbies, friends, family, and in general for what gives meaning to life (Csikszentmihalyi and Csikszentmihalyi 2006). It is becoming more and more important to develop the ability to select activities, relationships, needs and desires in a generative way, and give these a privileged space, making them emerge from an offer that becomes gradually more and more extensive and varied (Inghilleri et al. 2014).

The individuals actively build their own identity and do so in a harmonious way with the context, starting from their own biological basis and through their interaction with the culture (Massimini and Delle Fave 2000). So the quality of subjective experience is central for the construction of the personal Self and of personal behavior. The way we feel is related to a variety of causes: to our past; to the immediate experience; to the ability to connect the immediate experience with our intentions, our profound purposes, our projects. The focus of our knowledge and of our affections thus depends on the possibility that a specific mind/culture relationship provides an experience that the subject perceives as making sense and being organized in relation to the present situation, to the core of personal identity, and to future purposes. In this sense, the concept of *subjective experience* (Inghilleri 1999) may be defined as the sum of the information, originating either from the outer world or the inner world, that enters in the psychic system at a given point in time and its comprehensive interpretation by the consciousness. This conceptualization highlights how psychological processes (consciousness, attention, emotions) and cultural processes (social environment, the others) are part of a single system which the inner state of the individual and its development depend on: it is not possible to understand the psychological functions without considering the external culture as well (Inghilleri 2014).

The relationship between the individual and culture gives rise to two processes that are distinct and interacting at the same time: the Cultural evolution and the Individual psychological selection. The *Cultural evolution* is a historical cross-generational process of transmission of cultural information stored in extra-individual locations. The *Individual psychological selection*, on the other hand, is a process that relates to the single individual, and represents the selective internalization in the central nervous system of a part of the external cultural information. This process is associated with elaboration processes, construction of meanings and affective experience (Delle Fave et al. 2011). Cultural evolution and psychological selection are in a continuous relationship of reciprocal causality, in the sense that one influences the other. Culture co-determines the construction of the individual Self (think for example of all the educational and socialization activities) but it is the actions of individuals, their decision-making processes, the focus of attention and of behavior on certain purposes, the experiences and the emotions that make the different areas of our lives attractive or unpleasant, that cause certain elements of culture, and not others, to be transmitted in time.

Such elements of culture can be labeled as *artifacts*, a term widely used in cultural psychology that defines any entity not present in nature but constructed or produced by human beings (Inghilleri 2009). Artifacts are therefore the very constituents of the cultures. The category of artifact thus includes objects and material structures but also ideas, artistic products, technologies, institutions, political views, religions, rituals, daily practices and so on. Therefore it concerns both tangible and intangible entities. Artifacts are the result of the application, to the materials or the conceptual categories that constitute them, of outside forces originated by its authors: men and women who decide to create artifacts, to give them a meaning, to transmit or modify them. Artifacts therefore are a reflex of and can accept the trend towards complexity, organization, order and information typical of the living world itself, that is to say, proper to the people who choose them, use them and give them meaning. Culture is transmitted if there is an investment of psychic energy by the people on the artifacts of society and if these can produce *positive subjective experience* (Gardner et al. 2001). An element of culture draws our psychic energy (and so it will be adopted and kept) if it gives a good experience. The possibility of having positive states of experience is therefore the basis of the process of cross-generational transmission of human cultures. In this sense, the flow of consciousness theory takes a key position as explanatory model of subjective experience, and gives us a theoretical model able to explain the relation between subjective intrapsychic dynamics and socio-environmental features.

Self-development and cultural evolution are deeply related: the internalization of social values, ideologies, economic and material elements, brings to a specific identity, and, on the other side, the everyday behaviors and psychological processes maintain, transmit, and change culture. People tend to repeat behaviors and search for those elements of culture that allow the optimal experience as a positive and meaningful experience to the Self. The individual's inner world is thus built around nuclei and cultural practices that have been able to give them meaning and positive experience: the family, the members of the groups to which they belong, the places of everyday life, home, school and work. Society tends to organize itself in order to provide this type of complex and positive experience to the younger generations in the crucial moments of socialization such as, indeed, the family and school (Csikszentmihalyi 1993).

14.2 One Experience, Several Contexts: Applied Case Studies

In the following sections of this chapter we will show the main role of flow in three different areas of research in social psychology. First we will demonstrate the influence of flow experience in the consolidation of place attachment and environmental preference, suggesting a bio-cultural explanation as an alternative to the mainstream evolutionary framework in environmental psychology. Then we will show how flow theory can serve as theoretical cornerstone to understand social engagement, outlining group settings able to involve new citizens and sustain their commitment through time. Finally we will explain how, studying the daily experience of adolescents, flow can be used as a planned tool to trigger community renewal and social empowerment, reinforcing transgenerational artifact transmission and transcultural development of complex and creative identities.

14.2.1 Environment and Subjective Experience

14.2.1.1 Theoretical Issues and Empirical Data

To build new bridges between optimal experience and social psychology it would be useful to look at the disciplines that deal with the well-being in the environment. The link between socio-environmental context and this psychological experience can be a fertile meeting ground for both the domains, and could be expressed as follows:

The optimal experience is a meaningful experience of everyday life, which takes place, undoubtedly, living in a given body, acting in a given space and surrounded by a given social world. As evidence, its key element is a meaningful balance between external challenges and perceived skills. Then, such an experience is *inherently embodied* and, at the same time, *nestled in a socio-spatial framework*.

Following this approach, the main question becomes: *how does the optimal experience affect our perception of the socio-environmental context, and, at a higher level, the context itself?*

If we look at the context as a *macro-system*, that question is exhaustively answered by the process of psychological selection (Csikszentmihaly and Massimini 1985; Inghilleri 1999), according to which optimal experience is supposed to be able to change the cultural system as it is the main instrument of selection and progressive innovation of material and immaterial artifacts. At a *micro-level*, the question can be answered through a critical review of the already existing models in environmental psychology, which have long studied human environmental preferences and the positive effects of contemplating and/or enjoying certain environments. Since the 1970s, some research in this area has shown that specific environments, predominantly natural, may contribute significantly to psychological well-being, by reducing the levels of stress, supporting the attentional recovery and triggering a positive mood (*for a complete review see* Velarde et al. 2007; Berto 2014). Mainstream theories have focused on an evolutionary framework, postulating that the effects of well-being are attributable to *biophilia* (Wilson 1984), that is an innate affiliation between humans and other living things, developed as it would promote fitness and survival of the species. The two main existing theories, Stress Reduction Theory (SRT; Ulrich 1983) and Attention Restoration Theory (ART; Kaplan and Kaplan 1983) fall into this framework. Similarly, the environmental preference was also found to have a phylogenetic origin, and to be closely linked to the reported restorative effects (Hartig and Staats 2006). Rainisio and Inghilleri (2013) criticized those approaches, pointing out that they share an innatist and homeostatic vision about the psychological functioning, in which the cultural and experiential aspects are poorly treated. We deem it is possible to hybridize the mainstream in environmental psychology with the optimal experience, a construct that has so far been given little consideration by the discipline. In particular, it is possible to overlap the flow experience with the observed stress reduction and attention restoration phenomena, considering them as parts of a wider optimal experience, having in common many of their key issues. Just to mention the two main aspects (*for a detailed analysis see* Rainisio et al. 2014), both flow theory and ART share the crucial point of a conceptualization of the attentional process as effortless that is free from cognitive fatigue and therefore restorative. Flow theory and SRT are indeed supposed to be linked by a substantial stress reduction, since flow and stress share a u-shaped relationship.

Preference, Restorativeness and Flow An explorative study was conducted on a sample of students from Italy and Algeria (n = 169) to deepen our understanding of the relationship between optimal experience, restoration and environmental preferences. Nine pictures representing three different biomes (savannah, forest and desert) were shown to the participants, who evaluated them with the use of the following scales:

- Perceived Restorativeness Scale (PRS; Hartig et al. 1997): the most used tool for assessing place *restorativeness*, based on the ART's main constructs.
- Revised Restoration Scale (RRS; Han 2003): a tool that combines the main elements of ART and SRT
- Neighborhood Attachment Scale (NAS; Bonnes et al. 1997, adapted version): a scale focused on place attachment
- Flow in Environment Scale (FLIES; Rainisio 2012): this scale measures the perceived potential of a place to enable optimal experience, what we called *environmental flowability*. Using a well-known description of the optimal experience from the Flow Questionnaire (Csikszentmihalyi 1975/2000) as initial stimulus, the participants answered the following items:

  1. *Walking in a place like that I could feel this way*: perceived probability of flow
  2. *It happened to me to feel this way in places like that*: past flow experiences
  3. *Places like that can help me to feel this way*: perceived capability of the place as a trigger of optimal experiences
  4. *Sometimes I go to places like that to feel this way*: strategic use of the place as an activator of flow experiences

Data analysis showed a significant correlation between *environmental flowability* and aesthetic preferences (0.656), in both the restorativeness scales (PRS, 0.698; RRS, 0.773) and place attachment (NAS adapted, 0.690). Moreover, calculating a linear regression, it was found that the above correlation explains the 43 % of the preference variance (r 0.656; r^2 0.430; F. 123.57) and nearly 48 % of the NAS variance (r 0.690; r^2 0.476; F. 148.89).

Data also showed high multicollinearity values (tolerance 0.394; VIF 2.537) between FLIES, PRS and RRS. We would suggest that, as hypothesized above, it could be due to a wide overlapping between the two constructs, whereas optimal experience and restorative experience are supposed to share only some fundamental features.

14.2.1.2 Discussion

The data collected so far, even if they require further experimental verifications, allow some general reflections on the relationship between socio-physical environments and psychological well-being.

First of all, it can be assumed that the optimal experience is one of the organizing principles of human experience facing an environment, giving an alternative explanation to the positive outcomes observed in the past, and so far attributed to phylogenetic causes.

That leads to an evolution of the concept of flow, from a generative experience to an ordering principle of the daily individual and social behavior.

In fact, this experience seems to affect different levels in the social field, as it influences preferences and place attachment, that in turn are connected with the intensity of place frequentation, the conservational behaviors, and the ability to build meaningful local relationships. Also, as mentioned earlier, this means, at a macro-level, to select environments to be *passed down* to future generations.

Moreover, we suggest considering the optimal experience not only as a momentary experience, but as a cognitive system/process that continuously works by evaluating (in real time) the *flowability*, which is the perceived probability of an artifact (salient at a given moment) generating optimal experience.

According to this new conceptualization, the role of flow could be extended to all other objects and events observed in social reality (see Chap. 15 by Hout et al. in this volume). In conclusion, the optimal experience itself could be seen as a higher-level system that oversees the whole human activity within the social context.

14.2.2 Participation and Social Engagement

14.2.2.1 Theoretical Issues and Empirical Data

From the perspective of giving prominence to the social aspects of optimal experience, the research contributions offered by community psychology are a fruitful source of explanation for those mechanisms linking individual experiences and social contexts. Boffi et al. (2014) have recapitulated several constructs used in this field to explain the positive effects of participatory behaviors on individuals, highlighting their implicit connections with the flow theory. From their point of view having the opportunity to directly take part in one's community can support individual self-determination and self-efficacy, leading citizens to build personally meaningful aims and to integrate them in their own identity (Prilleltensky et al. 2001). Hence the sense of responsibility toward society at large, which underlies the initiatives of activists, is not an obligation nor merely empathic. It results from an individual evolution that has made activists more conscious and responsive, steadily incorporating such a sense of responsibility in their identity. In a similar way Klar and Kasser (2009) have shown that identifying ourselves as activists and enacting related initiatives are characteristics associated with higher levels of well-being both at the individual and social level. In their study the authors describe activism as an expression of intrinsic motivation, which is the basis for the promotion of positive personal development. In addition to such theoretical connections that suggest the importance of flow in describing civic engagement, optimal experience has been proven to be directly recognized by people in volunteering, even though less often in comparison to other free time activities (Delle Fave 2007; Delle Fave and Massimini 1992). The common idea of these studies is that participatory activities become a source of well-being for individuals, who tend to repeat them over time as they are gratifying.

Political Activists In a study addressed to explore the subjective experience of active citizens (Boffi 2012a) the author administered a questionnaire to political activists (N = 224) involved in structured groups, including national parties and university associations active in Italy. The questionnaire comprised four items adapted from the Flow Questionnaire (Csikszentmihalyi 1975/2000) aimed at exploring flow experience in life in general and in particular in the political field. It also included 36 items of the Flow State Scale (FSS) (Jackson and Marsh 1996) in its Italian version (Muzio 2004), addressing nine dimensions of flow: D1 challenge-skill balance (subjective perception of competence in the situation); D2 action-awareness merging (actions are done spontaneously without effort also when including complex tasks); D3 clear goals (to identify specific route of action); D4 unambiguous feedback (regular monitoring of how well one is going); D5 concentration on the task at hand (ignoring thoughts and environmental inputs not related with the performance itself); D6 sense of control (it transmits a feeling of mastery and self-confidence); D7 loss of self-consciousness (oneness with the environment that leaves no space for others' evaluation); D8 transformation of time (it seems to speed up or to slow down); D9 autotelic experience (the reward is the positive feeling itself, that is the ultimate aim of the activity: it is intrinsically motivated). Socio-demographic variables comprised questions about participatory activities (e.g. role in the group, frequency of political activity).

As for the Flow Questionnaire, 71.70 % of the activists recognize the state of flow in their lives in general and 71.52 % of them declare to experience it in politics. The χ^2 test shows a solid relation between these two experiences (χ^2 (1) = 46.91, $p < 0.001$), supporting the idea that given a general capability of recognizing flow it can be used to monitor specific sets of activities, such as political ones. The χ^2 test shows no significant association between experiencing flow in general and frequency, duration, or role in the political activity. On the contrary, experiencing flow in politics is associated with more frequent activities and higher roles in the group. When describing daily activities that most frequently give rise to optimal experiences, participants provide a clear picture. Political activities are frequently associated with flow: it is the third most cited activity after work/study and leisure. If added up in a single category referring to participation in general, civic and political engagement represents the second most cited activity after work/study. When asked to refer in detail to the most intrinsically rewarding activities among the political ones, activists mention actions referred to electoral campaigns (ranging from college initiatives to national events), debates (e.g. conventions, assemblies, public meetings) and organizational tasks (in initiatives with a political value but not strictly conventional, like concerts or cultural projects).

A closer look at FSS scores for each of the nine dimensions allows us to qualitatively describe the flow experience in politics. Autotelic experience (D9) is the most important dimension for political activists. It confirms that political engagement is highly intrinsically rewarding, also beyond practical results achieved, and that the reflection on the meaning of the performed activity is the key factor in this field. Clear goals (D3) is the second most relevant dimension, followed by Total concentration on the task at hand (D5), Challenge-skill balance (D1) and Sense of control (D6). This set of dimensions is over the mean value, suggesting that for political activists cognitive monitoring of action execution is more relevant than experiencing mental absorption.

Sustainability Awareness A study aimed at investigating the responsiveness to the topic of sustainability (Inghilleri et al. 2013) allowed us to understand the role of flow in raising awareness among a general population of youth (N=382) not specifically selected among activists. Participants from four different European countries (Croatia, Germany, Italy, Poland) had the chance to interact with a digital installation designed to offer them cognitive and emotional inputs regarding sustainability issues (e.g. through individual ecological footprint calculator, interactive videos and pictures, social networks interface). To assess the effects of such experience they completed a questionnaire including an adapted short scale of Sustainable Development Self-Efficacy (Hanss and Böhm 2010), an evaluation of satisfaction with the interactive experience, an item adapted from the Flow Questionnaire (Csikszentmihalyi 1975/2000) and behavioral measures.

After the digital interactive experience 67.70 % of participants reported a flow state, also referring to other dimensions like feeling positive emotions, a general state of well-being and a perception of engagement. It is not surprising that recognizing the flow experience is correlated with a general satisfaction with the interaction (0.204, $p<0.01$). A key point for the issues of this chapter is the correlation between flow experience and a form of social sharing represented by the will to recommend to friends the use of the digital interactive installation (0.193, $p<0.01$). Although flow is not directly correlated with a general increase in self-efficacy for sustainability, there are some significative relations with specific dimensions (e.g. an increased willingness to know more information about the topic and to be further involved).

14.2.2.2 Discussion

Data shows that activists recognize flow as a suitable description of their political engagement, offering a fruitful construct to explore the political field. In these cases the activities are a source of engagement and self-actualization, a rewarding autotelic experience (Csikszentmihalyi 1997) that individuals tend to repeat as often as possible. The replication of the process offers an explanation for the building of a life theme, which is the unique set of goals characterizing any individual (Inghilleri 1999).

Whereas young non-activists do not identify flow in short civic activities with the same percentages recorded in the previous study, it is recognized by the majority of participants. Data also confirms the importance of unconventional projects to sustain interest in participation. Research data shows that technology can foster the experience of flow (Ghani and Deshpande 1994) (see also Chap. 16 by Triberti et al. in this volume), hence lending more support to the idea of promoting online participation.

From such perspectives flow appears to be a precious theoretical and methodological resource. Building optimal environments for participation is a key aspect to be taken into account, in order to maximize the chances of youths having positive experiences. It is fundamental to provide clear goals, adequate feedback and motivational rewards: the inability of the political field to follow such guidelines is one of the reasons for youth withdrawal from participation (Boffi 2012b). Being in flow in these circumstances can drive them to engage more often and with a higher commitment.

14.2.3 Adolescents, Identity and Transgenerational Cultural Transmission

14.2.3.1 Theoretical Issues and Empirical Data

Adolescence is a crucial period during which the characteristics of personal identity and socio-relational skills of an individual are defined. Thanks to an ever more active and engaging relationship with social groups and the culturally shared norms, adolescents face an increasing complexity of the individual system (personal and psychological world) and a necessary relationship with the social system as a whole (groups and communities) (see Chap. 15 by Hout et al. in this volume). This process, which in Western culture is no longer comparable to a simple "rite of passage" circumscribed in a highly defined manner and time frame, ferries kids from the world of childhood to a personal and unique position in the reality of adults. Adolescence becomes a period of life when individuals come into contact with an increasing number and a growing variety of stimuli, objects, people, interpretations of events, and in which they are subjectively called to take a position in respect of each of these innovations. The psychic bonds that individuals create from time to time between the internal world and the external culture are representative of needs and desires with degrees of consistency with the Self (Delle Fave et al. 2011; Terranova and Riva 2015). Driven by the desire to communicate with others, teenagers use the information and cultural objects found in their contexts of interaction to acquire more and more socio-relational skills. The presence of other- culturally more expert- people, called by some authors "mentors" (Gardner 1993; Nakamura 2014), makes the experiential context interesting and simultaneously causes the adolescent's attention to be directed in a privileged way to certain cultural objects rather than others. In this stage of life the presence of mentors is considered an important variable supporting the internalization of symbolic meanings and tools for understanding and interacting, thus directing the development of personality and identity processes.

In the psychological and social situation just described, the optimal experience occupies a central position. It relates the teenagers, and their acquired skills and those yet to be acquired, with the external environment, outlining their degree of interest and emotional involvement. Flow also becomes central to the relationship with the mentor, creating the motivation for the teenager to associate with him. Flow becomes the experience that ferries the artifacts and the disciplines promoted by mentors and, more generally, by the socio-cultural context from the outside world into the mind of the adolescent. Thus it fosters both the creative development of the teenager's identity and the transgenerational transmission of culture (deCordova et al. 2010; Inghilleri 2014). The optimal experience then connects, each time in a unique way, the intra-psychic processes of identity development with the psychosocial processes of participation in relations and acquisition of norms, values and tools related to the specific culture to which the adolescent belongs. Following is a brief description of the findings from three different research studies involving groups of Italian teenagers, with a particular focus on the relationship between flow experience, transmission of culture and creative processes of identity development.

Study 1: Adolescents and Communication Tools The sample is composed by a group of second generation immigrant adolescents (n = 20), male and female, aged between 15 and 19 years old. The sample was collected in two high schools in Milan (Italy). The aim of this research was to investigate peer to peer communication practices mediated by digital technologies among adolescents belonging to the second generation of migrants in Italy, in order to highlight the role of new technologies in the process of cultural adaptation of adolescents and routes of definition of identity that they put in place (Caselli et al. 2011; de Cordova et al. 2010).

In recent research regarding the web environment (Chen 2006; Novak and Hoffman 1997, 1998; Novak et al. 2003) it has been demonstrated that the use of new media, because of their characteristics of interactivity, may promote flow situations (see Chap. 16 by Triberti et al. in this volume). Furthermore, the research data showed that a more widespread and varied use of mediated technology and communication, as is common in the adolescent generation, would enhance and reinforce subjective optimal experience. It emerged clearly that flow experience in the use of new technologies is not evoked simply by the mediated activity per se, but is elicited by the specific situation or activities that adolescents can achieve through new use of media. Therefore the activities themselves, made accessible to people through new media, give experience of flow, while the new media act as multipliers of experiences. This role is very important in modern and global society, because the ability to access the most numerous and diverse experiences by individuals automatically produces a greater opportunity to access the state of flow.

Most of the interviewees have been able to describe several situations of flow they experienced while using new media, in different kinds of activities. In particular, some participants identified their flow situations in *relational activities*, while others found them in individual tasks that require personal involvement, creativity and the improvement of knowledge/competences (Gardner 1993; Hunter and Csikszentmihalyi 2003), such as school research or the creation of informatics artifacts. Both in individual and relational activities, participants have felt actively involved in the construction of something new, significant and socially recognized. This direct link among new media activities, optimal experience and creative artifact construction promotes adolescents' mental integration and the development and reinforcement of a more complex personal, social and cultural Self (Csikszentmihalyi 1997; Csikszentmihalyi and Rathunde 1993; Inghilleri 1999, 2003). This specific identity construction process supports them in overcoming the social pressure that forces them to choose a cultural and social adaptation model between either the one ethnocentrically proposed by Italian society, or the one which embodies their parents' country of origin, and so develop a subjective identity that mixes cultural elements of each of the two groups of belonging in a unique and creative way.

Study 2: Adolescents and Creative Schooling The sample consists of a group of 370 adolescents, Italian and immigrant, male and female, aged between 14 and 19, attending a vocational high school in Milan. The research lasted 3 years and involved working with a group of ten teachers identified as mentors of the classes involved. The aim of this research was to investigate the educational experience of children, highlighting the limitations and strengths of the current educational model, and to solve a series of communicative and relational problems highlighted by teachers. Problems included a high level of student drop out and a high level of stress perceived by the teachers.

It has been shown that optimal learning environments can promote student engagement and also improve their level of performance in study (Csikszentmihalyi 1993; Shernoff 2013; Shernoff et al. 2003; Savio and Riva 2007). The construction of optimal learning environments however, depends on both situational features and the characteristics of the group of students and teachers who need to be involved in it. For this reason the research team first of all worked to analyze and understand the experiences that were perceived as the most positive and the most negative both by the students and by the group of teachers. To do this we used the constructs of optimal experience (Csikszentmihalyi 1990) and of creativity (Gardner 1993). The results showed that 74 % of the students had experienced flow and were able to define it and recognize it. Sixty-four percent claimed to often feel states of optimal experience and could describe specific activities in which they repeatedly experience flow. Twenty-seven percent of the students demonstrated the characteristics of autotelic personality. Some of the boys experienced flow during individual type of activities (30 %), while others emphasize social situations, often linked to leisure activities. In most cases the quoted activities, whether individual or group, are of a very concrete type (like playing soccer or disassembling an engine). Seventy-one percent of the sample live creative experiences on a regular basis and can describe one or more activities stimulating their creativity. Most of the activities listed are of a concrete type and require the construction of specific material artifacts, following the construction process from the beginning to the end. These creative experiences are mostly lived in extra-curricular environments. Seventy percent of the teenagers who experienced creative situations claimed to have been in a state of flow at that moment. Forty percent of the students were able to identify the presence of one or more mentors in their personal experience. Paradoxically the persons identified as mentors are in most cases peers and only on rare occasions teachers or educators. Consequently, the results of the study have brought to the creation of learning environments where teamwork is the most valued element. Here learning takes place by doing concrete activities, and the creative work of the individual is emphasized through a peer review process.

Study 3: Adolescents, Environment and Cultural Transmission The sample consisted of Italian adolescents living in the archeological town of Tarquinia (n=84), male and female, aged between 15 and 19 years old. The 3-year project, which aimed to promote the territory and local culture, directly involved the teenagers in the experience of archaeological excavations carried out by the University of Milan. Archeology students from the university were involved as mentors. The aim of this research was to promote activities that involved the younger generation of the citizens of Tarquinia. By collaborating with the local high school, the researchers intention was to recreate a positive relationship with the environment and allow the local population to recover the value of the history and artifacts of the Etruscan culture present in the city.

Secondary school students were hosted at the archaeological site of Civita, in the city of Tarquinia, during the annual excavation of the Equipe of Etruscan studies, for three consecutive years. During the excavation the students joined the archaeologists in their daily activities. Afterwards the students completed a questionnaire assessing their experience. The questionnaires showed that 68 % of the participants had experienced flow during the excavation. Those who had not experienced flow during the excavation said that they had never experienced it elsewhere. Only 20 % of the group that had experienced flow during the excavation reported previous experiences in which they perceived similar feelings, and almost all were situations involving sports. But the most interesting data is that 80 % of the Tarquinian adolescents said they experienced flow for the first time during the archeological excavation. The activities that have been identified as triggers of states of flow are concrete activities, carried out in person, requiring a task divided into phases and often producing a result of a material type, like digging with a pick in search of shards or cleaning and classifying relics. The proportion of individuals experiencing flow in this sample is in line with the data from other studies and with the literature, but showed a special feature nonetheless (Bassi et al. 2012; de Cordova et al. 2010; Freire 2013). The participation in the excavation represented for many of the adolescents the opportunity to live that optimal experience which they had not been able to recognize in other situations. In other words, whereas the ability to experience flow falls within the average for that age, the much less rich social and environmental context compared to that of the city of Milan, does not offer a sufficient variety of situations in which the students can experience flow. So, because of an environmental understimulation, the great potential for optimal experience of this sample often does not emerge. The results show that concrete activities, such as the manipulation of real artifacts, not only introduce the teenagers directly to the history and ancient culture of their territory, but also are highly stimulating in terms of emotional involvement and in activating the states of intense well-being and intrinsic motivation. This situation promotes the development of a more profound attachment to the places where the students live and a more lively and genuine interest in the Etruscan history and culture of which the citizens of Tarquinia are custodians.

14.2.3.2 Discussion

Data shows that teenagers have a high capacity to live and identify situations of optimal experience, regardless of the context in which they live and the situations they have to deal with. The environmental variable is still extremely significant in this age group. Living in a big city, or having access to multiple virtual worlds through new technologies, are situations which offer young people the opportunity to be involved in various and creative activities, which transforms the potential of adolescents to experience flow in real situations. In contrast, poor social and environmental stimulation tends not to develop the potential of optimal experience. However, in poorly stimulating contexts teenagers welcome concrete and innovative experiences with great enthusiasm and invest all of their intrinsic motivation in these experiences and are able to find flow in a creative way.

Teenagers tend to prefer a concrete type of activity with peers, whether social or individual or productive, among tasks promoting flow and tend to prefer, as activities promoting flow, concrete types of activity, often social activities or activities that are produced, even individually, in contexts where there are other peers. Besides being material, these activities must propose a process that at the end is recognizable by the person who performs them as a tangible product, and thus evaluable in terms of goodness or creativity. These activities must have an important meaning, either for the personal story of the participant, or for the history and culture of the social group and the territory in which the young person belongs. The presence of a mentor, whether an adult or a peer, is important in recognizing the meaning and value of the artifacts produced by the activity generating flow. The role of the mentor is to make clear the links between the socio-environmental system and the artifact in question, or to enhance the quality and uniqueness of the work of the adolescent.

14.3 Conclusions

The results of the data reported in the three areas of research reveal how close the relationship is between experience of subjective well-being and socio-cultural environment. We propose considering the flow experience as an ordering principle of the daily individual and social behavior. From this perspective flow experience can be fruitfully conceived as a key selective principle guiding human subjective relationships with the environment. It is through flow experience that we enhance place attachment, select favorite places, develop intrinsic motivation to enter certain places and not others. Flow not only promotes engagement in the environment, it also prompts social involvement, participation in political or social actions and fosters activities strictly connected to social values. In order to build an optimal environment it is fundamental to provide clear goals, adequate feedback and motivational rewards, so as to encourage a rewarding autotelic experience. Finally, environment seems to be an extremely significant variable in the developmental age as it is a key element in the selection of activities that promote flow. The experience of flow will in turn allow a better use of the artifacts that culture proposes and a better transgenerational transmission of culture itself. Socio-cultural environments such as a virtual space, a school classroom, heritage sites, are all places rich in stimuli, artifacts, experiences and meanings that are available to the new generations for them to create a bond between their individual and culture identity and the complex changes of the world around them.

References

Bassi, M., Ferrario, N., Ba, G., Delle Fave, A., & Viganò, C. (2012). Quality of experience during psychosocial rehabilitation: A real-time investigation with experience sampling method. *Psychiatric Rehabilitation Journal, 35*, 447–453.

Berto, R. (2014). The role of nature in coping with psycho-physiological stress: A literature review on restorativeness. *Behavioral Sciences, 4*(4), 394–409.

Boffi, M. (2012a). *Flow as a measure of political engagement*. ECPP 2012. 6th European conference on positive psychology. 26–29 June, Moscow.

Boffi, M. (2012b). Politicians as cultural selectors: favoring or discouraging youth participation. *Human Affairs: Postdisciplinary Humanities & Social Sciences Quarterly*, *22*(3), 325–334.

Boffi, M., Riva, E., & Rainisio, N. (2014). Positive change and political participation: Well-being as an indicator of the quality of citizens' engagement. In P. Inghilleri, G. Riva, & E. Riva (Eds.), *Enabling positive change. Flow and complexity in daily experience* (pp. 105–122). Warsaw: De Gruyter.

Bonnes, M., Bonaiuto, M., Aiello, A., Perugini, M., & Ercolani, P. (1997). A transactional perspective on residential satisfaction. In C. Despres & D. Pichè (Eds.), *Housing surveys: Advances in theory, and methods* (pp. 75–99). Quebec: CRAD Universitè Laval.
Caselli, M., de Cordova, F., Riva, E., & Vittadini, N. (2011). Tecnologie digitali e pratiche identitarie tra gli adolescenti figli di famiglie immigrate (numero monografico). *Ikon : forme e processi del comunicare*, 58/59.
Chen, H. (2006). Flow on the net–detecting web users positive affects and their flow states. *Computers in Human Behavior, 22*, 221–233.
Csikszentmihalyi, M. (1975/2000). *Beyond boredom and anxiety*. San Francisco: Jossey-Bass.
Csikszentmihalyi, M. (1990). *Flow: The psychology of optimal experience*. New York: Harper & Row.
Csikszentmihalyi, M. (1993). *The evolving self: A psychology for a third millennium*. New York: HarperCollins.
Csikszentmihalyi, M. (1997). *Finding flow. The psychology of engagement with everyday life*. New York: Basic Books.
Csikszentmihalyi, M., & Csikszentmihalyi, I. (2006). *A life worth living: Contributions to positive psychology*. New York: Oxford University Press.
Csikszentmihalyi, M., & Massimini, F. (1985). On the psychological selection of bio-cultural information. *New Ideas in Psychology, 3*(2), 115–138.
Csikzentmihalyi, M., & Rathunde, K. (1993). The measurement of flow in everyday life. Toward a theory of emergent motivation. In *Nebraska symposium of motivation, 40*. Lincoln: University of Nebraska Press.
de Cordova, F., Riva, E., & Vittadini, N. (2010). Emerging communication practices and how they affect immigrant adolescents in their developmental process. In N. Billias (Ed.), *Proceedings of the 5th Global Conference of Cybercultures*. Salzburg:Interdisciplinary Net.
Delle Fave, A. (2007). Individual development and community empowerment: Suggestions from studies on optimal experience. In J. Haworth & G. Hart (Eds.), *Well-being: Individual, community, and societal perspectives* (pp. 41–56). London: Palgrave McMillan.
Delle Fave, A., & Massimini, F. (1992). The ESM and the measurement of clinical change: A case of anxiety disorder. In M. W. de Vries (Ed.), *The experience of psychopathology: Investigating mental disorders in their natural settings* (pp. 280–289). New York: Cambridge.
Delle Fave, A., Massimini, F., & Bassi, M. (2011). *Psychological selection and optimal experience across cultures: Social empowerment through personal growth* (Vol. 2). New York: Springer Science & Business Media.
Freire, T. (2013). *Positive leisure science: From subjective experience to social context*. Dordrecht: Springer.
Gardner, H. (1993). *Multiple intelligences: The theory in practice*. New York: Basic Books.
Gardner, H., Csikszentmihalyi, M., & Damon, W. (2001). *Good work: When excellence and ethics meet*. New York: Basic Books.
Ghani, J. A., & Deshpande, S. P. (1994). Task characteristics and the experience of optimal flow in human—computer interaction. *The Journal of Psychology, 128*(4), 381–391.
Han, K. T. (2003). A reliable and valid self-rating measure of the restorative quality of natural environments. *Landscape & Urban Planning, 995*, 1–24.
Hanss, D., & Böhm, G. (2010). Can I make a difference? The role of general and domain-specific self-efficacy in sustainable consumption decisions. *Umweltpsychologie, 14*, 46–74.
Hartig, T., & Staats, H. (2006). The need for psychological restoration as a determinant of environmental preferences. *Journal of Environmental Psychology, 26*, 215–226.
Hartig, T., Korpela, K., Evans, G. W., & Garling, T. (1997). A measure of restorative quality in environments. *Scandinavian Housing & Planning Research, 23*, 3–26.
Hunter, J. P., & Csikszentmihalyi, M. (2003). The positive psychology of interested adolescents. *Journal of Youth and Adolescence, 32*(1), 27–35.
Inghilleri, P. (1999). *From subjective experience to cultural change*. New York: Cambridge University Press.

Inghilleri, P. (2003). *La "buona vita". Per l'uso creativo degli oggetti nella società dell'abbondanza*. Milano: Guerini e Associati.
Inghilleri, P. (Ed.). (2009). *Psicologia Culturale*. Milano: Raffaello Cortina Editore.
Inghilleri, P. (2014). Phenomenology of positive change: Social growth. In P. Inghilleri, G. Riva, & E. Riva (Eds.), *Enabling positive change. Flow and complexity in daily experience* (pp. 6–17). Warsaw: De Gruyter.
Inghilleri, P., Boffi, M., Rainisio, N., & Pola, L. (2013). The sustainable lightness of participating: New paths of civic engagement for youth. In *Beyond the crisis. Building community and critical visions to achieve justice, fairness and wellbeing*. 6–7 Nov, Naples.
Inghilleri, P., Riva, G., & Riva, E. (2014). Introduction. Positive change in global world: Creative individuals and complex societies. In P. Inghilleri, G. Riva, & E. Riva (Eds.), *Enabling positive change. Flow and complexity in daily experience* (pp. 1–5). Warsaw: De Gruyter.
Jackson, S. A., & Marsh, H. W. (1996). Development and validation of a scale to measure optimal experience: The flow state scale. *Journal of Sport & Exercise Psychology, 18*, 17–35.
Kaplan, S., & Kaplan, R. (1983). *Cognition and environment: Functioning in an uncertain world*. Ann Arbor: Ulrich's.
Klar, M., & Kasser, T. (2009). Some benefits of being an activist: Measuring activism and its role in psychological well-being. *Political Psychology, 30*(5), 755–777.
Massimini, F., & Delle Fave, A. (2000). Individual development in a bio-cultural perspective. *American Psychologist, 55*, 24–33.
Muzio, M. (Ed.). (2004). *Sport: Flow e Prestazione Eccellente*. Milano: Franco Angeli Editore.
Nakamura, J. (2014). Positive change and mentoring in adulthood. In P. Inghilleri, G. Riva, & E. Riva (Eds.), *Enabling positive change. Flow and complexity in daily experience* (pp. 166–182). Warsaw: De Gruyter.
Novak, T. P., & Hoffman, D. L. (1997). Measuring the flow experience among web users. *Interval Research Corporation*, 31 July.
Novak, T. P., & Hoffman, D. L. (1998). *Modeling the structure of the flow experience among web users*. INFORMS Marketing Science and the Internet Mini-Conference MIT, Mar 1998.
Novak, T. P., Hoffman, D. L., & Duhachek, A. (2003). The influence of goal-directed and experiential activities on online flow experiences. *Journal of Consumer Psychology, 13*(1&2), 3–16.
Prilleltensky, I., Nelson, G., & Peirson, L. (2001). The role of power and control in children's lives: An ecological analysis of pathways toward wellness, resilience and problems. *Journal of Community & Applied Social Psychology, 11*(2), 143–158.
Rainisio, N. (2012). *Nature del benessere. Gli effetti psicologici dell'ambiente naturale in una prospettiva bio-culturale*. Unpublished doctoral thesis, Università degli Studi di Milano.
Rainisio, N., & Inghilleri, P. (2013). Culture, environmental psychology, and well-being: An emergent theoretical framework. In A. Delle Fave & H. Knoop (Eds.), *Well-being and cultures* (pp. 103–116). The Netherlands: Springer.
Rainisio, N., Boffi, M., & Riva, E. (2014). Positive change in environment: Aesthetics, environmental flowability and well-being. In P. Inghilleri, G. Riva, & E. Riva (Eds.), *Enabling positive change: Flow and complexity in daily experience* (pp. 91–104). Warsaw: De Gruyter.
Savio, A., & Riva, E. (2007). La città policentrica: il ruolo dei servizi nella definizione dei processi identitari. *Passaggi. Rivista Italiana di Scienze Transculturali, 14*(7), 15–53.
Shernoff, D. J. (2013). *Optimal learning environments to promote student engagement*. New York: Springer.
Shernoff, D. J., Csikszentmihalyi, M., Schneider, B., & Shernoff, E. S. (2003). Student engagement in high school classrooms from the perspective of flow theory. *School Psychology Quarterly, 18*, 158–176.
Terranova Cecchini, R., & Riva, E. (2015). Dalla psiche africana a una visione transculturale dell'uomo: l'apporto di Ibrahima Sow. In E. D'Ippolito (Ed.), *Ibrahima Sow: L'io culturale. Dall'etnopsichiatria alla transcultura* (pp. 9–15). Rome: Armando Editore.

Ulrich, R. S. (1983). Aesthetic and affective responses to natural environments. In I. Altman & J. F. Wohlwill (Eds.), *Human behavior and environment: Behavior and the natural environment* (Vol. 6, pp. 85–125). New York: Plenum.
Velarde, M. D., Fry, G., & Tveit, M. (2007). Health effects of viewing landscapes-landscape types. *Environmental Psychology. Urban Forestry & Urban Greening, 6*, 199–212.
Wilson, E. O. (1984). *Biophilia*. Cambridge: Harvard University Press.

Chapter 15
The Application of Team Flow Theory

Jef J.J. van den Hout, Orin C. Davis, and Bob Walrave

Abstract Despite the noted potential for 'team flow' to enhance a team's effectiveness, productivity, performance, and capabilities, studies on the construct are scarce. Most research on flow has been conducted either at the individual level, which generally constitutes the experience of complete absorption while working on a task, or at the artistic ensemble level, which reflects a gestalt group experience. But, team flow in the work environment, where teams differ from performance groups, has not yet been studied or reported. One of the reasons for this is the difficulty applying theories of flow to the team level, because the research on flow, group flow, and team dynamics does not readily gel. In this chapter, however, we will briefly discuss the precursors and components of team flow and its consequences. We will also describe how these precursors and components work by giving some examples of team flow experiences in different environments. Our analysis provides both theoretical insights into the causes of the emergence of team flow and practical suggestions for work teams to foster team flow experiences.

15.1 Introduction

Concurrent with Csikszentmihalyi's delineation of flow (for a review, see Csikszentmihalyi 1990) was the idea that flow might also be connected with the dynamics of a cohesive group. Researchers like Keith Sawyer (2003, 2006, 2007) have developed this theory into a conception of 'group flow' that describes how the group, as a unit, experiences an analog of the flow state. Much of their work, however, focuses on group creativity and the development of innovation. Sawyer's

J.J.J. van den Hout (✉) • B. Walrave
School of Industrial Engineering, Eindhoven University of Technology,
P.O. Box 513, 5600 MB Eindhoven, The Netherlands
e-mail: j.j.j.v.d.hout@tue.nl; b.walrave@tue.nl

O.C. Davis
City University of New York, Baruch College, New York, NY, USA

University of Massachusetts Boston, Boston, MA, USA
e-mail: davisoc@gmail.com

L. Harmat et al. (eds.), *Flow Experience*, DOI 10.1007/978-3-319-28634-1_15

work was developed through the study of groups engaged in the arts, especially musicians and thespians. As noted by Snow (2010), there is little work that reviews the dynamics of team flow experiences in the workplace outside the context of creative production.

Flow is a subjective experience in which people report performing their best; when in flow, the individual operates at full capacity (Nakamura and Csikszentmihalyi 2002). The defining feature of flow is intense experiential involvement in moment-to-moment activity; attention is fully invested in the task at hand, and the person functions at his or her fullest capacity. A host of studies have found a strong positive relationship between flow and performance. Even more compelling are the developmental implications of flow: as individuals master challenges in an activity, they develop greater levels of skill, and the activity ceases to be as involving as before. To continue experiencing flow, they must identify increasingly greater challenges. Thus, over time, the balance between challenges and skills enhances competence, and even mastery (Csikszentmihalyi et al. 2005).

Consistent with Kozlowski and Klein's (2000) multilevel approach, as well as Gully et al.'s (2002) contention that constructs experienced at the individual level can be aggregated when they are being assessed at the team level, we maintain that when *all* team members are experiencing flow concomitant with pursuing the team's common purpose, there is a collective flow experience which we define as *team flow*.

Here, our aim is to investigate which organizational climates foster the collective flow experiences for collaborating team members, and which constructs are experienced when the collective team flow experience occurs. We introduce an integrated theory of team flow, which extrapolates the construct of individual flow to the team level. We then turn to the precursors (climates) and components (constructs) of team flow, after which we propose interventions that could ignite the team flow experience.

15.2 Flow Theory in a Team Context

During the individual experience of flow when being part of a team, a team member perceives the original nine conditions of flow, which are (1) clear proximal goals every step of the way, (2) immediate feedback to one's actions, (3) balance between challenges and skills, (4) no worry of failure, (5) distractions excluded from consciousness, (6) a merging of action and awareness, (7) the disappearance of self-consciousness, (8) distorted sense of time, (9) the activity is done for its own sake (intrinsically rewarding [autotelic]) (Csikszentmihalyi 1996). For a team environment, the nine conditions of the original flow theory can be distinguished into antecedents, scaffolds, and components, but they appear in modified forms at the team level, as we will discuss.

The first five can be coined as antecedents (external conditions) that foster flow and the latter four as components (internal conditions) that indicate flow

(Csikszentmihalyi 1994; Hamilton and Hurford 2007). Yet, the antecedent 'no worry of failure' can also be seen as a component of flow if thought of as 'a sense of control'. The same goes for 'distractions excluded from consciousness' if it is interpreted as 'concentration' (Hamilton and Hurford 2007; Nakamura and Csikszentmihalyi 2002). Because these two *antecedents* can be created by the individual and subsequently arise as a *component*, we refer to them as *scaffolds* of the individual flow experience in a team context rather than antecedents or components. That is, they create the bridge necessary for the individual to cross into a flow experience.

A key facet of this conception is that the antecedents, and to some extent the scaffolds, are within the control of the individual, such that (s)he can directly influence if or how these antecedents are created. In fact, in team contexts, individuals can affect the development and/or progress of these antecedents for other team members, and thus make it possible for the components (which are outside the control of the individual) to emerge.

15.3 The Team Flow Theory

15.3.1 The Precursors for Team Flow

We expect that team flow creates a group-level state in which all participating team members are completely involved in their common activity, and are working together intuitively and synergistically towards the common purpose (cf. Sawyer 2006, 2007). Therefore, while experiencing team flow, individual team members are experiencing the mental state of flow simultaneously by executing their personal task for the team. The question this raises is how a team can establish a dynamic in which this is possible, and we posit that the establishment of such a dynamic requires a set of baseline conditions, or *precursors*.

We argue that the precursors follow from the collective ambition that all team members share (Posner et al. 1985; Ready and Truelove 2011; Weggeman 2007), particularly insofar as it is the starting point and *raison d'être* of the team. Starting from the existence of a collective ambition we distill six precursors. (1) *Common goal*: The presence of a common goal that is shared by all team members (cf. Sawyer 2007). The common goal of the team should be clear and meaningful to all team members, compatible with members' individual goal(s), internalized by all team members and growth-promoting. (2) *Aligned personal goals*: The presence of personal goals that contribute to achieving the common goal. The personal goals established are clearly defined, meaningful and specific, and also provide growth and development for the individual team member (Locke and Latham 2006; O'leary-kelly et al. 1994). The personal goals unite the individual team members and create a 'clear proximal goal' for each of them. As noted, a clear proximal goal is one of the antecedents of individual flow. (3) *High skill integration*: The integration of complementary, high-level skills present within each individual team member.

In the distribution of tasks all team members are deployed on a challenging task/role that suits their preferences, talents, knowledge, and skills (Katzenbach and Smith 1992; Salas et al. 2008). For this to happen, everyone on the team must have roughly comparable [high] levels of skill, along with some specific unique skills, which together are representative for his/her specific role in the team. In this way, the individual forces are optimally utilized and combined to create a degree of synergy (win-win) through their collaboration. (4) *Open communication*: Open and transparent communication ensures that all team members know exactly how each delivers his/her contribution to the team (Sawyer 2007). In this way each team member has his/her perspective broadened by the other members of the team, which is also one of the conditions of interpersonal flow (Snow 2010). To achieve this, feedback is required on each individual's personal task, the joint team task, and the process of collaboration. The feedback given must be clear, constructive, and encouraging. This kind of feedback helps team members to build on their interactions and achieve the common goal in the most efficient and effective way (Guzzo and Salas 1995). This implies that team members listen to each other and achieve familiarity with each other (cf. Sawyer 2007). A form of open communication within the team environment gives each individual team member the requisite 'immediate feedback' about the joint progress that is being made. (5) *Safety*: A psychologically safe environment to perform personal tasks in the interest of the team. To achieve a safe environment, unnecessary and unacceptable risks are eliminated, but the possibility of failure still exists for each team member. The goal is, after all, set at a challenging level to release high skills. Therefore, failure is seen as an opportunity for growth and team members support each other in achieving these challenging goals without worrying about what others think (cf. Snow 2010). Safety within the team environment decreases each individual team member's worries about his/her performance on the task at hand. As Sawyer (2007) notes, this uses the potential for failure to push the group towards the flow state rather than being intimidated by it. Having 'no worries of failure' is defined as a scaffold of individual flow that can be partly designed or structured in the work environment and thus can act as an antecedent. Safety is therefore an important contributor to our proposed team flow component *sense of shared trust* (see below). (6) *Mutual commitment*: The responsibility to engage with each other to achieve the desired common goal with devotion and dedication. Everyone is aware of how the tasks are distributed, the process of pursuing the target (goal), and the current state of the project. Team members support each other in creating the ideal team dynamics to achieve the common goal with task-oriented behavior and accountability for fulfilling responsibilities (Katzenbach and Smith 1993). Mutual commitment within the team environment decreases the availability of distractions for each team member (Aubé and Rousseau 2005), which makes it possible for everyone to concentrate on the task at hand (Csikszentmihalyi 1996; Sawyer 2007). The degree of commitment of the individuals is often mentioned as a potential mediating mechanism to performance (Aubé et al. 2014; Landhäußer and Keller 2012; Nakamura and Csikszentmihalyi 2009). When mutually committed, team members are intensely involved in a shared, meaningful activity and are able to remain concentrated on this activity as long as necessary to achieve the common goals.

15.3.2 The Components of Team Flow

Once team flow is achieved, one shares a number of experiences at the team level, which we term the components: (1) *Shared identity*: The collective ambition of the team, constituting the reason of team existence, is the first component of team flow, and is about the shared sense of intrinsic motivation to operate and to perform as a team based on shared values and recognition of complementary skills. This feeling and recognition forms the basis for a shared identity, which is also mentioned as a condition for interpersonal flow (Snow 2010). In addition, other components could also be shared with each other, if the precursors are optimally derived from the collective ambition. (2) *A sense of unity*: A shared feeling that together the team forms a unity by expressing the collective ambition of the team. The feeling of unity is partly the result of setting aligned personal goals that each contribute to the common goal, which in turn is derived from the collective ambition. Team members experience a sense of unity that is also consistent with Csikszentmihalyi's (1990) notion of a loss of self-consciousness in the sense that one is not paying attention to one's own needs in favor of focusing on the activity at hand. Concordantly, Snow (2010) describes this effect as not feeling self-conscious with each other, and Sawyer (2007) views it as a true blending of egos. (3) *Trust*: The shared feeling of trust to accomplish the joint task together. This feeling arises because people feel safe to act (i.e., no worry of failure) and they know exactly how they are doing through the open form of communication that delivers the required feedback. This feeling of being in control is described by Sawyer (2007) as having the autonomy to take any ideas which come out and run with them based on their merits rather than on being granted permission. Formally, trust is mostly defined as: "the willingness to be vulnerable" (Mayer et al. 1995, 712), which reflects the willingness to accept a limited degree of control over the final outcome and thus the readiness to depend on the other team member(s). When there is trust, team members do not worry about failure, and instead feel confident to act because of the acceptance and support they receive to do their job (see also safety). They trust that their joint actions will have a positive outcome whatever happens next. A team flow experience feeds team members' perceptions of a safe climate in which to act, because they have experience trusting each other's capabilities to achieve a common task. This is in line with the findings of Salanova et al. (2014) that believe in collective efficacy predicts collective flow over time, and that they are reciprocally related. (4) *Sense of joint progress*: The shared feeling of making progress together in achieving the goals and the cooperation with each other. This feeling arises because people join forces (high skill integration) and communicate openly with each other. Because of the open form of communication everybody knows exactly how they are doing and what should be the next joint action (integration of high skills) in achieving both their common and personal goals. (5) *Holistic Focus*: The realization that there is a collective consciousness among team members to promote the collective ambition, resulting in a shared focus on their cooperation and achievement of the goals set. This form of 'holistic focus,' which is comparable with Snow's (2010) condition 'having total concentration on the shared activity,' arises from a mutual

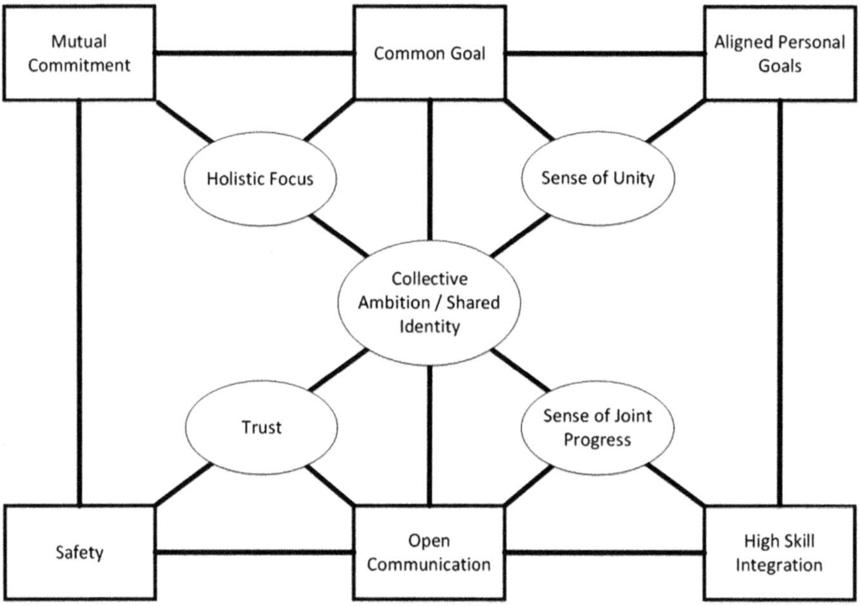

Fig. 15.1 Precursors and components of team flow

commitment to the common goal and from that the concentration on allocated tasks (Katzenbach and Smith 1993). The presence of the components for team flow determine whether and to what extent team flow occurs.

Figure 15.1, summarizing the discussion so far, shows the six precursors (rectangles) to achieve team flow and the components (ovals) that characterize the shared experienced of team flow. This figure illustrates the relationships between the precursors and the components. Taking into consideration team flow theory, we expect that a team first needs to determine their *collective ambition*, which operates as starting point of flow and turns into a component (shared identity) when all precursors are met. The precursors mutual commitment and common goal primarily determine the presence of the shared component *holistic focus*, the precursors common goal and aligned personal goals mainly determine the presence of the shared component *sense of unity with the team*, the precursors high skill integration and open communication mainly determine the presence of the shared component *sense of joint progress*, and the precursors open communication and safety mainly determine the presence of the shared component *trust*.

15.4 Consequences of Team Flow

Team flow provides team members with several consequences. In flow, one is fully dedicated to the task(s) at hand, with an intense focus and full concentration. The performance of the task seems to go spontaneously without any effort (effortless action) (Csikszentmihalyi 1990, 1996; Nakamura and Csikszentmihalyi 2009). This optimal experience in which one is intrinsically motivated to persist in their activities will logically lead to *a better performance* (Landhäußer and Keller 2012). Experiencing flow also provides *satisfaction* (Csikszentmihalyi 1990, 1996, 2004).

If flow experiences go together (integrate) in a team environment, its members help each other and to excel as a unit. In this respect, Aubé et al. (2014) found that the flow experience is positively related to team performance and this relationship is mediated by team goal commitment and moderated by the level of information exchange between team members. When team members share this feeling with each other it intensifies the feeling (Walker 2010) and binds the team members together more tightly (i.e., cohesion) (cf. Sawyer 2007; Widmeyer et al. 1986).

Perhaps most important: In flow, people proceed in a situation of high challenge where they have to show high (new) skills to control the situation (Asakawa 2004). In these situations their ability to learn new things is greater because they have to develop their skillset further in order to carry out the task to control the situation. The presence of teammates greatly enhances such *development* by the direct possibility of task feedback. The team members can correct themselves at both the individual and team levels and, as such, there is development on both levels. Experiencing flow creates a desire for a new challenge (Abuhamdeh and Csikszentmihalyi 2009). In a team, the desire for a new collective challenge can be even more intense because the team flow experience is of great significance (meaning) and therefore delivers more intense satisfaction. When there are opportunities to fulfill these desires for new challenges, this could result in a great level of *positive energy* among team members.

15.5 Examples of the Team Flow Experience

Csikszentmihalyi (1990) has given several examples of flow experiences while being part of a team. The following example is about the work of surgeons (Csikszentmihalyi 1990, p. 65): "*Surgeons say that during a difficult operation they have the sensation that the entire operating team is a single organism, moved by the same purpose; they describe it as a "ballet" in which the individual is subordinated to the group performance, and all involved share in a feeling of harmony and power.*"

To provide more face-validity to our model of team flow, and understand better how the flow conditions work in team environments we conducted several in depth interviews and conducted case studies in different areas. In this chapter we will briefly report some relevant citations that exemplify the team flow theory. (Note that, for privacy reasons, all names have been anonymized.)

15.5.1 Interview with a Member of a Successful Orchestra

In 2011 a group of musicians appeared in the Netherlands who were sold out for all their concerts, performed at all important festivals and won almost every prize that could be won in the Dutch music industry. Newspapers described the band as a bunch of musicians who were bouncing with optimal mutual chemistry, which also characterizes our concept of team flow. To find out what happened in this group, we conducted an in-depth interview with one of their musicians who was one of the rappers of the band. He recognized and agreed to our definition of team flow and confirmed this with words as: "*As you describe it, we have certainly experienced it. Both within the group and externally. There was a clear gradient in, because we knew it was a temporary project; we do it now, then quit and go on to the next project. Afterwards, we pulled back together and we found that we are more a band than we thought we were.*" This quote also suggests that the team flow experience gives most team members the desire to reconvene as a team again. The rapper confirmed that he experienced the band more as a team rather than a group. This is because of the mutual accountability of a team that is not always present in a group. He said: "*At such times you are creating moments where everybody feels that you must be present and capture the moment. This feeling reaches everyone as a domino effect, you can go on then until five o'clock in the night. Whatever happens, this kind of experiences triggers the feeling again, that these moments will happen more often, because everyone then realizes again what the strength of such a moment is. Living this way is a prerequisite to make beautiful things!*" About a safe environment he continues: "*You must have trust in feedback, so that there is a connection which you can build on.*" This last statement exemplifies the relation between open communication and trust within the team flow model. Moreover: "*The willingness to bring the group to a higher level should always be more important than individual progress. Of course there are 'egos' in the band, but they are extremely well good positioned. The whole is more important than the individual in the group. This allows you to grow as an individual. The band had everyone feel this way, the different energy of all different members made sure that things were created by them that they had never achieved before.*" He also clearly mentioned that the context where they play together is of great importance to achieve team flow. "*It is a gathering of variables, it has to do with the people in the group. Openness within the group, spontaneity of yourself and your peers and simplicity of the moment are all very important. It requires something for people who are part of the group not to be too anxious, and dare to have a certain surrender to the moment. That is very important to enforce that context again and again where 'things' happen.*"

15.5.2 Interview with a CEO of a Successful Team-Based Organization

This example is a home-care organization with small teams, consisting of (district) nurses and nurses providing care at home. They started in 2006 and have grown to a home care organization with more than 650 teams and 8,000 employees. The decision to work with small, professional self-managing teams who focus on the relationship with their client is the main reason for their success. We conducted an interview with their business leader, and asked him how team flow emerges in the context of the self-managing teams: "*Flow in teams happens when you pursue the same [goal] with each other, you do that with people who like to see each other, trust each other, then the energy goes to the right things, and then you do not have to invest energy in all kind of things that do not matter. If you look at the people I work with, these are all friendly relations, where there is a shared work experience with each other, where we know each other well and can rely on each other, which brings you very quickly to the essentials. We don't have to talk about policy that you see happening in a lot of organizations. You can work very instrumentally, and we do not want to develop policies. So what we do is: If there is a problem which must be solved, you look for the right people and set them together to do something meaningful and then we get started*". The reason why they have chosen for self-managing teams is to create an optimal work environment for their employees. "*The most optimal environment for our employees is one without bureaucracy. We try just to be specific in why we are there* [i.e., *raison d'être*], *so that our employees can focus on what they encounters. The context is guiding, and we try not to distract our employees with too much overflowing top-down communication.*" To support teams in their work the organization has not employed team leaders but only coaches, which can be consulted on request. They do not want to lead teams but only support them when needed. "*We continuously try to move along with our teams. There is a great diversity among teams and you need to connect to the process of each team. The coach needs to listen and ask on the basis of what is wise to do for the team. By doing this, you see that teams in our organization develop their capacity to resolve thing themselves. What we do need is a very clear framework on vision, content, and way of working and we try to reach a clear shared understanding on those items with our teams.*"

In the examples above, you can read that during team flow experiences members are set challenging situations. Team members experience themselves as a unit with one purpose [collective ambition] and where the individual is subordinated to the team [aligned personal goals to the common goal] and all are contributing by delivering with their unique skillset [high skill integration]. The outcome is during a team flow experience often more than their expectations of it before, together with intense satisfaction and a desire to reconvene.

For organizations, it is important to create an context together where people feel safe to give themselves to the moment. Where they can be open and spontaneous with their complementary skills, and where everybody commits to the common purpose. In the next paragraph, we will discuss how to create an environment for team flow experiences.

15.6 The Team Flow Environment

It is difficult to build wellbeing at work, in large part because it is challenging to find meaning in work (Wrzesniewski et al. 2003); it is important for people to care about what they are doing and decide for themselves the contexts in which they will apply their effort, attention, care and connection. As such, a key component of productivity in knowledge work is the creation of meaning. In teams, such meaning has the potential to develop into an internalized *raison d'etre* that can translate into a foundation for team flow. Consequently, employers should invest in developing and aligning collective, team, and personal ambitions for their organizations, and make sure that this fit is a constant in the workplace.

For team flow experiences, members of teams have to create an environment where they are all committed to a collective ambition [common purpose] in a manner that they all are able to experience flow. Then, together they define the precursors that fit to their collective ambition and support one another to keep each other on track. Teamwork is not as easy as one thinks and organizations should be aware that they need to invest extra resources to create a good performance climate.

From this, the precursors for team flow help to derive guidelines and interventions that could spark the presence of the team flow experience. The precursors for team flow foster an environment (social system) for joint flow experiences in teams. To foster team flow experiences in the workplace environment, it is useful to consider which key precursors can be most easily facilitated by the team itself or the employer. Therefore we extracted nine steps that teams could follow to design a team flow environment where the chance for team flow experiences is more likely to occur.

1. Identify team members' underlying motivations, shared values, and unifying strengths that united them as a team and formulate *a collective ambition*.
2. Align from the collective ambition a concrete *common goal* that is achievable and challenging *and* can be reached in a foreseeable period of time.
3. Set for each member of the team an *aligned personal goal* that also fosters meaning, growth, and intrinsic motivation for each person.
4. Derive from the common and personal goals the tasks (roles) and responsibilities into a clear process (strategy) in which each team member is able to execute his or her personal strengths where together those strengths form a unified force (*integration of high skills*).
5. Optimize mutual feedback on process and outcome so that everyone knows how (s)he is doing, as well as the team as a whole (*open communication*).
6. Create an environment in which one feels safe to act by eliminating unacceptable risks and supporting each other with positive and encouraging feedback (safety).
7. Hold each other accountable to accomplish the tasks successfully with dedication and vigor. Keep each other on track by coaching each other on the task (feed forward) and take care of the presence of the precursors for team flow. (*mutual commitment*).
8. Allow the team to function on its own (autonomous) and share experiences of unity, trust, focus, progress, and identity and sometimes magic moments like team flow.
9. Evaluate, reflect, and enjoy the moments of team flow and reconvene for new collective ambitions and shared goals.

The above steps can help to create a team flow environment for business teams. In addition, we have developed an instrument to measure the conditions and components of team flow. The name of this questionnaire is the Team Flow Monitor

(TFM). By utilizing the TFM participants can determine which precursors are present within their team and which are not. Together with their supervision or support they can decide which interventions will be included in an action plan to build a team flow environment. Also, these results help to decide upon which precursors a team should start to intervene. For instance, when a team scores low on the component 'trust' they might consider employing interventions that support 'safety' and/or 'open communication'.

15.7 Discussion and Future Research

As noted above, the individual can generate the external conditions of flow during a solo activity (Csikszentmihalyi 1994). If we view external conditions as being created by a participant in an activity, then an extension to the team level would suggest that everyone participating in the activity has the ability to facilitate the creation of the external conditions for flow. For example, team members can set goals, give and receive feedback on each other's progress, and try to remove distractions and unacceptable risks to maintain team members' concentration and focus. All these activities concern team interactions that involve members directing, aligning, coordinating, and monitoring task work to achieve collective goals (Marks et al. 2001), which is consistent with prior research that defines teamwork as comprising interpersonal interactions that are necessary to accomplish team goals, such as exchanging information and coordinating actions (Bowers et al. 1997). Teamwork differs from taskwork in that the latter implies an interaction with tasks, tools, machines, and systems and teamwork interacts with other team members (Bowers et al. 1997).

If the formation of a team is founded by the collective ambition of its members, and together the team members design an environment to collaborate, team members will instantiate the precursors for team flow by themselves (if not, this is readily guided). The precursors for team flow can in turn help team members to express their collective ambition in an efficient, effective, and personally-meaningful way, which results in a better performance. As such, we conclude that the presence of a strongly shared 'collective ambition' of a team has strong positive correlations with the presence of all precursors for team flow. Of course, future empirical studies should be directed toward confirming such a conclusion.

So far, we focused on external conditions for individual flow and precursors for team flow experiences. The multilevel theory of flow suggests that individual flow is the foundation for team flow and may exert a unique influence on it, distinct from team processes. So, the next step is to conceptualize a mechanism that may explain this relationship. According to our view of flow theory in a team context, individuals, as living open systems, need to perceive the external conditions to experience flow internally. In teams, fellow team members can help each other to create this optimal environment for flow experiences. The external conditions for flow can be designed and structured in the work environment by the individual, team members, and/or management, which is consistent with Katzenbach and Smith's (1993, p. 112) definition of a team: "*a small number of people with complementary skills who are committed to a common purpose, set of performance goals, and approach for which they hold themselves mutually accountable*". From this perspective, team members are responsible for each other's flow experiences, and the interdependent team members provide the external conditions for each other. This suggests that when individual team members engage in opportunities for action, they spark flow experiences for each other by setting a social action system in which every single team member in his/her personal task environment is surrounded by the external conditions for flow. The precursors prevent each individual's set external conditions from conflicting with the establishment of others' external conditions. In this way, it is possible that everyone involved in the same activity is experiencing flow during the execution of his or her personal task.

Once team flow emerges, a climate has a reality that is partly independent of the individual actions that gave rise to it, and, as a collective property, it guides individual and collective actions (Morgeson and Hofmann 1999). In the domain of flow, a supportive climate for flow experiences may enhance team flow and thus acts as the process linking individual flow and team flow. To summarize we propose that the average level of individual flow in a team is positively related to the experience of the components of team flow via a supportive climate (the presence of the precursors altogether) for team flow. This conclusion also provides an interesting starting point for future research.

15.8 Conclusion

In conclusion, team flow is characterized by a situation in which all the team members are completely involved in their common activities as part of a collaboration toward the common purpose. *Team flow* can be considered a function of an individual's experience of flow during the execution of one's personal task in a team context with three core aspects: (1) it is an individual team member who experiences the mental state of flow by executing his/her personal task; (2) the team member derives flow from the team dynamic which is structured by a collective ambition that set the precursors which are shared goals (team and personal), high skill integration, open communication, safety, and mutual commitment; and (3) team members share a dynamic that reflects a state of flow as a whole, which is characterized by five specific components: trust, holistic focus, a sense of unity, a sense of joint progress, and a shared identity [that expresses the collective ambition]. The occurrence of team flow leads to a meaningful experience and satisfaction for the individual team members, which is probably stronger than experiencing solitary flow. Also, a desire to reconvene as a team and an extension of the team's capability are further consequences of team flow.

To help people to experience more flow it is important to build the conditions for entering flow in people's work but also to teach and train them to be aware of conditions to let flow be more likely to emerge. The whole in this case is definitely more than the sum of its parts. In addition, one must respect the fact that there are personal and internal factors, over which limited control can be exercised, limiting the emergence of the internal conditions. As such, a key point is that flow cannot occur on demand – indeed, attempts to control or force it often backfire (Csikszentmihalyi 1997; Gardner et al. 2001), but it is possible to set an environment where team flow experiences are more likely to occur.

It is our hope that this theory can provide a common language for scholars and practitioners, and shed light on unanswered questions in the literature relevant to flow and work teams. We submit this model to the research and practitioner communities in the hopes that they will partner with us to find the most effective ways to enable the highest levels of team performance.

References

Abuhamdeh, S., & Csikszentmihalyi, M. (2009). Intrinsic and extrinsic motivational orientations in the competitive context: An examination of person–situation interactions. *Journal of Personality, 77*(5), 1615–1635. doi:10.1111/j.1467-6494.2009.00594.x.

Asakawa, K. (2004). Flow experience and autotelic personality in japanese college students: How do they experience challenges in daily life? *Journal of Happiness Studies, 5*(2), 123–154. doi:10.1023/B:JOHS.0000035915.97836.89.

Aubé, C., & Rousseau, V. (2005). Team goal commitment and team effectiveness: The role of task interdependence and supportive behaviors. *Group Dynamics: Theory, Research, and Practice, 9*(3), 189–204. doi:10.1037/1089-2699.9.3.189.

Aubé, C., Brunelle, E., & Rousseau, V. (2014). Flow experience and team performance: The role of team goal commitment and information exchange. *Motivation and Emotion, 38*(1), 120–130. doi:10.1007/s11031-013-9365-2.

Bowers, C. A., Braun, C. C., & Morgan, B. B., Jr. (1997). Team workload: Its meaning and measurement. In M. T. Brannick, E. Salas, & C. Prince (Eds.), *Team performance assessment and measurement: Theory, methods, and applications* (pp. 85–108). Mahwah: Lawrence Erlbaum Associates Publishers.

Csikszentmihalyi, M. (1990). *Flow: The psychology of optimal experience*. New York: Harper & Row, Publishers.

Csikszentmihalyi, M. (1994). *The evolving self: A psychology for the third millennium* (Reprint.). Harper Perennial.

Csikszentmihalyi, M. (1996). *Creativity: Flow and the psychology of discovery and invention* (4 TRA.). New York: Harper & Row.

Csikszentmihalyi, M. (1997). *Finding flow: The psychology of engagement with everyday life*. New York: Basic Books.

Csikszentmihalyi, M. (2004). *Good business: Leadership, flow, and the making of meaning* (Reprint.). New York: Harper & Row.

Csikszentmihalyi, M., Abuhamdeh, S., & Nakamura, J. (2005). Flow. In A. J. Elliot & C. S. Dweck (Eds.), *Handbook of competence and motivation* (pp. 598–608). New York: Guilford Publications.

Gardner, H. E., Csikszentmihalyi, M., & Damon, W. (2001). *Good work*. New York: Basic Books.

Gully, S. M., Incalcaterra, K. A., Joshi, A., & Matthew, J. (2002). A meta-analysis of team-efficacy, potency, and performance: Interdependence and level of analysis as moderators of observed relationships. *Journal of Applied Psychology, 87*(5), 819–832. doi:10.1037/0021-9010.87.5.819.

Guzzo, R. A., & Salas, E. (1995). *Team effectiveness and decision making in organizations*. San Francisco: Jossey-Bass.

Hamilton, E., & Hurford, A. (2007). Combining collaborative workspaces with tablet computing: Research in learner engagement and conditions of flow. In *Frontiers in education conference – global engineering: Knowledge without borders, opportunities without passports, 2007. FIE'07. 37th Annual* (pp. T3C–3 –T3C–8). Presented at the Frontiers In Education Conference – Global Engineering: Knowledge Without Borders, Opportunities Without Passports, 2007. FIE'07. 37th Annual. doi:10.1109/FIE.2007.4418151

Katzenbach, J. R., & Smith, D. K. (1992). *The wisdom of teams: Creating the high-performance organization*. Harvard Business Press.

Katzenbach, J. R., & Smith, D. K. (1993). The discipline of teams. *Harvard Business Review, 71*(2), 111–120.

Kozlowski, S. W. J., & Klein, K. J. (2000). A multilevel approach to theory and research in organizations: Contextual, temporal, and emergent processes. In K. J. Klein & S. W. J. Kozlowski (Eds.), *Multilevel theory, research, and methods in organizations: Foundations, extensions, and new directions* (pp. 3–90). San Francisco: Jossey-Bass.

Landhäußer, A., & Keller, J. (2012). Flow and its affective, cognitive, and performance-related consequences. In S. Engeser (Ed.), *Advances in flow research* (pp. 65–85). New York: Springer.

Locke, E. A., & Latham, G. P. (2006). New directions in goal-setting theory. *Current Directions in Psychological Science, 15*(5), 265–268. doi:10.1111/j.1467-8721.2006.00449.x.

Marks, M. A., Mathieu, J. E., & Zaccaro, S. J. (2001). A temporally based framework and taxonomy of team processes. *The Academy of Management Review, 26*(3), 356–376. doi:10.2307/259182.

Mayer, R. C., Davis, J. H., & Schoorman, F. D. (1995). An integrative model of organizational trust. *Academy of Management Review, 20*(3), 709–734. doi:10.5465/AMR.1995.9508080335.

Morgeson, F. P., & Hofmann, D. A. (1999). The structure and function of collective constructs: Implications for multilevel research and theory development. *Academy of Management Review, 24*(2), 249–265. doi:10.5465/AMR.1999.1893935.

Nakamura, J., & Csikszentmihalyi, M. (2002). The concept of flow. In C. R. Snyder & S. Lopez (Eds.), *Handbook of positive psychology* (pp. 89–105). Oxford: Oxford University Press.

Nakamura, J., & Csikszentmihalyi, M. (2009). Flow theory and research. In S. Lopez & C. R. Snyder (Eds.), *Handbook of positive psychology* (pp. 195–206). New York: Oxford University Press.

O'leary-kelly, A. M., Martocchio, J. J., & Frink, D. D. (1994). A review of the influence of group goals on group performance. *Academy of Management Journal, 37*(5), 1285–1301. doi:10.2307/256673.

Posner, B. Z., Kouzes, J. M., & Schmidt, W. H. (1985). Shared values make a difference: An empirical test of corporate culture. *Human Resource Management, 24*(3), 293–309. doi:10.1002/hrm.3930240305.

Ready, D. A., & Truelove, E. (2011). The power of collective ambition. *Harvard Business Review, 89*(12), 94–102.

Salanova, M., Rodríguez-Sánchez, A. M., Schaufeli, W. B., & Cifre, E. (2014). Flowing together: A longitudinal study of collective efficacy and collective flow among workgroups. *The Journal of Psychology, 148*(4), 435–455. doi:10.1080/00223980.2013.806290.

Salas, E., Cooke, N. J., & Rosen, M. A. (2008). On teams, teamwork, and team performance: Discoveries and developments. *Human Factors: The Journal of the Human Factors and Ergonomics Society, 50*(3), 540–547. doi:10.1518/001872008X288457.

Sawyer, R. K. (2003). *Group creativity: Music, theater, collaboration*. Mahwah: Lawrence Erlbaum Associates.

Sawyer, R. K. (2006). Group creativity: Musical performance and collaboration. *Psychology of Music, 34*(2), 148–165. doi:10.1177/0305735606061850.

Sawyer, R. K. (2007). *Group genius: The creative power of collaboration*. New York: Basic Books.

Snow, K. Y. (2010). *Work relationships that flow: Examining the interpersonal flow experience, knowledge sharing, and organizational commitment*. Ann Arbor: The claremont graduate university.
Walker, C. J. (2010). Experiencing flow: Is doing it together better than doing it alone? *The Journal of Positive Psychology, 5*(1), 3–11. doi:10.1080/17439760903271116.
Weggeman, M. (2007). *Leidinggeven aan Professionals? Niet Doen!: Over Kenniswerkers, Vakmanschap en Innovatie*. Schiedam: Scriptum.
Widmeyer, W. N., Brawley, L. R., & Carron, A. V. (1986). *Measurement of cohesion in sport teams: The group environment questionnaire*. London: Sports Dynamics.
Wrzesniewski, A., Dutton, J. E., & Debebe, G. (2003). Interpersonal sensemaking and the meaning of work. *Research in Organizational Behavior, 25*, 93–135. doi:10.1016/S0191-3085(03)25003-6.

Chapter 16
New Technologies as Opportunities for Flow Experience: A Framework for the Analysis

Stefano Triberti, Alice Chirico, and Giuseppe Riva

Abstract New technologies present remarkable opportunities for flow experience. We provide an integrated theoretical framework for the study of flow in Human-Technologies Interaction referring to two specific cognitive processes – presence and social presence – whose goals are the control of the activity of the Self (presence) and the understanding of the activity of the Other (social presence). On the individual level, the chance for a technology user to enter a state of flow depends on how much the technology addresses the user's hierarchy of intentions (presence): I am present in a real or virtual space if I manage to put my intentions into action (enacting them). On this basis, we elaborate on a new model aimed to describe how a "Perfect Interaction" (P.I.M.) takes place. On the collective level, research shows that a peculiar type of flow state could be reached by creative groups. Central to the presented model is the definition of a shared intersubjective space, which we identify with (highest level of) social presence. When this is achieved, participants can experience networked flow, an optimal state that maximizes the creative potential of the group.

16.1 Introduction

According to recent studies in cyber psychology (Riva et al. 2012, 2014), the quality of experience should become the main principle orienting design decisions while developing new technologies. This means, not only the technologies of the future should be analyzed to evaluate their ease of use, but they should also be able to guarantee positive, engaging and self-actualizing experiences to the users. Consider the following examples. A user has to write a chapter for an edited book. He is given

S. Triberti (✉) • A. Chirico
Department of Psychology, Università Cattolica del Sacro Cuore, Milan, Italy
e-mail: stefano.triberti@unicatt.it

G. Riva
Department of Psychology, Università Cattolica del Sacro Cuore, Milan, Italy

Applied Technology for NeuroPsychology Lab, Istituto Auxologico Italiano, Milan, Italy

L. Harmat et al. (eds.), *Flow Experience*, DOI 10.1007/978-3-319-28634-1_16

a document template, along with additional informational material about how to prepare his own contribution. In the end, the user is able to write the chapter. However, his computer skills being at a medium-low level, and the template not completely optimized for his text editor program, he often has to consult the additional material and make numerous attempts with the program interface in order to correctly edit the manuscript.

Another user has to write a chapter for the same book. Differently from the first, this user has high computer skills and a more adequate program for text editing. She simply opens the template and *writes*. She can concentrate on the content of her contribution only, so that the writing task results in a continuous stream of intention and action, which is inherently pleasant, engaging and effective.

In the end, it is possible to say that both these examples referred to a usable technology, since both the users were finally able to achieve their goals (writing) and to obtain desirable results (the chapters). Despite this, the two interaction examples profoundly differ for what regards the *subjective experiences*. It is easy to see that the experience of the second user is preferable from many points of view.

Indeed, it appears a satisfying experience if you consider fundamental theories in Human-Computer Interaction (Winograd and Flores 1986), which sustained that interactive technology, should be "ready-to-hand" instead of easy to understand.

Precisely, the interaction with a technology can be really satisfying if no need to initiate a problem solving process arises. In these cases, the user is able to fluently act with no need to consciously think about how to achieve his/her own single interaction goals, the actions on the interface following one another in the context of a profound involvement within the task.

This example shows that usability is not an ultimate goal for design, but a starting point. What is important to achieve is a technology that is able to properly correspond to the intentions and actions of its users, this way guaranteeing the possibility to engage oneself into fluid streams of interaction.

Moving a step forward to the content of the present contribution, it is easy to see how the described "fluid interaction" calls to mind the *experience of flow*. Indeed, the flow construct made its way through the field of new technologies study and design. The role of flow, usually depicted as a fundamental feature of successful and satisfying interactions, has been pointed out in the context of many human-technology interaction scenarios, such as e-commerce (Koufaris 2002; Bilgihan et al. 2014), e-learning (Liu et al. 2009; Ho and Kuo 2010), video-gaming (Pavlas et al. 2010; Argenton et al. 2014; Triberti and Argenton 2013), social network activities (Mauri et al. 2011), virtual reality (Riva et al. 2004, 2011).

However, we cannot say that a particular type of flow is related to the experience of any technology. As suggested by Finneran and Zhang (2003, 2005), who were the first to review the studies on flow in the context of human-technologies interaction, flow is related to the experience of the user with the task he/she is trying to complete. Indeed, I can experience flow surfing the web, but this is not generated by the web itself: I may surf the web for different purposes, ranging from finding information, buying products or staying in contact with my friends. In this sense, considering flow in the context of human-technology interactions does not mean to identify technologies that are able to generate a state of flow but, on the contrary, to understand what aspects of a technology may be useful to properly respond to the users' goals.

Pace (2004) conducted a grounded theory study to analyze the flow experience of users who surfed the internet looking for general information. He found the most important characteristics of flow (Csikszentmihalyi and Csikszentmihalyi 1992) actually emerging from the interviews with the users (balance between the challenges of an activity and the users' skills; clear goals and feedback; concentration on the task at hand; sense of control; a "merging" of action and awareness; a loss of self-consciousness; a distorted sense of time; the autotelic experience).

Moreover, he provided some suggestions for the design of websites adequate to promote the emergence of flow, such as exploiting curiosity, focusing attention with interesting content and avoiding distracting interface elements.

Indeed, these suggestions make sense only if we consider the task of the user which, in this particular case, is the information finding. If Pace or other scholars would have focused their attention on other tasks, they would have provided different guidelines for the design.

Starting from these premises, it seems quite impossible to provide shared guidelines for the design of technologies, unless every possible technology-task bond would is studied as a unique monad.

On the contrary, we argue that a general framework can be introduced to guide design decisions in the context of different tasks and different technologies. We propose that this could be made referring to (1) theoretical premises which are based on fundamental experiential processes and (2) deriving general models from them that would be adequate to analyze different human-technology interaction situations. In the end, basing design decisions on similar considerations would augment the chances for a given technology to promote a flow state in its users.

Firstly, in the next subsection, we will introduce the theoretical basis of the framework focusing on the individual (i.e. interaction situation with a user completing a task using a technology) and on the collective level (i.e. interaction situation with a group/network of users completing a task using a technology which maintains them in contact with each other). Then, we will introduce models to analyze the two situations, providing methodological guidelines to apply them in design contexts.

16.2 The Individual Level: Presence and Intentions

The construct of presence has emerged in the 1990s in the field of virtual reality studies: numerous scholars tried to understand how is it possible to feel the sensation of "being-there" while interacting with 3D environments generated by a computer. Then, these technology focused studies led to more fundamental questions (Riva et al. 2011): why would a human subject have a mental function devoted to the sensation of presence? What is its role in daily life, beyond the experience within simulation technologies such as virtual reality?

Answering to these questions, the studies on presence defined it as a fundamental component of human experience. According to this vision, presence is a neuropsychological phenomenon, evolved from the interplay of our biological and cultural inheritance (Riva et al. 2012, 2004, 2011; Riva and Mantovani 2014). The feeling of "being there" in a given environment allows one to locate him or herself not in the sense of mere spatial coordinates, but in the sense of a situation made of opportunities and limits to action. Precisely, presence is the intuitive perception of successfully transforming intentions into action (see Chap. 14 by Boffi et al. in this volume) (*enaction*) (Riva 2009; Riva and Waterworth 2014; Riva et al. 2011), and it has two fundamental functions: firstly, it "locates" the Self in an external physical and/or cultural space: the Self is "present" in a space if he/she can act in it; secondly, presence provides feedback to the Self about the status of its activity: the Self perceives the variations in presence and tunes its activity accordingly.

Indeed, a feeling of presence can be interrupted and/or reduced. In the first example we provided earlier, about the user who wrote his chapter, but often had to consult the informational material to adapt his own work, numerous interruptions in the sense of presence (*breakdowns*) occurred. Differently, the second user experienced a continuous stream of writing and was fully absorbed by the task, in other words she was experiencing an optimal experience/flow. Indeed, optimal experiences are the situations featuring the highest possible level of sense of presence (Riva et al. 2006, 2011).

But what does it mean that we feel present "enacting our intentions"? What exactly are intentions? According to Pacherie (2006, 2008), the mental antecedents of our actions can be represented in hierarchies, since a given intention can have different characteristics and a peculiar relation with the action and the external world. Consider the following example. Paul is a young boy in love with a girl named Sarah. One day, he decides to call her on the cell phone to ask her out on a date.

This is nothing more than the brief story of a simple action, involving the interaction with a technology. However, if we carefully consider the intention of Paul, we can see its complexity and how it comprises multiple and different antecedents for the action.

One is the intention of Paul to win Sarah's love, that is, his desire of himself becoming her boyfriend. This intention is oriented to the future and refers to a (for now) abstract concept, which is the representation of a possible reality; moreover, this intention is not limited by the conditions of the present situation, that is, it is not context-specific (Paul dreams about Sarah's love independently of what he is doing or not-doing at the present moment).

Another intention is the one related to ask Sarah out on a date. This intention is present-oriented, since Paul decides to do it *now*. Of course, this intention comes from the first one (second level of the hierarchy), but it is perceptual, since Paul will know he has achieved it when he would be able to see that he is actually talking with her; moreover, this intention is context-specific, because its existence and also its achieving are strictly dependent on the here-and-now situation (the cell phone is functional; Paul is in a condition that allows him to speak; Sarah answers to the call; and so on).

Table 16.1 Levels of the intentional hierarchy, each with associated characteristics and layer of presence

The intention of the subject	Hierarchy position and type of intention	Characteristics	Layer of presence
"I desire that Sarah will become my girlfriend"	1. Distal intention	Future-oriented; conscious of the world; not context-specific; conceptual in nature	Extended
"So, today I want to call her to ask her out on a date"	2. Proximal intention	Present-oriented; conscious of here and now; context-specific; perceptual in nature	Core
"So, I'm about to move my thumb down-up on the screen on my cell phone to find her number in the phone book"	3. Motor intention	Micro-present oriented; mostly unconscious; micro-context specific; proprioceptive in nature	Proto

In the end, the last intention refers to the use of the cell phone; Paul intends to move his fingers on the interface in order to (for example) find Sarah's number in the phone book. This intention develops at a micro-present level and guides the mere movements, and, differing from the other two, is *mostly unconscious*.

The hierarchy of intentions as explained by Pacherie (2006, 2008) allows us to understand in what sense the intuitive perception of intention enacting (presence) can be distorted and interrupted. Precisely, a subject such as Paul can have the impression he is fluidly using the interface of his cell phone, immediately finding Sarah's number and calling her. However, the successful enacting of this motor intention does not assure that the stream of action will be entirely addressed by the interaction; Sarah may not answer to the call (the proximal intention "asking her out" is not enacted) or, sadly, she may not be interested in Paul (distal intention "becoming Sarah's boyfriend" is not enacted). Similarly, assume that Paul's cell phone is not working; Paul would be in need of finding another way to contact Sarah, this way experiencing a breakdown at the motor level of his intentional hierarchy (see Table 16.1 for a resume of the hierarchical structure of intentions).

According to presence theory, a high level of presence, which enhances the probability of the rising of an optimal experience if the interaction is characterized by a positive emotion (Riva et al. 2006), can be reached when the hierarchical structure of intentions is addressed in its entirety. Precisely (Riva et al. 2011; Riva and Mantovani 2014), the user achieves a level of *proto presence* successfully coupling sensory inputs and movements, for example interacting with a technology interface; he/she achieves a level of *core presence* when able to focus his/her attention on the environment features which can respond to what he/she wants to obtain in the here-and-now; and in the end, he/she achieves a level of *extended presence* when able to conceptually represent/prefigure future/possible events in the environment, which may respond to his/her intentions and which can be pursued through the enacting of proximal and motor intentions.

16.3 The Collective Level: Social Presence and We-Intentions

Attempting to provide a general model to orient design decisions in the field of technology, it is necessary to consider the collective level of interaction.

Indeed, sociality is a fundamental characteristic of new technologies since the 2.0 era rising. According to Katz (2002), on the one hand technologies became more and more integrated with our clothes, body and Self, enhancing our abilities to communicate; on the other hand, they give us new opportunities and instruments to represent ourselves to others, for example as avatars in digital environments.

More precisely, recent literature shows that new technologies are able to assist groups while they are networking and collaborating in order to generate a creative product.

Moreover, as we will show, while the group/network is working, it can achieve a peculiar type of optimal experience, namely the *networked flow* (Gaggioli et al. 2011, 2013b) which is able to optimize the performance of the group itself and the well-being experience of its members. The first and fundamental aspect generate this experience is a high level of *social presence*. Short and colleagues (1976) introduced this term referring to the degree of salience of the other person in a mediated environment and the consequent salience of the interpersonal interaction with him or her. According to Biocca and colleagues (2003), numerous factors influence the sense of social presence in the context of a mediated environment: some of them are the sensory perception of body shapes (or their digital representations), the psychological involving with another intelligence and the behavioral engagement in the context of interaction and synchronization. Social presence is highly influenced by the media richness, which is the sum of the properties of a given medium able to convey and exchange social information (Davide et al. 2014; Liu et al. 2009).

Social presence can also be defined referring to the role of intentions in communication scenarios. Indeed, social presence may be understood as the sensation of being with other selves in an environment, resulting from the ability to recognize the intentions of others in the surroundings (Riva et al. 2004).

Suppose that you are in a room with an incredibly realistic statue; although its appearance may mislead you for some seconds, you will soon understand it is not a real person, because it is not engaged in an action, it is not expressing a human intention. In contrast, a small line of text inside a web-chat, such as a series of footprints on the sand of a beach, can be sufficient to generate a quite strong sense of social presence. Indeed, they are indices of intentions somebody expressed in the environment through his/her own behavior.

Why are intentions important in the context of social presence too? Interestingly, if you recognize the intentions of others in the environment, you can also synchronize your own intentions to them. This is what happens when groups and collaborative work environments are created and maintained. Indeed, collective intentionality is a peculiar phenomenon that is not simply a sum of individual intentions. Imagine that two artists are collaborating to paint a big mural. One of them is painting the background, while the other is painting some figures at the opposite side of the wall.

"Painting the background" and "painting the figures" are the individual intentions, but "painting the mural" is another intention which can't be attributed to one of the two artists at the current moment. Despite this, the last intention is the one that promotes the individual ones as components of itself.

This we-intention (Searle 1990; Gaggioli et al. 2013b) has to be conceived as the most important outcome of a high-level sense of social presence, and should be addressed by a human (group) – technology interaction in the same way as individual intentions.

16.4 Methods

In the present section, we will introduce the fundamental methodological frameworks and related instruments to provide new technology design and evaluation. In the end, we will discuss their application and their effect in promoting technology-related flow experiences.

16.4.1 The Individual Level: The Perfect Interaction Model

On the individual level, the first step for a technology design method oriented to the promotion of optimal experiences is the consideration of the technology from the point of view of the intentional hierarchy. A technology designer or analyst should not simply consider the interface of the technology, since that is just the last step of a new technology design. According to User Centered Design (UCD) (Lowdermilk 2013; Garrett 2010), a designer has to *delineate* the technology users before the design process starts. Doing so, he/she can assure that not only the technology will be easy to use, but also it will adequately respond to the users' needs.

The Perfect Interaction Model (P.I.M.) (Triberti and Riva 2015) is based on the assumption that a *natural isomorphism* exists between the intentional hierarchy of the user and the characteristics of the technology. That is, when the user starts using the technology, a *dovetailing process* begins, in which every step of the intentional hierarchy interlocks with a precise level of the technology. In Fig. 16.1, three arrows symbolize the steps of the interaction.

Arrow 1: the distal intention of the user dovetails with the goal of the application/technology that is the scope for which it has been created. That is, the user wants to achieve something ("X") and the technology represents an opportunity to extend the user's action in order to reach that purpose in an immediate or distant future.

Arrow 2: the proximal intention of the user transforms the distal intention that is the general objective to be pursued, in one or more actions to be performed now ("Y"). The proximal intention dovetails with the structure of the technology, which is the set of functions that it allows. The structure is composed by temporal and spatial constrains that imply an order and an organization for the action.

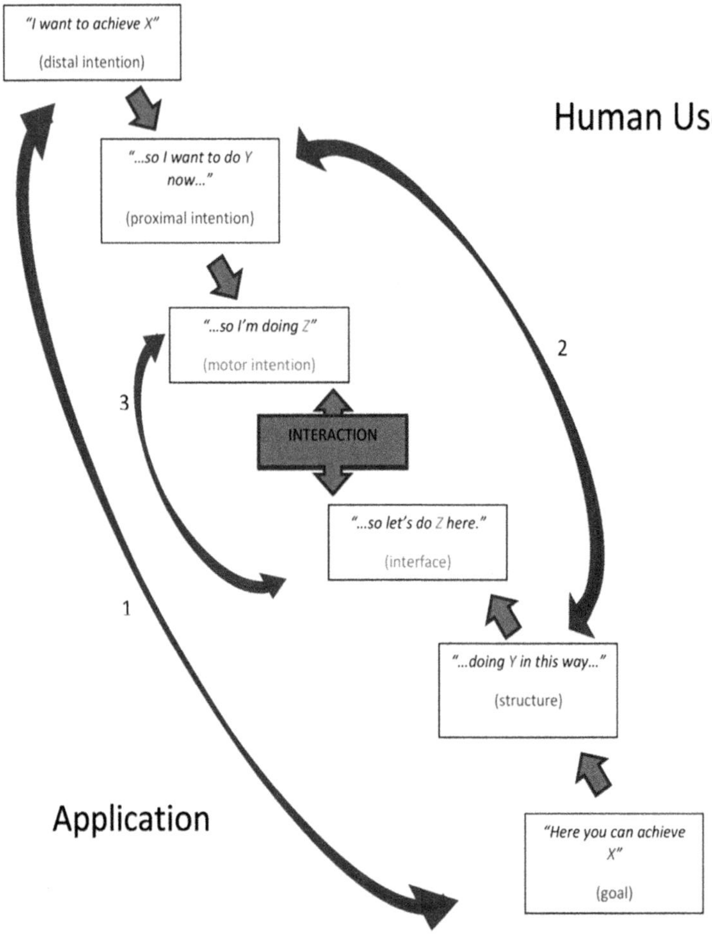

Fig. 16.1 The perfect interaction model (Source: Triberti and Riva 2015)

Arrow 3: the motor intention describes the fine-grained aspects of the action (e.g.: you have to move your fingers in *this* way, "Z"). It dovetails with the interface of the technology, which is the physical representation of the structure and is composed by a number of interactive devices that make the technology work.

The three arrows of P.I.M. allow us to identify six design errors that will possibly affect the interaction with the technology. These errors are showed in Table 16.2.

Basing on P.I.M. as a methodological reference, it is possible to provide general methods and instruments, most of them coming from User Centered Design and User Experience (Triberti and Liberati 2014; Triberti and Riva 2015), which can be used to avoid the design errors, or, if they already affect an interaction situation, to identify their sources and guide the intervention to repair them.

Table 16.2 The six errors possibly happening in a human-technology interaction at the intentional level

P.I.M. arrow	User	Application/technology
1. Distal intention and goal	The user doesn't know what he/she wants	The application has not got a clear Goal
2. Proximal intention and structure	The user doesn't know how to act to obtain what he/she wants	The functions are not adequately expressed in a Structure
3. Motor intention and interface	The user isn't able to move	The interface is not usable

Adapted from Triberti and Riva (2015)

The errors affecting Arrow 1 concern the distal intention of the user and/or the way in which the technology communicates its own goal. A common example is the user who is "just surfing" the internet without a clear goal, jumping from a web-link to another for pure time-killing. This type of user may ignore a given website/application independently of it being useful and usable, because he/she does not have a precise intention at the moment of browsing. Arrow 1 errors can be solved through qualitative methods of research, such as user-centred semi-structured interviews (Wilson 2013; Wood 1997). These methods allow the creation of personas (Miaskiewicz and Kozar 2011), which are complex profiles of the possible users for a technology to be designed. Personas are rich descriptions of users that entail physical and personality characteristics, personal data and story. Design based on personas allows us to produce technologies that would be centered on their users starting from their most general desires and needs.

The errors affecting Arrow 2 regards the proximal intention of the user, that is, what he/she wants to achieve at the present moment, and the adequacy of the technology's functions that can be reached by his/her action. A classic structure design error is the one involving vehicle horns. Created and commercialized around 1910, they were intended to signal the vehicle approaching in possibly dangerous situations. Despite that, drivers still use them to express emotions (usually anger), for example in the context of traffic jams. This is an example of a technology which had been created for a certain purpose, but later became associated to another behavioral intention that was not imagined by the designers.

Methods useful to avoid Arrow 2 errors should be able to (1) carefully take into account the behavior of users during their here-and-now interaction and (2) do not underestimate the role of the context(s) of use (see Chap. 14 by Boffi et al. in this volume). In this sense, interviews can still be useful, but only to a limited extent; indeed, users may also not be aware of the complexity of an interaction situation before being actively involved in it.

Contextual inquiry (Da Silva et al. 2011; Garrett 2010) is a design/research method which entails an in depth interview that is conducted with the user during a preliminary exploration of one or more contexts of use, the user and the designer identifying opportunities and obstacles for the technology implementation together.

Moreover, paper and virtual prototyping (Snyder 2003; Bordegoni et al. 2013) allow the designers to understand what basic functions have to be included in a technology.

Arrow 3 errors concern the mere motor interaction with a technology interface.

As the last step of a user centered design process, usability studies (Albert and Tullis 2013) involving interacting subjects allow to identify the possible difficulties affecting the direct interaction with a device. Moreover, another user profiling focused on limits and abilities is very important (this is mandatory especially while designing for users who may have physical or mental disabilities).

16.4.2 The Collective Level: Networked Flow

Research shows that a peculiar type of flow state can be reached by creative groups, (Gaggioli et al. 2011, 2013a, b). While Csikszentmihalyi studied flow mainly at the individual level, Sawyer (2007, 2014) considered flow as a peak experience also typical of a group performing at its top level of activity. Conditions which facilitate the occurrence of a group flow include definition of a common mission; well defined and stable group identity; close listening among the members; equal participation and complete concentration; "moving it forward" (members are able to provide new contribution based on others' ideas); and "potential of failure" (the activity the group is involved in should be adequately challenging) (see Chap. 15 by Hout et al. in this volume). Moreover, Sawyer also emphasizes the fact that the emerging collective state of mind cannot be easily reduced to the subjective experiences of the individual group members. However, possible limitations of Sawyer's contribution are related to the lack of focus on the developmental dynamics, which lead a group to the experience of a shared flow, and the analysis, which was limited to the face-to-face interactions (excluding the mediated ones).

On the contrary, as we previously stated, high levels of sense of social presence are an important pre-condition for achieving group flow (Gaggioli et al. 2011), which is able to support the development of the experience of networked flow.

In contrast to Sawyer, this could happen in the context of mediated interactions too. Indeed, a high level of social presence identifies a situation in which the intentions of others are not only perceived and understood, but also shared. The we-intention (Searle 1990) develops and is enacted through a process that can be represented in six phases.

At the time of **phase 1** (*meeting-persistence*) some individuals are present in an environment (real or virtual/mediated). Every individual has his/her own intentional structure but, through a process of communication, the diverse intentional hierarchies start to overlap, assuming the form of an objective to be commonly pursued.

Phase 2 is labelled "*reduction of distances*". The individuals start to express their preference for interacting with people they recognize having an intentional hierarchy similar to their own. In this phase a we-intention starts to develop and grow.

Phase 3 (*liminality-parallel action*) is the one where the new-born group starts to balance internally (leaders may emerge; roles may be appointed; etc.) and to define its own boundaries and characteristics.

Phase 4 is the one where *networked flow* is able to manifest itself. The leaders initiate the transformation of common goals into distributed actions, clarifying sub-objectives and plans. In this phase, networked flow can be inferred by the quality of the experience (state of mind featuring high concentration, involvement, control of the situation, intrinsic motivation and a positive emotional state).

Other characteristics are typical of networked flow establishing: balance between resources, collective intention internalized as directed to the future and the group frame made explicit and recognized by the members at the time.

Phase 5, the second phase of networked flow after its establishment, is characterized by the *creation of an artefact*. Indeed, the group/network that is experiencing an optimal experience is not inert. On the contrary, it is engaged in an activity which will generate some sort of product. The artefact can be an object, but also an idea, a strategy, a theory… in any case it is something physical or abstract that did not exist before the group activity. At the time of phase 5, the artefact was relevant only to the group itself.

Phase 6 entails the *application of the artefact* to the social context, that is, the sharing of it. This phase is particularly important because, despite networked flow developed at the time of the previous phases, it's only in the present one that the network properly "exists". Indeed, (1) the artefact "embodies" the collective intention in something perceivable/understandable; moreover, (2) thanks to the creation of the artefact, the frame of a group can be extended out of its boundaries, reaching the more complex social network and creating communities of practice.

How is it possible to measure/analyse networked flow? How can we know if a given technology characterizing a context of creative work is promoting a networked flow evolutionary dynamic, exploiting its probabilities of reaching desirable outcomes?

Social network analysis (SNA) constitutes the more adequate candidate as a method to analyse networked flow not as a static phenomenon, but as a dynamic process (Gaggioli et al. 2015).

This method is based on the graphical representation of group/network units and relationships between them. Usually, when the interaction between members is based on communication technologies (online social networks, web-chats, Massive Multiplayer Online Learning Environments or Games, etc.), it is also possible to derive algebraic indices that allow evaluators to keep traces of the interaction and collaboration activities occurring inside the group. For example, a diagram that represents a social network usually depicts the individuals as dots and the links between them as lines that connect the dots. Visual characteristics such as dimension of the lines can be used to express characteristics of the network, such as number of connections related to a given link. From the point of view of mathematical computation of social network indices, SNA is a field in continuous evolution to the point that it is impossible to provide here a complete rendition of its methods and advances (Kossinets and Watts 2006), especially from the point of view of dynamical analyses

(Scott 2011). However, we provide at least a preliminary example to show how networked flow can be analyzed and monitored.

Gaggioli and colleagues (2013a) were able to observe the activity of five groups of students developing an application during 11 weeks of a course assignment. The students were in contact via a dedicated web platform. In the end, the products of the groups were evaluated by expert judges using the creative product semantic scale (O'Quin and Besemer 1989) and the SNA was carried out using the method described by Manca et al. (2009). First of all, the analyses showed different patterns of interaction among the groups, with the most intense interactions appearing during the first weeks (initial phases of defining the product) and the last ones (providing the final prototype/relation). However, other analyses showed that during the central weeks there was not a lack of collaboration but, on the contrary, the interactions appeared more centralized toward single members, according to a process of role-assigning and/or leaders emerging. This is consistent with the networked flow model, in which the central phases of the process are devoted to the internal structuring of the creative group. Moreover, when confronted with the outcomes of the creative product evaluation, it clearly emerged that the groups that achieved the best results were also the ones with highest scores in SNA indices related to social presence and best trends regarding decentralized control of the group activity and neighbor interactions.

Although preliminary, this kind of observation shows how a group interaction devoted to the development of creative products can be observed in its activity and behavior, and that measurable features of it can be interpreted as indices of a shared flow experience manifesting itself.

16.5 Discussion and Conclusion

In the present contribution, we explored a general framework useful to orient design decisions and analysis while developing new technologies. This framework would be numbered among the User Experience and User Centred Design approaches, since its main objective is to guide the design of technologies not only towards ease of use, but also to enable more users to engage in fluid, pleasant and effective streams of interaction, in other words optimal experiences.

The recent literature on flow showed that, in addition to the intrinsic characteristics of optimal experience, numerous factors can contribute to the emergence of flow states in various contexts, ranging from cognitive strategies to contextual variables, and even personality traits (Bassi et al. 2013a; b; Cavanagh and Shernoff 2014; Schmidt et al. 2014). In line with these approaches, we argue that, in the context of human-technology interactions, a fundamental factor for the rise of optimal experiences relies on the high level of sense of presence that the interaction itself is able to guarantee its users. This strongly depends on the capacity of the technology to address users' intentions at every level of their complex hierarchies. For this reason, we provided a model showing how a "perfect interaction" should be designed, and added the methods and instruments associated to the assessment of every intention-technology dovetailing level.

Moreover, we elaborated on the peculiar type of flow experience that it is possible to observe in the context of the creative groups' activity, especially when they are interacting by means of a computer-mediated communication. Despite the study of networked flow is still in its infancy, its theoretical rendition allows designers and evaluators to consider what developmental phases should be observed when monitoring a group that is expected to reach a shared optimal experience.

According to our opinion, the insights and methods provided by this theoretical framework may lay the groundwork for the design and evaluation of future technologies, which would become more and more devoted to engage users into optimal frames of interaction.

References

Albert, W., & Tullis, T. (2013). *Measuring the user experience: Collecting, analyzing, and presenting usability metrics*. Indianapolis: Morgan Kaufmann.

Argenton, L., Triberti, S., Serino, S., Muzio, M., & Riva, G. (2014). Serious games as positive technologies for individual and group flourishing. In A. L. Brooks, S. Brahnam, & L. C. Jain (Eds.), *Technologies of inclusive well-being* (pp. 221–244). New York: Springer.

Bassi, M., Bacher, G., Negri, L., & Delle Fave, A. (2013a). The contribution of job happiness and job meaning to the well-being of workers from thriving and failing companies. *Applied research in quality of life, 8*(4), 427–448.

Bassi, M., Steca, P., Monzani, D., Greco, A., & Delle Fave, A. (2013b). Personality and optimal experience in adolescence: Implications for well-being and development. *Journal of Happiness Studies, 15*(4), 829–843.

Bilgihan, A., Okumus, F., Nusair, K., & Bujisic, M. (2014). Online experiences: Flow theory, measuring online customer experience in e-commerce and managerial implications for the lodging industry. *Information Technology & Tourism, 14*(1), 49–71. doi:10.1007/s40558-013-0003-3.

Biocca, F., Harms, C., & Burgoon, J. (2003). Toward a more robust theory and measure of social presence: Review and suggested criteria. *Presence, 12*(5), 456–480.

Bordegoni, M., Ferrise, F., & Cugini, U. (2013). Development of virtual prototypes based on visuo/tactile interaction for the preliminary evaluation of consumer products usage. In *CIRP design 2012* (pp. 149–158). New York: Springer.

Cavanagh, R., & Shernoff, D. (2014). Positive change and scholastic education. In P. Inghilleri, G. Riva, & E. Riva (Eds.), *Enabling positive change: Flow and complexity in daily experience*. Berlin: De Gruyter Open.

Csikszentmihalyi, M., & Csikszentmihalyi, I. S. (1992). *Optimal experience: Psychological studies of flow in consciousness*. Cambridge: Cambridge University Press.

Da Silva, T. S., Martin, A., Maurer, F., & Silveira, M. S. (2011). User-centered design and agile methods: A systematic review. In *AGILE, 2011* (pp. 77–86).

Davide, F., Triberti, S., & Collovà, F. (2014). Exchanging social information in online social games. In M. C. Angelides & H. Agius (Eds.), *Handbook of digital games* (pp. 197–234). Hoboken: John Wiley & Sons.

Finneran, C. M., & Zhang, P. (2003). A person–artefact–task (PAT) model of flow antecedents in computer-mediated environments. *International Journal of Human-Computer Studies, 59*(4), 475–496.

Finneran, C. M., & Zhang, P. (2005). Flow in computer-mediated environments: Promises and challenges. *Communications of the Association for Information Systems, 15*(1), 4.
Gaggioli, A., Milani, L., Mazzoni, E., & Riva, G. (2011). Networked flow: A framework for understanding the dynamics of creative collaboration in educational and training settings. *Open Education Journal, 4*(1), M3.
Gaggioli, A., Riva, G., Milani, L., & Mazzoni, E. (2013a). Analyzing the experience of networked flow through social network analysis. In *Networked flow* (pp. 71–99). New York: Springer.
Gaggioli, A., Riva, G., Milani, L., & Mazzoni, E. (2013b). The emergence of networked flow. In *Networked flow* (pp. 55–70) New York: Springer.
Gaggioli, A., Mazzoni, E., Milani, L., & Riva, G. (2015). The creative link: Investigating the relationship between social network indices, creative performance and flow in blended teams. *Computers in Human Behavior, 42*, 157–166.
Garrett, J. J. (2010). *Elements of user experience, the: User-centered design for the Web and beyond*. New York: Pearson Education.
Ho, L.-A., & Kuo, T.-H. (2010). How can one amplify the effect of e-learning? An examination of high-tech employees' computer attitude and flow experience. *Computers in Human Behavior, 26*(1), 23–31.
Katz, J. E. (2002). *Machines that become us: The social context of personal communication technology*. Piscataway: Transaction Publishers.
Kossinets, G., & Watts, D. J. (2006). Empirical analysis of an evolving social network. *Science, 311*(5757), 88–90.
Koufaris, M. (2002). Applying the technology acceptance model and flow theory to online consumer behavior. *Information Systems Research, 13*(2), 205–223.
Liu, S.-H., Liao, H.-L., & Pratt, J. A. (2009). Impact of media richness and flow on e-learning technology acceptance. *Computers & Education, 52*(3), 599–607.
Lowdermilk, T. (2013). *User-centered design: A developer's guide to building user-friendly applications*. Sebastopol: O'Reilly Media.
Manca, S., Delfino, M., & Mazzoni, E. (2009). Coding procedures to analyse interaction patterns in educational web forums. *Journal of Computer Assisted Learning, 25*(2), 189–200.
Mauri, M., Cipresso, P., Balgera, A., Villamira, M., & Riva, G. (2011). Why is facebook so successful? Psychophysiological measures describe a core flow state while using facebook. *Cyberpsychology, Behavior and Social Networking, 14*(12), 723–731.
Miaskiewicz, T., & Kozar, K. A. (2011). Personas and user-centered design: How can personas benefit product design processes? *Design Studies, 32*(5), 417–430.
O'Quin, K., & Besemer, S. P. (1989). The development, reliability, and validity of the revised creative product semantic scale. *Creativity Research Journal, 2*(4), 267–278.
Pace, S. (2004). A grounded theory of the flow experiences of Web users. *International Journal of Human-Computer Studies, 60*(3), 327–363.
Pacherie, E. (2006). Toward a dynamic theory of intentions. In S. Pockett, W. P. Banks, & S. Gallagher (Eds.), *Does consciousness cause behavior?* (pp. 145–167). Cambridge: MIT Press.
Pacherie, E. (2008). The phenomenology of action: A conceptual framework. *Cognition, 107*(1), 179–217.
Pavlas, D., Heyne, K., Bedwell, W., Lazzara, E., & Salas, E. (2010). Game-based learning: the impact of flow state and videogame self-efficacy. In *Proceedings of the human factors and ergonomics society annual meeting, 2010* (Vol. 54, pp. 2398–2402, Vol. 28). Thousand Oaks: SAGE Publications
Riva, G. (2009). Is presence a technology issue? Some insights from cognitive sciences. *Virtual Reality, 13*(3), 159–169.
Riva, G., & Mantovani, F. (2014). Extending the self through the tools and the others: A general framework for presence and social presence in mediated interactions. In G. Riva, J. Waterworth, & D. Murray (Eds.), *Interacting with presence: HCI and the sense of presence in computer-mediated environments*. Berlin: De Gruyter Open.

Riva, G., & Waterworth, J. (2014). Being present in a virtual world. In M. Grimshaw (Ed.), *The oxford handbook of virtuality* (p. 205). Oxford: Oxford University Press.
Riva, G., Waterworth, J. A., & Waterworth, E. L. (2004). The layers of presence: A bio-cultural approach to understanding presence in natural and mediated environments. *CyberPsychology & Behavior, 7*(4), 402–416.
Riva, G., Castelnuovo, G., & Mantovani, F. (2006). Transformation of flow in rehabilitation: The role of advanced communication technologies. *Behavior Research Methods, 38*(2), 237–244.
Riva, G., Waterworth, J. A., Waterworth, E. L., & Mantovani, F. (2011). From intention to action: The role of presence. *New Ideas in Psychology, 29*(1), 24–37.
Riva, G., Banos, R. M., Botella, C., Wiederhold, B. K., & Gaggioli, A. (2012). Positive technology: Using interactive technologies to promote positive functioning. *Cyberpsychology, Behavior and Social Networking, 15*(2), 69–77.
Riva, G., Gaggioli, A., Villani, D., Cipresso, P., Repetto, C., Serino, S., et al. (2014). Positive technology for healthy living and active ageing. *Studies in Health Technology and Informatics, 203*, 44–56.
Sawyer, R. K. (2007). *Group genius: The creative power of collaboration*. New York: Basic Books.
Sawyer, R. K. (2014). *Group creativity: Music, theater, collaboration*. Mahwah: Lawrence Erlbaum Associates.
Schmidt, J. A., Shernoff, D. J., & Csikszentmihalyi, M. (2014). Individual and situational factors related to the experience of flow in adolescence. In *Applications of flow in human development and education* (pp. 379–405). New York: Springer.
Scott, J. (2011). Social network analysis: Developments, advances, and prospects. *Social Network Analysis and Mining, 1*(1), 21–26.
Searle, J. (1990). Collective intentionality. In P.R. Cohen, J. Morgan & M.E. Pollack (Eds.), *Intentions in Communication*. Cambridge: MIT Press.
Short, J., Williams, E., & Christie, B. (1976). *The social psychology of telecommunications*. New York: Wiley.
Snyder, C. (2003). *Paper prototyping: The fast and easy way to design and refine user interfaces*. Indianapolis: Morgan Kaufmann.
Triberti, S., & Argenton, L. (2013). *Psicologia dei videogiochi*. Milan: Apogeo.
Triberti, S., & Liberati, E. G. (2014). Patient centered virtual reality: An opportunity to improve the quality of patient's experience. In P. Cipresso & S. Serino (Eds.), *Virtual reality: Technologies medical applications and challenges*. New York: Nova Science.
Triberti, S., & Riva, G. (2015). Engaging users to design positive technologies for patient engagement: The perfect interaction model. In G. Graffigna, S. Barello, & S. Triberti (Eds.), *Patient engagement: A consumer-centered model to innovate healthcare*. Berlin: De Gruyter Open.
Wilson, C. (2013). *Interview techniques for UX practitioners: A user-centered design method*. Indianapolis: Morgan Kaufmann.
Winograd, T., & Flores, F. (1986). *Understanding computers and cognition: A new foundation for design*. Menlo Park: Addison-Wesley.
Wood, L. E. (1997). Semi-structured interviewing for user-centered design. *Interactions, 4*(2), 48–61.

Part VII
Flow and Personality

Chapter 17
Flow and Individual Differences – A Phenotypic Analysis of Data from More than 10,000 Twin Individuals

Fredrik Ullén, László Harmat, Töres Theorell, and Guy Madison

Abstract Earlier studies suggest that individual differences in flow experiences depend on both situational variables, e.g. the environmental opportunities to engage in flow promoting activities, and personal traits. Here, we present results of phenotypic analyses of associations between flow proneness and five major modalities of individual differences, i.e. personality, cognitive abilities, motivation, emotional competence (alexithymia) and performance on chronometric tasks. The data was collected using self-report questionnaires in a cohort of more than 10,000 Swedish twin individuals. The aim of the study was partly exploratory, but we also addressed three specific hypotheses suggested by earlier literature, i.e. that flow proneness is (i) correlated with personality, specifically with traits reflecting emotional stability (low neuroticism) and conscientiousness; (ii) unrelated to cognitive ability; and (iii) correlated with trait intrinsic motivation. The results confirmed all three hypotheses. Additional main findings were that flow proneness is related to extraversion, agreeableness, openness to experience, low schizotypy, and emotional competence (low alexithymia). Sex differences in flow proneness were mostly negligible, but flow proneness increased weakly with age. In summary, individual differences in flow proneness show substantial relations to personality related traits but appear essentially independent of cognitive abilities. We conclude that the results taken together support the notion of flow proneness being related to an autotelic personality, and discuss the potential implication of relations between the observed correlates of flow proneness and outcomes related to health and well-being.

The original version of this book was revised. An erratum can be found at http://dx.doi.org/10.1007/978-3-319-28634-1_23

F. Ullén (✉) • L. Harmat Ph.D. • T. Theorell
Department of Neuroscience, Karolinska Institutet, Retzius väg 8, SE-171 77 Stockholm, Sweden

G. Madison
Department of Psychology, Umeå University, SE-901 87 Umeå, Sweden

L. Harmat et al. (eds.), *Flow Experience*, DOI 10.1007/978-3-319-28634-1_17

17.1 Introduction

Flow can been studied using both experimental and differential approaches. As several contributions in the present volume illustrate (see the *Preface* of this volume) experimental studies of flow focus on the flow experience as a psychological state, and investigate e.g. how this state relates to situational variables and performance measures, or its underlying physiological mechanisms. In differential studies, a main interest is rather the variation between individuals in *flow proneness* (FP), i.e. a dispositional tendency to experience flow. Several self-report questionnaires have been developed to measure FP, e.g. Jackson and Eklund's Dispositional Flow Scale-2 (DFS-2) (Jackson and Eklund 2004), which also exists in a shorter form (Jackson et al. 2008); Csikszentmihalyi's Flow Questionnaire (Csikszentmihalyi 1975/2000); and the Swedish Flow Proneness Questionnaire (SFPQ) (Ullén et al. 2012a). Studies using such instruments have demonstrated that, although flow as such may well be a universal human experience, there is indeed a considerable individual variation in FP (Csikszentmihalyi and Schneider 2000; Asakawa 2010; Moneta 2004; Csikszentmihalyi and Csikszentmihalyi 1988; Ullén et al. 2012a).

The sources of this variability in FP are of interest theoretically but also from a practical and social perspective. FP is correlated with many positively valued outcomes, such as self-esteem and perceived ability (Asakawa 2010; Jackson et al. 2001; Adlai-Gail 1994; Jackson et al. 1998), life satisfaction (Asakawa 2010) and psychological well-being (Asakawa 2004, 2010; Ishimura and Kodama 2006), intrinsic motivation (Jackson et al. 1998), and lower anxiety (Asakawa 2010; Jackson et al. 1998) (see Chapter 19 by Riva et al. in this volume). Understanding the reasons for individual differences in FP could thus potentially be important for the development of means to increase flow and well-being.

In more recent years, there has been a growing research interest in the biological basis of FP, and its relations to other psychological traits (see Part VIII in this volume). Mosing and coworkers (2012b) investigated genetic influences on FP in a cohort of adult twins using the SFPQ, which provides separate estimates of the frequency of flow experiences in three domains of life, i.e. work, maintenance, and leisure time. Multivariate classical twin modelling indicated a moderate heritability of FP and, furthermore, that the same genetic factors influenced all three SFPQ domains. This suggests that genetic influences on FP could be related to global traits, such as personality. Indeed, Ullén and coworkers (2012a) found that FP is correlated with the Big Five personality traits emotional stability (i.e. low neuroticism) and conscientiousness. Relations to intelligence, on the other hand, were insignificant or very weak. Support for common genetic influences on FP and personality was found by Mosing et al. (2012a), who showed that FP is related to lower behavioral inhibition and an internal locus of control – two traits that are associated with emotional stability – and that these relations were mainly driven by genetic influences. Finally, de Manzano and coworkers (2013) used positron emission tomography (PET) to investigate relations between FP and dopamine D2 receptors in the brain. A positive relation between FP and D2 receptor availability was found in the striatum. The authors proposed that these differences in the dopamine system could reflect personality differences, i.e. a lower impulsivity which is correlated with both higher emotional stability and conscientiousness, in individuals with higher FP.

In summary, existing studies suggest that FP is related to personality rather than cognitive ability, and that these associations have a biological basis. However, some of the studies have used relatively small study groups and no more comprehensive study has so far mapped associations between FP and a wide range of individual difference variables in a large cohort. Here, we use data collected from more than 10,000 twin individuals to characterize correlations between FP, age, sex, and five main modalities of individual differences, i.e. (i) personality, (ii) cognitive abilities, (iii) motivation, (iv) emotional competence, and (v) chronometric tasks. Personality was investigated using both global personality (Big Five) dimensions and more specific traits, i.e. schizotypy and gender role related personality traits. Cognitive abilities included measures of general IQ as well as musical abilities. Motivation was assessed using the Global Motivation Scale, which includes several subscales tapping into various forms of intrinsic and extrinsic motivation. Emotional competence was operationalised as alexithymia. In alexithymia there is an impaired awareness and regulation of emotions, which may reflect a poor ability to represent emotions mentally (Taylor et al. 1991). The administered chronometric tasks included simple and choice reaction time and a motor timing task. Further details on the employed questionnaires and tasks are provided in the Sect. 17.2. in the current chapter.

Many of these variables had been collected for the purpose of investigating various specific questions relating to music, learning, creativity and health in other projects (see e.g. Mosing et al. 2014, 2015; Theorell et al. 2014, 2015). Here, we utilized the extensive dataset in a more exploratory way, in order to locate FP in the larger landscape of individual differences. However, we also tested three specific hypotheses suggested by earlier studies. First, previous results showing relations between FP and general personality were based on a relatively small sample (n = 137) (Ullén et al. 2012a). One aim of the present study was therefore to see whether we could replicate these findings, i.e. a negative relation between FP and neuroticism and a positive relation between FP and conscientiousness, in a new and much larger cohort. Secondly, earlier studies found very weak or non-significant associations between intelligence and FP in a sample of 2,539 twins (Ullén et al. 2012a). Since this is essentially a negative finding using a single measure of cognitive performance, it was of interest to investigate if it could be replicated and extended in an even larger sample, from which we had data on general IQ, specific cognitive abilities (musical) as well as performance on chronometric tasks (reaction time, motor timing accuracy) that are related to cognitive ability (Jensen 2006; Madison et al. 2009). Finally, earlier studies and flow theory suggest that individuals who spend much time with challenging, flow promoting activities tend to have an *autotelic personality*, which is characterized by a tendency to perform activities for their own sake, i.e. because they are intrinsically enjoyable (Csikszentmihalyi 1997a, b). This suggests that FP should be related to a high level of intrinsic rather than extrinsic motivation. We therefore predicted that FP would correlate negatively with the External subscale of the Global Motivation Scale, but positively with the Intrinsic subscale, as well as with the Relative Autonomy Index, which provides an overall measure of an individual's degree of self-determination.

17.2 Methods

17.2.1 Participants

The data presented here were collected as part of a web-survey sent out to a cohort of approximately 32,000 twins (the STAGE cohort) in the Swedish Twin Registry (STR). More information on the STAGE cohort can be found in (Lichtenstein et al. 2006). In total, 11,543 individuals participated in the web-survey. For further details on the data collection, see e.g. (Mosing et al. 2014). All participants gave informed consent and the study was approved by the Regional Ethics Review Board in Stockholm (Dnr 2011/570–31/5, 2012/1107/32).

17.2.2 Study Sample

The aim of the study was to analyse FP and its covariates on the phenotypic level. Ten thousand two hundred sixty participants had provided answers to the FP questionnaire. From this group, a sample of unrelated participants was constructed, that included all twins from incomplete pairs (i.e. where pairs where only on of the two twins had participated) and one randomly selected twin from each complete twin pair. This final sample was used in all analyses and consisted of 7,793 individuals (3,346 men and 4,447 women), aged between 27 and 54 years. However, due to attrition the number of participants was smaller for tests towards the end of the survey. A summary of the number of participants in the various tests is provided in Table 17.1.

17.2.3 Tests

17.2.3.1 Flow Proneness

FP was measured using the Swedish Flow Proneness Questionnaire (SFPQ) (Ullén et al. 2012a). The SFPQ has three subscales, in which the participants self-rate of how frequently they have flow experiences in three different situations: work, maintenance, and leisure time, respectively. The flow at work subscale is only answered by individuals that are employed. Each subscale consists of seven items, which were chosen to capture the main dimensions of a flow experience (Csikszentmihalyi and Csikszentmihalyi 1988), i.e. a subjective sense of concentration, balance between

Table 17.1 Included tests and number of participants

Measure	Test	Number of participants
Flow proneness	Swedish Flow Proneness Questionnaire (SFPQ)	7,793
Motivation	Global Motivation Scale (GMS)	7,792
Big Five Personality	Big Five Inventory (BFI-44)	7,434
IQ	Wiener Matrizen Test (WMT)	6,398
Personality: gender roles	Bem Sex Role Inventory (BSRI)	6,247
Emotional competence	Toronto Alexithymia Scale (TAS-20)	6,057
Personality: schizotypy	Community Assessment of Psychic Experiences (CAPE-42), positive symptoms scale	4,972
Reaction time	Simple reaction time	5,211
	Choice reaction time	5,166
Motor timing	Isochronous Serial Interval Production (ISIP)	5,128

Tests have been sorted in order of administration, i.e. from highest to lowest number of participants

skills and the challenge of a task, explicit goals, clear feedback, sense of control, lack of a sense of boredom and enjoyment. All items have five response alternatives ranging from 1 ('Never') to 5 ('Every day, or almost every day'). For further details on the psychometric properties of the SFPQ, see (Ullén et al. 2012a). Mean scores of the seven items in each subscale are used to calculate separate measures of FP in professional life (FP-Work), maintenance (FP-Mainten), and leisure time (FP-Leisure). The mean of all items is used as a measure of overall FP (FP-Total).

17.2.3.2 General Personality (Big Five)

Personality was measured with a Swedish translation (Zakrisson 2010) of the 44-item Big Five Inventory (BFI-44) (John et al. 1991). Items consist of descriptions of various personal characteristics that may or may not apply to the respondent. Responses are given on a five-point Likert scale, ranging from 1 ('Do not agree at all') to 5 ('Agree completely'). There are five subscales, which correspond to the Big Five personality traits Openness to Experience (ten items), Conscientiousness (nine items), Extraversion (eight items), Agreeableness (nine items), and Neuroticism (eight items). The score on each subscale is the average of the responses to the corresponding items; 16 of the items are reverse scored.

17.2.3.3 Gender Roles (Personality)

Nine items from the Bem Sex Role Inventory (BSRI) were used to assess behavioural tendencies associated with biological sex. Bem (1974) proposed that masculinity, tendencies more pronounced amongst males, and femininity, those more pronounced amongst females, be considered two independent dimensions rather than opposite poles along one continuum. Several review and factor-analytic studies (summarized in Choi et al. 2009) further indicate two masculinity dimensions, one social and one personal, in addition to femininity. Because short response time was important, we selected the three items with the largest effects sizes for each dimension, as reported by Holt and Ellis (1998). In relation to their order in the original 60-item instrument, the selected items were 32, 35, and 44 for Femininity, 1, 7, and 43 for Personal Masculinity, and 13, 37, 46 for Social Masculinity (Bem 1974).

17.2.3.4 Schizotypy

Schizotypy was assessed with the 20 items of the positive symptoms subscale of the CAPE-42 (Community Assessment of Psychic Experiences) (Stefanis et al. 2002). A Swedish translation verified with back-translation was administered (Therman et al. 2014). This instrument was explicitly designed to probe subclinical psychotic experiences. Items describe psychic experiences or beliefs and responses are given on a frequency scale ranging from 1 ('Never') to 4 ('Almost always'). The final score consists of the mean value of the responses to all 20 items.

17.2.3.5 Intelligence

Intelligence was measured using the Wiener Matrizen Test (WMT; Formann and Piswanger 1979). This is a non-verbal matrix test that is similar in construction to Raven's Progressive Matrices, with which it is highly correlated ($r=0.92$) (Formann and Piswanger 1979). The WMT consists of 24 multiple choice questions and is administered with a 25 min time limit. The total score (General IQ) is the number of correctly answered items.

17.2.3.6 Musical Abilities

Musical abilities were measured using the Swedish Musical Discrimination Test, which includes three subscales: Melody (18 items), Rhythm (18 items), and Pitch (27 items) (Ullén et al. 2014). In all test items, the task of the participant is to discriminate between two consecutively presented stimuli. Each subscale is constructed so that items become progressively more difficult. In the Melody subscale, stimuli consist of isochronous sequences of piano tones that range between four and nine tones in length. The pitch of one randomly selected tone is different in the second stimulus as compared to the first stimulus, and the task of the participant is to indicate which tone. In Rhythm, stimuli consist of rhythmic sequences of brief sine tones (5–7 tones per stimulus sequence). In 11 out of the 18 Rhythm item the two stimuli differ, and in the remaining items they are identical. The task of the participant is to judge whether the two stimuli are the same or different. In the Pitch subscale, stimuli consist of single sine tones. The frequency of one of the tones in an item is always 500 Hz, whereas the frequency of the other tone varies between 501 and 517 Hz. The standard tone (500 Hz) is presented first in some items and last in the others, and the participant indicates whether the first tone was higher or lower in pitch than the second tone. A detailed description of the test can be found in (Ullén et al. 2014).

17.2.3.7 Motivation

Motivation was measured using a Swedish translation of the General Motivation Scale (GMS) (Guay et al. 2003). The GMS consists of six subscales, tapping into different dimensions of motivation: Intrinsic, Integrated, Identified, Introjected, External and Amotivation. Each subscale has 3 items, giving a total of 18 items. Items are rated on a seven-point Likert-type scale, ranging from 1 ('Do not agree at all') to 7 ('Completely agree'). The Relative Autonomy Index is a global score, which is assumed to represent a higher-order index of the extent to which an individual feels self-determined (Vallerand and Bissonnette 1992). It was calculated as a weighted summary of the subscales, using the following weights: Intrinsic, 3; Integrated, 2; Identified, 1; Introjected, −1; External, −2; and Amotivation, −3.

17.2.3.8 Emotional Competence

Emotional competence was operationalised as low alexithymia. Alexithymia was measured using a back-translated and psychometrically validated Swedish version (Simonsson-Sarnecki et al. 2000) of the Toronto Alexithymia Scale (TAS-20) (Bagby et al. 1994, 2014). The TAS-20 contains three subscales that reflect a poor ability to describe emotions (Difficulty Describing, seven items), a poor ability to recognize feelings (Difficulty Identifying, five items), and a tendency for mismatches between coping behaviour and emotions due to a tendency to focus attention externally (Externally Oriented, eight items). The full scale (Global Alexithymia) gives a measure of overall alexithymia. Items are rated on a scale from 1 ('Strongly disagree') to 5 ('Strongly agree'); five items are reverse scored. The score on each is the subscale is the sum of the scores on the individual items of the subscale.

17.2.3.9 Reaction Time

Simple and choice auditory reaction time (RT) was measured with a computer-based task. In Simple RT the stimulus was a cowbell sound, after which the participants had to press the space bar on their computer as fast as possible. In the Choice RT condition the participant heard either the sound of a car horn or of breaking glass, and was instructed to press a key to the left of the keyboard with the left hand or a key to the right with the right hand accordingly. After each response the next sound was presented after a time interval that varied between 2.5 and 4.0 s from a rectangular distribution. An initial 10 runs were given for training before each RT trial proper, which consisted of 25 runs for each condition. Reaction times and their variability for the following analysis were the median and the inter-quartile range across all 25 runs.

17.2.3.10 Motor Timing

The ability to produce consistent time intervals was assessed with an isochronous serial interval production task (ISIP; e.g. Madison et al. 2013) in which the participant was instructed to first entrain to a series of regular sounds by pressing the spacebar 30 times in synchrony with the sounds, and then continue to press it at the same rate for another 30 intervals when the sounds ceased. This was done for four different inter onset intervals (IOI), 524, 655, 819, and 1,024 ms. The ISIP variability measure was the mean proportional variability across all four trials, consisting of the SD across the 30 response intervals divided by the inter onset interval.

17.3 Results

Relations between FP, sex and age are summarized in Table 17.2 Females reported higher FP on all scales, but the effect sizes were very small, except for FP-Mainten, for which a slightly higher effect was seen (Cohen's $d=0.24$). For FP-Leisure there was only a trend for a sex difference at $p=0.04$. Age showed weak positive correlations with all flow scales ($r=0.057$–0.15).

In line with our first hypothesis, FP showed substantial associations with personality. Partial correlations between FP and personality variables (controlling for sex and age) are shown in Table 17.3 Relations were similar for the three FP scales. For the Big Five dimensions, FP correlated positively with Openness to Experience, Conscientiousness, Extraversion, and Agreeableness and negatively with Neuroticism. The strongest correlations were seen with Conscientiousness and Neuroticism. In a multiple regression of FP-Total on all five Big Five dimensions, the latter together explained 33 % of the total variance in FP-Total. Weak to moderate positive correlations were also found with the Femininity and Personal Masculinity subscales of the BSRI, while relations with Social Masculinity were very weak (Table 17.3). Finally, FP was weakly negatively related to Schizotypy (Table 17.3). Adding the BSRI scales and Schizotypy to the multiple regression model only gave a marginal increase in the explained variance in FP-Total, which increased from 33 % to 35 %. FP thus appeared to be mainly related to general personality traits (Big Five).

The second hypothesis was also confirmed by the data, i.e. FP showed negligible correlations with both general intelligence and more narrow cognitive abilities (musical aptitudes) (Table 17.4). Partial correlations were in the range $r=-0.03$–

Table 17.2 Flow proneness, sex and age

		FP-Work	FP-Mainten	FP-Leisure	FP-Total
Males		3.82 (0.54)	3.54 (0.58)	3.70 (0.56)	3.68 (0.45)
Females		3.86 (0.55)	3.68 (0.57)	3.72 (0.58)	3.75 (0.46)
Sex difference	η^2	0.0014	0.014	0.00057	0.0053
	Cohen's *d*	0.076	0.24	0.048	0.15
	p value	0.001	<0.0001	0.04	<0.0001
Age	Pearson *r*	0.15	0.057	0.053	0.10
	p value	<0.0001	<0.0001	<0.0001	<0.0001

Mean values for the different flow proneness variables are shown separately for males and females. Values in parentheses are standard deviations. Females reported higher values for all variables, but the effect sizes (η^2) were very small. Age showed a weak positive correlation with all flow proneness variables

Table 17.3 Personality and flow proneness

	FP-Work	FP-Mainten	FP-Leisure	FP-Total
Big Five Inventory (BFI-44)				
Openness to experience	0.10	0.07	0.14	0.13
Conscientiousness	0.42	0.36	0.36	0.48
Extraversion	0.29	0.22	0.28	0.33
Agreeableness	0.25	0.23	0.25	0.31
Neuroticism	−0.37	−0.27	−0.33	−0.41
Bem sex role inventory				
Femininity	0.17	0.20	0.19	0.23
Personal masculinity	0.29	0.22	0.27	0.33
Social masculinity	0.09	0.07	0.09	0.10
Community Assessment of Psychic Experiences (CAPE-42)				
Schizotypy	−0.12	−0.12	−0.12	−0.16

Numbers are *r* values of partial correlations, controlling for age and sex. All correlations were highly significant ($p<0.0001$)

0.06, with the majority of the correlations not reaching significance at $p<0.01$. A multiple regression of FP-Total on general IQ and the three musical aptitudes further corroborated that the cognitive ability measures explained essentially no variance in FP (multiple $R^2=0.0023$).

Associations with motivational variables (Table 17.5) were in line with predictions from flow theory (hypothesis 3). Correlations were thus weakly or moderately positive with the Intrinsic, Integrated, and Identified subscales, while negative correlations were seen with the subscales Introjected, Extrinsic, and Amotivated. The Relative Autonomy Index, which is a weighted summary of the subscales and represents a higher-order index of the extent to which an individual feels self-determined, correlated $r=0.39$ with FP-Total, supporting that FP is related to a high degree of self-determination. A multiple regression of FP-Total on the six motiva-

Table 17.4 Flow proneness and cognitive abilities

	FP-Work	FP-Mainten	FP-Leisure	FP-Total
Wiener Matrizen Test				
General IQ	0.05*	0.03	0.06*	0.06*
Swedish Music Discrimination Test (SMDT)				
Melody	−0.02	−0.03	−0.01	−0.03
Rhythm	0.01	−0.02	0.04*	0.01
Pitch	0.02	−0.02	−0.01	−0.00

Numbers are *r* values for partial correlations, controlling for age and sex
Correlations significant at $p<0.01$ are indicated with an asterisk

Table 17.5 Flow proneness and motivational scales

	FP-Work	FP-Mainten	FP-Leisure	FP-Total
Global Motivation Scale (GMS)				
Intrinsic	0.24	0.22	0.31	0.32
Integrated	0.20	0.19	0.25	0.27
Identified	0.19	0.16	0.24	0.25
Introjected	−0.11	−0.08	−0.12	−0.13
External	−0.09	−0.08	−0.11	−0.11
Amotivated	−0.15	−0.14	−0.16	−0.19
Relative autonomy index	0.30	0.27	0.36	0.39

Numbers are *r* values for partial correlations, controlling for age and sex. All correlations were highly significant ($p<0.0001$)

tion scales gave a multiple R^2 of 17 %, confirming that motivation explains a substantial amount of variance in FP.

Table 17.6 summarizes correlations between FP and emotional competence, operationalized as alexithymia. Global alexithymia showed weak to moderate negative relations with all FP scales, i.e. FP was related to higher emotional competence. These relations were somewhat stronger for the Difficulty Describing and Difficulty Identifying subscales, which correlated $r=-0.34$ and $r=-0.28$ with FP-Total, respectively, than for External Orientation ($r=-0.17$). A multiple regression showed that the three alexithymia subscales together explained 14 % of the variance in FP-Total.

Finally, Table 17.7 summarizes correlations between FP and the various chronometric tasks, which included reaction time tasks and a motor timing task. As for cognitive abilities, these correlations were mostly non-significant and in all cases negligible in magnitude. A multiple regression of FP-Total on all the chronometric variables gave a multiple R^2 of 0.005.

In summary, significant correlations with FP were thus found for three of the investigated domains: personality, motivation, and emotional competence. To investigate how well FP is predicted by these three domains together, we regressed FP-Total on the nine personality variables (Table 17.3), the six motivational variables (Table 17.5), and the three alexithymia variables (Table 17.6). The multiple R^2 of this regression was 39 %, suggesting that unique contributions from motivational

Table 17.6 Flow proneness and emotional competence

	FP-Work	FP-Mainten	FP-Leisure	FP-Total
Toronto Alexithymia Scale (TAS-20)				
Difficulty describing	−0.28	−0.24	−0.28	−0.34
Difficulty identifying	−0.20	−0.23	−0.23	−0.28
Externally oriented	−0.11	−0.14	−0.15	−0.17
Global alexithymia	−0.25	−0.26	−0.29	−0.34

Numbers are *r* values for partial correlations, controlling for age and sex. All correlations were highly significant ($p<0.0001$)

Table 17.7 Flow proneness and performance on chronometric tasks

	FP-Work	FP-Mainten	FP-Leisure	FP-Total
Reaction time				
Simple RT (median)	−0.01	−0.01	−0.04*	−0.03
Simple RT (interquartile range)	−0.05*	−0.03	−0.05*	−0.06
Choice RT (median)	−0.00	−0.01	−0.03	−0.02
Choice RT (interquartile range)	−0.03	−0.03	−0.04*	−0.05*
Motor timing				
Isochronous Serial Interval Production (ISIP)	−0.01	0.00	−0.03	−0.02

Numbers are *r* values for partial correlations, controlling for age and sex. Correlations significant at $p<0.01$ are indicated with an asterisk

and emotional variables, over and above general personality (Big Five), are relatively small.

17.4 Discussion

The present study represents, to our knowledge, the most extensive investigation to date of how individual differences in flow experiences relate to psychological traits. The overall pattern of the findings is clear: FP is related to personality, emotional competence, and motivation, but essentially unrelated to cognitive abilities and performance on chronometric tasks. The specific hypotheses based on earlier studies were all confirmed, i.e. FP is (i) correlated with emotional stability and conscientiousness, (ii) essentially unrelated to IQ, and (iii) correlated with intrinsic motivation and self-determination.

17.4.1 Flow, Sex and Age

Sex differences in mean FP were negligible (Cohen's $d<0.1$) during work and leisure, while females reported somewhat higher flow during maintenance (Cohen's $d=0.24$). For both males and females, FP was highest during work, followed by leisure and then maintenance. The participants in the present study were in the age range 27–54 years, but the same pattern (i.e. FP-Work > FP-Leisure > FP-Mainten) was previously observed in a cohort of older twins (age 51–68 years) (Ullén et al. 2012a). For Swedish adults with an employment it thus appears typical that the most flow promoting situations occur at work rather than during leisure time, while household work and other maintenance is perceived as least flow promoting. This finding is in line with results from studies from the US, where flow in everyday life was studied using experience sampling; participants were found to spend proportionately more work than leisure time in flow (LeFevre 1988). We found a positive correlation between age and FP-Work, possibly reflecting that work related tasks tend to get more flow promoting with age, as individuals advance in their careers. In line with this, the previously studied twins in the 51–68 years age range reported somewhat higher mean FP-Work (3.95–3.98) than the present, younger participants (Ullén et al. 2012a). However, these effects have to be interpreted with caution, since age and cohort effects are obviously confounded in cross-sectional data.

17.4.2 Flow Proneness and Personality

In line with previous studies we find substantial associations between flow proneness and personality. The five Big Five dimensions together explained 33 % of the variance in FP and the incremental predictive value of variables related to motivation and emotional competence was comparatively small (6 %). Global personality is thus an important influence on how often an individual experiences flow. As predicted from earlier, smaller studies the strongest relations were seen with Neuroticism and Conscientiousness. The negative correlation between Neuroticism and FP could reflect several mechanisms. The negative affect typical of high neuroticism (Gray and McNaughton 2000) is likely to interfere with affective aspects of the flow experience. Furthermore, the emotional and cognitive instability associated with neuroticism (Eid and Diener 1999; Flehmig et al. 2007) could increase the risk for attentional lapses and reduce the sense of control and skill during performance. Finally, neuroticism could have a negative influence on an individual's tendency to participate in challenging activities that are conducive to flow (Ullén et al. 2012a). In line with this, neuroticism is related to an external locus of control (Clarke 2004), a personality trait which in turn is genetically correlated with FP (Mosing et al. 2012a). Conversely, a high conscientiousness appears likely to involve emotional and cognitive mechanisms that enable an individual to engage successfully in flow promoting activities. Conscientiousness is thus related to positive affect and well-being (Marrero Quevedo and Carballeira Abella 2011) as well as active problem coping (D'Zurilla et al. 2011). Conscientious individuals may be more likely to spend time on activities that increase their competence and thereby their ability to take on challenging and flow promoting tasks (Kappe and van der Flier 2010). A neuropsychological key component in the associations between FP, neuroticism and conscientiousness may be impulse control. Neuroticism is related to higher impulsivity, while conscientiousness and impulsivity are negatively related (Whiteside and Lynam 2001). One brain imaging study using positron emission tomography has found that FP is related to individual differences in dopamine systems that are of importance for impulse control and emotional regulation (de Manzano et al. 2013).

The present results extend previous work on FP and personality by showing positive associations with Extraversion, Agreeableness, and Openness to Experience in the Big Five model, the Personal Masculinity and Feminity subscales of the BSRI, as well as negative relations with Schizotypy, i.e. the positive symptoms subscale of the CAPE-42. The associations with both Personal Masculinity and Feminity would appear to be in line with the very weak effects of biological sex on FP. Individual variability in FP thus appears to be minimally influenced by both biological sex and differences in gender role related personality traits as measured by the BSRI.

Measures of Big Five personality dimensions are often non-orthogonal, and models that include higher-order personality factors have been proposed to explain these intercorrelations (see e.g. Digman 1997; Musek 2007). One of the most discussed models in the recent literature includes a general factor of personality (GFP) that sits at the top of a hierarchical structure of personality traits, thus capturing positive correlations between extraversion, conscientiousness, agreeableness and openness to experience, and negative correlations between these four dimensions and neuroticism (Musek 2007). Interestingly, the pattern of correlations between FP and Big Five dimensions observed here suggests that FP may be correlated with the GFP. The GFP has been interpreted as a tendency to act in a socially well-adapted way that promotes personal growth and well-being (Davies et al. 2015). Notably, both the GFP and FP are related to measures of self-esteem (Erdle et al. 2010; Asakawa 2010). These findings certainly appear to suggest interesting possible avenues for future work on FP and personality. However, one should note that there is still considerable controversy around to what extent the GFP exists a substantive higher-order personality trait, and to what extent it rather reflects response set artefacts and social desirability bias (for a recent metaanalysis and discussion see e.g. Davies et al. 2015).

Finally, the observed associations between FP and personality are of interest in relation to potential associations between FP, psychological well-being and health. We find negative correlations between FP and Schizotypy, operationalised as the positive symptoms subscale of the CAPE-42. This measure is in turn associated with a higher risk for depressive episodes or generalized anxiety disorder (Therman et al. 2014). Many studies have investigated relations between Big Five personality traits and psychiatric diseases. Quantitative reviews of this literature support that many forms of depressive, anxiety, and substance-abuse disorders are associated with high neuroticism and low conscientiousness; low extraversion has also found in several disorders (Spinhoven et al. 2013; Kotov et al. 2010). All these traits are associated with lower FP (see Table 17.3).

17.4.3 Flow Proneness and Cognitive Abilities

The present results replicate our previous findings of negligible relations between FP and IQ (Ullén et al. 2012a) in an even larger sample and using more cognitive ability measures. The general IQ test employed here, the WMT, is a matrix test which is similar to, and highly correlated with Raven's Progressive Matrices (Formann and Piswanger 1979) – a commonly used single test proxy for general IQ (Jensen 1998). Standard psychometric models represent human cognitive abilities as a hierarchical structure of factors, with the single factor at the highest level (*g*) corresponding to general cognitive ability, and a number of broad but more specific, second-order cognitive abilities in a second stratum (McGrew 2009; Carroll 1993; Jensen 1998). The weak relations between FP and WMT both here and our previously studied cohort, as well as the negligible relations between FP and the other cognitive ability measures in the present study provide a strong indication that FP is essentially unrelated to *g*. Whether FP is related to other broad abilities remains partly an open question, since we have data from a limited set of cognitive tasks and have not performed any factor analysis of their correlation structure. Most notably, perhaps, we lack measures of Comprehension-knowledge ("crystallized intelligence", Gc), a broad ability factor that reflects language-based and procedural competencies acquired through acculturation (McGrew 2009; Cattell 1987). To investigate whether Gc is related to FP, e.g. by allowing the individual to engage more successfully in challenging activities, would be an interesting question for further studies. However, one can note that tests employed here would be expected to tap into several other broad abilities. Matrix IQ tests of the WMT/Raven type typically load on both Fluid Reasoning (Gf), which is strongly related to *g*, and Visual Processing (Gv) (Gustafsson 1984). The musical discrimination tests (SMDT) would be expected to load on the ability factor Auditory Processing (Ga) and reaction time tasks tap into Reaction and Decision Speed (Gt) (McGrew 2009; Carroll 1993). While more detailed studies would be of interest, the nil relations in the present data could thus be seen as a first indication that FP may be relatively independent of both general intelligence and several of the more well-defined specific human cognitive abilities in the second stratum.

The lack of a relation between FP and intellectual abilities could be seen as surprising for at least two reasons. First, cognitive ability is correlated with a host of real life variables, including outcomes such as scholastic achievement and job complexity (Jensen 1998; Hunt 2011), which could be expected to correlate with the opportunity and capacity to engage in challenging and flow promoting activities. In line with this, we found in our previous study a trend for a slightly higher relation between IQ and FP-Work (regression $\beta=0.11$), than the other SFPQ subscales (Ullén et al. 2012a). However, this was not replicated here. Perhaps the solution to this paradox is simply that individuals with different psychological trait profiles find flow in different activities. Flow research has from the beginning emphasized that the flow experience can occur in a wide range of activities, with very different physical, emotional and cognitive demands, as long as there is appropriate balance between challenge and skills (Csikszentmihalyi and Csikszentmihalyi 1988).

A second reason to expect FP-intelligence correlations is that flow is characterized by high concentration on the performed task, and attention is substantially correlated with intelligence (Schweizer and Moosbrugger 2004; Schweizer et al. 2005). One possibility is that the subjectively effortless attention characteristic of a flow state has different neuropsychological underpinnings, and hence different relations to cognitive ability, than the various form of effortful attention that are typically studied in attention paradigms (Ullén et al. 2010; Bruya 2010). However, an important caveat in this context is that we currently do not have methods that allow us to study the temporal characteristics of state flow in an experimental setting, and we therefore do not know whether the detailed characteristics of flow states (e.g. their stability, intensity, or duration) correlate with cognitive abilities or other traits.

17.4.4 Flow Proneness and Motivation

The associations between FP and the various motivation subscales of the GMS were as predicted and entirely in line with flow theory, i.e. flow prone individuals tend to be intrinsically motivated (Csikszentmihalyi 1997b). The GMS test is constructed based on the self-determination theory of motivation (Deci and Ryan 1985). The highest correlations with FP were consistently seen for the Intrinsic subscale but a weighted index of all the subscales which is intended to give an overall measure of an individual's degree of self-determination, the Relative Autonomy Index, showed somewhat larger associations with FP than any of the individual subscales. Correlations between FP and motivation were essentially the same for FP-Work, FP-Leisure, and FP-Mainten suggesting that the observed relations reflect a general tendency that affects flow in all domains of life.

Earlier work by Csikszentmihalyi has suggested that intrinsic motivation and flow may be important factors underlying creative achievement (Csikszentmihalyi 1997a). One important focus in self-determination theory based research has been the prediction of physical activity, which is correlated with many health-related outcomes. The literature indeed demonstrates that physical activity is correlated with self-determined motivation, although the reported effect sizes generally are weak or modest (Owen et al. 2014).

It can be noted that the GMS subscales refer to general forms of motivation rather than domain or task specific motivation. We have recently found that engagement in voluntary music practice is substantially predicted by the frequency of flow experiences specifically during musical activities (i.e. "musical flow proneness"), while relations to general flow proneness (i.e. the SFPQ subscales employed here) were considerably weaker (Butković et al. 2015). An interesting question is therefore whether stronger associations than those observed here, would be seen between flow experiences in a particular domain or activity and intrinsic motivation for that particular activity. It does not appear unlikely that there could be important domain-specific differences in both flow proneness and motivation.

17.4.5 Flow Proneness and Emotional Competence

The terms "emotional competence" or "emotional intelligence" are commonly used for a variety of constructs that are related to skills and abilities of importance for emotional processing, e.g. the identification and understanding of emotions, emotional expression, attention to emotions and emotional regulation (for a recent discussion see e.g. Keefer 2015). Here, we evaluated emotional competence using a measure of alexithymia. The term "alexithymia" (literally, "no words for feelings") was introduced by Sifneos (1973) who observed that patients with psychosomatic disorders had difficulties in recognizing and finding appropriate words for emotions and feelings. Self-report measures such as the Toronto Alexithymia Scale employed here (Bagby et al. 1994, 2014) treat alexithymia as a dimensional, continuous trait and investigations on population representative samples have found that alexithymia is normally distributed (Salminen et al. 1999). High alexithymia thus indicates a deficiency in emotional processing, and the negative associations with FP seen in the present study suggest that individuals experiencing more flow tend to have a higher emotional competence. These associations were seen for all three TAS-20 subscales as well as Global Alexithymia, although the correlations were somewhat weaker for the External Orientation subscale, indicating that FP is particularly related to a higher ability to identify and describe emotions.

One interesting aspect of these associations is that alexithymia is related to various health outcomes. The prevalence of alexithymia is higher in chronic pain patients than in the general population (Mendelson 1982). Other clinical outcomes related to alexithymia are depression (Honkalampi et al. 2000) and hypertension (Jorgensen and Houston 1986; Grabe et al. 2010). Early stage hypertensive subjects have also shown poor ability to describe feelings (Theorell et al. 1984). One suggestion is that these associations reflect a poor regulation of emotions in persons with a high level of alexithymia (Taylor et al. 1991). Causal mechanisms underlying the relations between FP, alexithymia, and health outcomes are likely to be complex but the observed correlations suggest the possibility that FP may be of importance for both psychological and physical well-being.

17.4.6 Flow Proneness and Chronometric Tasks

Cognitive ability shows weak to moderate relations with both reaction time (Deary et al. 2001) and accuracy of motor timing (Madison et al. 2009; Ullén et al. 2012b). The close to nil relations between these tasks and FP thus further support that FP is essentially unrelated to cognitive ability.

However, intertrial variability in reaction time (Robinson and Tamir 2005) as well as motor timing (Forsman et al. 2009) have also been found to be related to neuroticism. Given the robust correlations between FP and emotional stability (low neuroticism), one could therefore have predicted a negative relation between FP and chronometric task variability that was mediated by this personality trait. However, one should note that the reported correlations between variability in chronometric tasks and neuroticism in the earlier, relatively small literature on this topic are weak, with some studies finding no significant relation at all (Colom and Quiroga 2009). In general, the correlations between FP and variability of reaction time and motor performance observed here tended to be slightly less than 0, although the effect sizes were so minute that they often failed to reach significance even in this large sample (see Table 17.7). This could possibly be seen as weak support for that flow prone individuals have somewhat lower variability in chronometric tasks, although associations of this magnitude, if present, are unlikely to have any practical significance.

17.4.7 Conclusion

Earlier flow research has provided ample evidence for that flow experiences depend on situational variables, most prominently the opportunity to engage in tasks that are neither too simple, nor too challenging relative to the skills of the individual (Csikszentmihalyi 1975/2000, 1997a; Csikszentmihalyi and Csikszentmihalyi 1988). The present data shows unequivocally that individual differences also matter for how much flow we experience, and that these influences primarily are related to personality, in the broad sense, rather than cognitive abilities. To summarize, the typical flow prone individual appears to be emotionally stable, conscientious, agreeable, extravert, open to new experiences, emotionally competent and intrinsically motivated. We note that this overall picture is quite consonant with the concept of the autotelic personality as discussed by Csikszentmihalyi (1997b). Given the strong influence of task variables, i.e. environment, on flow it might at first glance be seen as surprising that the traits analysed here, taken together, explain as much as 39 % of the variance in FP. However, it should be noted that the interactions between personal and environmental variables in this context are likely to be very complex. In particular, it would be incorrect to assume that the observed associations only reflect trait-dependent differences in how individuals react to identical situations. Rather, the correlations are likely to be in part mediated by environmental differences, since flow prone, autotelic individuals actively select and create environments that have beneficial effects on their long-term possibilities to experience flow (Csikszentmihalyi 1997b) (See Chapter 14 Boffi at al. in this volume; for a general discussion of active trait-environment covariation see also e.g. Scarr 1996).

As in any study of this kind, we were only able to analyse some of the myriad of individual differences variables that potentially could be relevant for FP. As noted, we had a limited sampling of cognitive abilities and more narrow personality traits.

For certain individual difference modalities – e.g. interests, religious beliefs, and social attitudes – we had no data at all. Nevertheless, the results taken together make a strong case for that individual differences related to FP largely belong in the personality domain. The study was purposely designed as a broad, exploratory mapping of a larger psychological territory. Follow-up studies that address more specific hypotheses using multivariate modelling techniques would obviously be valuable. An important consideration is that several of the traits that correlate with FP are socially desirable (e.g. openness, emotional stability and emotional competence). In principle, the observed correlations could thus be influenced by both social desirability related response biases and true correlations between desirable traits. However, independent support for that the association between FP and personality is substantial, i.e. due to shared mechanisms, is provided by neuropsychological studies demonstrating genetic overlaps between FP and personality traits (Mosing et al. 2012a), and associations between FP and neural systems involved in personality (de Manzano et al. 2013). Finally, a particularly interesting general observation is that – as discussed – several of the correlates of flow proneness found here have in turn been found to be related to well-being, an active lifestyle, and health. The positive correlates of a life with frequent flow experiences could thus be manifold and wide ranging.

Acknowledgement This work was supported by the Bank of Sweden Tercentenary Foundation (M11-0451:1).

References

Adlai-Gail, W. (1994). *Exploring the autotelic personality*. Unpublished doctoral dissertation, University of Chicago.

Asakawa, K. (2004). Flow experience and autotelic personality in Japanese college students: How do they experience challenges in everyday life? *Journal of Happiness Studies, 5*, 123–154.

Asakawa, K. (2010). Flow experience, culture, and well-being: How do autotelic Japanese college students feel, behave, and think in their daily lives? *Journal of Happiness Studies, 11*, 205–223.

Bagby, R. M., Parker, J. D., & Taylor, G. J. (1994). The twenty-item Toronto Alexithymia Scale–I. Item selection and cross-validation of the factor structure. *Journal of Psychosomatic Research, 38*(1), 23–32.

Bagby, R. M., Ayearst, L. E., Morariu, R. A., Watters, C., & Taylor, G. J. (2014). The internet administration version of the 20-item Toronto Alexithymia Scale. *Psychological Assessment, 26*, 16–22.

Bem, S. L. (1974). The measurement of psychological androgyny. *Journal of Consulting and Clinical Psychology, 42*, 155–162.

Bruya, B. (Ed.). (2010). *Effortless attention*. Cambridge, MA: The MIT Press.

Butković, A., Ullén, F., & Mosing, M. A. (2015). Personality and related traits as predictors of music practice: Underlying environmental and genetic influences. *Personality and Individual Differences, 74*, 133–138.

Carroll, J. B. (1993). *Human cognitive abilities. A survey of factor-analytic studies*. New York: Cambridge University Press.

Cattell, R. B. (1987). Intelligence: Its structure, growth, and action. Amsterdam: North-Holland
Choi, N., Fuqua, D. R., & Newman, J. L. (2009). Exploratory and confirmatory studies of the structure of the Bem sex role inventory short form with two divergent samples. *Educational and Psychological Measurement, 69*, 696–705.
Clarke, D. (2004). Neuroticism: Moderator or mediator in the relation between locus of control and depression? *Personality and Individual Differences, 37*, 245–258.
Colom, R., & Quiroga, M. A. (2009). Neuroticism, intelligence, and intra-individual variability in elementary cognitive tasks: Testing the mental noise hypothesis. *Psicothema, 21*(3), 403–408.
Csikszentmihalyi, M. (1975/2000). *Beyond boredom and anxiety*. San Francisco: Jossey-Bass.
Csikszentmihalyi, M. (1997a). *Creativity: Flow and the psychology of discovery and invention*. New York: Harper Perennial.
Csikszentmihalyi, M. (1997b). *Finding flow: The psychology of engagement with everyday life*. New York: Basic Books.
Csikszentmihalyi, M., & Csikszentmihalyi, I. (1988). *Optimal experience. Psychological studies of flow in consciousness*. Cambridge: Cambridge University Press.
Csikszentmihalyi, M., & Schneider, B. (2000). *Becoming adult: How teenagers prepare for the world of work*. New York: Basic Books.
D'Zurilla, T. J., Maydeu-Olivares, A., & Gallardo-Pujol, D. (2011). Predicting social problem solving using personality traits. *Personality and Individual Differences, 50*(2), 142–147.
Davies, S. E., Connelly, B. S., Ones, D. S., & Birkland, A. S. (2015). The general factor of personality: The "Big One," a self-evaluative trait, or a methodological gnat that won't go away? *Personality and Individual Differences, 81*, 13–22. doi:10.1016/j.paid.2015.01.006.
de Manzano, Ö., Cervenka, S., Jucaite, A., Hellenäs, O., Farde, L., & Ullén, F. (2013). Individual differences in the proneness to have flow experiences are linked to dopamine D2-receptor availability in the striatum. *NeuroImage, 67*, 1–6.
Deary, I. J., Der, G., & Ford, G. (2001). Reaction times and intelligence differences – a population-based cohort study. *Intelligence, 29*(5), 389–399.
Deci, E., & Ryan, R. (1985). *Intrinsic motivation and self-determination in human behavior*. New York: Plenum.
Digman, J. M. (1997). Higher-order factors of the Big Five. *Journal of Personal and Social Psychology, 73*, 1246–1256.
Eid, M., & Diener, E. (1999). Intraindividual variability in affect: Reliability, validity, and personality correlates. *Journal of Personal and Social Psychology, 76*, 662–676.
Erdle, S., Irwing, P., Rushton, J. P., & Park, J. (2010). The general factor of personality and its relation to self-esteem in 628,640 internet respondents. *Personality and Individual Differences, 48*, 343–346.
Flehmig, H. C., Steinborn, M., Langner, R., & Westhoff, K. (2007). Neuroticism and the mental noise hypothesis: Relationships to lapses of attention and slips of action in everyday life. *Psychological Science, 49*, 343–360.
Formann, A. K., & Piswanger, K. (1979). *Wiener Matrizen-Test. Ein Rasch-skalierter sprachfreier Intelligenztest*. Beltz, Weinheim.
Forsman, L., Madison, G., & Ullén, F. (2009). Neuroticism is correlated with drift in serial time interval production. *Personality and Individual Differences, 47*(3), 229–232.
Grabe, H. J., Schwahn, C., Barnow, S., Spitzer, C., John, U., Freyberger, H. J., et al. (2010). Alexithymia, hypertension, and subclinical atherosclerosis in the general population. *Journal of Psychosomatic Research, 68*(2), 139–147. doi:10.1016/j.jpsychores.2009.07.015.
Gray, J. A., & McNaughton, N. (2000). *The neuropsychology of anxiety: An inquiry into the functions of the septo-hippocampal system*. Oxford: Oxford University Press.
Guay, F., Mageau, G. A., & Vallerand, R. J. (2003). On the hierarchical structure of self-determined motivation: A test of top-down, bottom-up, reciprocal, and horizontal effects. *Personality and Social Psychology Bulletin, 29*, 992–1004.
Gustafsson, J.-E. (1984). A unifying model for the structure of intellectual abilities. *Intelligence, 8*, 179–203.

Holt, C. L., & Ellis, J. B. (1998). Assessing the current validity of the Bem sex-role inventory. *Sex Roles, 39*, 929–941.

Honkalampi, K., Hintikka, J., Tanskanen, A., Lehtonen, J., & Viinamaki, H. (2000). Depression is strongly associated with alexithymia in the general population. *Journal of Psychosomatic Research, 48*(1), 99–104. doi:10.1016/s0022-3999(99)00083-5.

Hunt, E. (2011). *Human intelligence*. Cambridge: Cambridge University Press.

Ishimura, I., & Kodama, M. (2006). Dimensions of flow experience in Japanese college students: Relation between flow experience and mental health. *Japanese Journal of Health Psychology, 13*, 23–34.

Jackson, S. A., & Eklund, R. C. (2004). *The flow scales manual*. Morgantown: Publishers Graphics.

Jackson, S. A., Kimiecik, J. C., Ford, S., & Marsh, H. W. (1998). Psychological correlates of flow in sport. *Journal of Sport and Exercise Psychology, 20*, 358–378.

Jackson, S. A., Thomas, P. R., Marsh, H. W., & Smethurst, C. J. (2001). Relationships between flow, self-concept, psychological skills, and performance. *Journal of Applied Sport Psychology, 13*, 129–153.

Jackson, S. A., Martin, A. J., & Eklund, R. C. (2008). Long and short measures of flow: The construct validity of the FSS-2, DFS-2, and new brief counterparts. *Journal of Sport and Exercise Psychology, 30*(5), 561–587.

Jensen, A. R. (1998). *The g factor (The g factor)*. Westport: Praeger Publishers.

Jensen, A. R. (2006). *Clocking the mind: Mental chronometry and individual differences*. Oxford: Elsevier.

John, O. P., Donahue, E. M., & Kentle, R. L. (1991). *The Big Five Inventory-Versions 4a and 54*. Berkeley: Institute of Personality and Social Research.

Jorgensen, R. S., & Houston, B. K. (1986). Family history of hypertension, personality pattern, and cardiovascular reactivity to stress. *Psychosomatic Medicine, 48*, 102–117.

Kappe, R., & van der Flier, H. (2010). Using multiple and specific criteria to assess the predictive validity of the Big Five personality factors on academic performance. *Journal of Research in Personality, 44*(1), 142–145.

Keefer, K. V. (2015). Self-report assessments of emotional competencies: A critical look at methods and meanings. *Journal of Psychoeducational Assessment, 33*(1), 3–23. doi:10.1177/0734282914550381.

Kotov, R., Gamez, W., Schmidt, F., & Watson, D. (2010). Linking "Big" personality traits to anxiety, depressive, and substance use disorders: A meta-analysis. *Psychological Bulletin, 136*, 768–821.

LeFevre, J. (1988). Flow and the quality of experience during work and leisure. In M. Csikszentmihalyi & I. S. Csikszentmihalyi (Eds.), *Optimal experience: Psychological studies of flow in consciousness* (pp. 307–318). Cambridge: Cambridge University Press.

Lichtenstein, P., Sullivan, P. F., Cnattingius, S., Gatz, M., Johansson, S., Carlström, E., et al. (2006). The Swedish twin registry in the third millenium: An update. *Twin Research and Human Genetics, 9*(6), 875–882.

Madison, G., Forsman, L., Blom, Ö., Karabanov, A., & Ullén, F. (2009). Correlations between general intelligence and components of serial timing variability. *Intelligence, 37*(1), 68–75.

Madison, G., Karampela, O., Ullén, F., & Holm, L. (2013). Effects of practice on variability in an isochronous serial interval production task: Asymptotical levels of tapping variability after training are similar to those of musicians. *Acta Psychologica, 143*, 119–128.

Marrero Quevedo, R. J., & Carballeira Abella, M. (2011). Well-being and personality: Facet-level analyses. *Personality and Individual Differences, 50*, 206–211.

McGrew, K. S. (2009). CHC theory and the human cognitive abilities project: Standing on the shoulders of the giants of psychometric intelligence research. *Intelligence, 37*, 1–10.

Mendelson, G. (1982). Alexithymia and chronic pain – prevalence, correlates and treatment results. *Psychotherapy and Psychosomatics, 37*(3), 154–164.

Moneta, G. (2004). The flow model of intrinsic motivation in Chinese: Cultural and personal moderators. *Journal of Happiness Studies, 5*, 181–217.

Mosing, M. A., Cesarini, D., Johannesson, M., Magnusson, P. K. E., Pedersen, N. L., Nakamura, J., et al. (2012a). Genetic and environmental influences on the relationship between flow proneness, locus of control and behavioral inhibition. *PLoS One, 7*(11), e47958.
Mosing, M. A., Magnusson, P. K., Pedersen, N. L., Nakamura, J., Madison, G., & Ullén, F. (2012b). Heritability of proneness for psychological flow experiences. *Personality and Individual Differences, 53*(5), 699–704.
Mosing, M. A., Madison, G., Pedersen, N. L., Kuja-Halkola, R., & Ullén, F. (2014). Practice does not make perfect: No causal effect of music practice on music ability. *Psychological Science, 25*(9), 1795–1803.
Mosing, M. A., Madison, G., Pedersen, N. L., & Ullén, F. (2015). Investigating cognitive transfer within the framework of music practice: Genetic pleiotropy rather than causality. *Developmental Science*. doi:10.1111/desc.12306.
Musek, J. (2007). A general factor of personality: Evidence for the Big One in the five-factor model. *Journal of Research in Personality, 41*, 1213–1233.
Owen, K. B., Smith, J., Lubans, D. R., Ng, J. Y. Y., & Lonsdale, C. (2014). Self-determined motivation and physical activity in children and adolescents: A systematic review and meta-analysis. *Preventive Medicine, 67*, 270–279. doi:10.1016/j.ypmed.2014.07.033.
Robinson, M. D., & Tamir, M. (2005). Neuroticism as mental noise: A relation between neuroticism and reaction time standard deviations. *Journal of Personality and Social Psychology, 89*(1), 107–114.
Salminen, J. K., Saarijarvi, S., Aarela, E., Toikka, T., & Kauhanen, J. (1999). Prevalence of alexithymia and its association with sociodemographic variables in the general population of Finland. *Journal of Psychosomatic Research, 46*(1), 75–82. doi:10.1016/s0022-3999(98)00053-1.
Scarr, S. (1996). How people make their own environments: Implications for parents and policy makers. *Psychology, Public Policy, and Law, 2*, 204–228.
Schweizer, K., & Moosbrugger, H. (2004). Attention and working memory as predictors of intelligence. *Intelligence, 32*(4), 329–347.
Schweizer, K., Moosbrugger, H., & Goldhammer, F. (2005). The structure of the relationship between attention and intelligence. *Intelligence, 33*, 589–611.
Sifneos, P. E. (1973). The prevalence of 'alexithymic' characteristics in psychosomatic patients. *Psychotherapy and Psychosomatics, 22*(2), 255–262.
Simonsson-Sarnecki, M., Lundh, L. G., Torestad, B., Bagby, R. M., Taylor, G. J., & Parker, J. D. (2000). A Swedish translation of the 20-item Toronto Alexithymia Scale: Cross-validation of the factor structure. *Scandinavian Journal of Psychology, 41*, 25–30.
Spinhoven, P., van der Does, W., Ormel, J., Zitman, F. G., & Penninx, B. (2013). Confounding of Big Five personality assessments in emotional disorders by comorbidity and current disorder. *European Journal of Personality, 27*(4), 389–397. doi:10.1002/per.1885.
Stefanis, N. C., Hanssen, M., Smirnis, N. K., Avramopoulos, D. A., Evdokimidis, I. K., Stefanis, C. N., et al. (2002). Evidence that three dimensions of psychosis have a distribution in the general population. *Psychology and Medicine, 32*(2), 347–358.
Taylor, G. J., Bagby, R. M., & Parker, J. D. (1991). The alexithymia construct: A potential paradigm for psychosomatic medicine. *Psychosomatics, 32*, 153–164.
Theorell, T., Alfredssson, L., Knox, S., Perski, A., Svensson, J., & Waller, D. (1984). On the interplay between socioeconomic factors, personality and work environment in the pathogenesis of cardiovascular disease. *Scandinavian Journal of Working Environment and Health, 10*, 373–380.
Theorell, T., Mosing, M. A., Lennartsson, A.-K., & Ullén, F. (2014). Musical activity and emotional competence – a twin study. *Frontiers in Psychology, 5*, 744.
Theorell, T., Lennartsson, A.-K., Madison, G., Mosing, M. A., & Ullén, F. (2015). Predictors of continued music practice – from childhood and adolescence to adult years. *Acta Paediatrica, 104*(3), 274–284.

Therman, S., Suvisaari, J., & Hultman, C. M. (2014). Dimensions of psychotic experiences among women in the general population. *International Journal Methods in Psychiatric Research, 23*(1), 62–68. doi:10.1002/mpr.1427.

Ullén, F., de Manzano, Ö., Theorell, T., & Harmat, L. (2010). The physiology of effortless attention. In B. Bruya (Ed.), *Effortless attention* (pp. 205–218). Cambridge, MA: The MIT Press.

Ullén, F., de Manzano, Ö., Almeida, R., Magnussson, P. K. E., Pedersen, N. L., Nakamura, J., et al. (2012a). Proneness for psychological flow in everyday life: Associations with personality and intelligence. *Personality and Individual Differences, 52*, 167–172.

Ullén, F., Söderlund, T., Kääriä, L., & Madison, G. (2012b). Bottom-up mechanisms are involved in the relation between accuracy in timing tasks and intelligence – further evidence using manipulations of state motivation. *Intelligence, 40*, 100–106.

Ullén, F., Mosing, M. A., Holm, L., Eriksson, H., & Madison, G. (2014). Psychometric properties and heritability of a new online test for musicality, the Swedish musical discrimination test. *Personality and Individual Differences, 63*, 87–93.

Vallerand, R. J., & Bissonnette, R. (1992). Intrinsic, extrinsic, and amotivational styles as predictors of behavior – a prospective-study. *Journal of Personality, 60*(3), 599–620.

Whiteside, S. P., & Lynam, D. R. (2001). The Five Factor Model and impulsivity: Using a structural model of personality to understand impulsivity. *Personality and Individual Differences, 30*(4), 669–689.

Zakrisson, I. (2010). Big Five Inventory (BFI): Utprövning för svenska förhållanden. *Social Science Reports from Mid Sweden University 3*: Mid Sweden University.

Chapter 18
Optimal Experience and Optimal Identity: A Multinational Examination at the Personal Identity Level

Yanhui Mao, Scott Roberts, and Marino Bonaiuto

Abstract The present chapter provides evidence for the association between flow and identity via quantitative examinations based on Eudaimonistic identity theory, where an individual is seen to recognize elements of his or her true self, including interests, talents, and abilities, through participating in a range of personally salient (identity-related) and therein self-defining activities. Specifically, salient characteristics of activity experiences, i.e., feelings of personal expressiveness and flow, are seen to facilitate an individual's personal growth in the process of solidifying self-definition. On these bases, a relationship between flow experience and personal identity strength is hypothesized and confirmed via a multinational investigation, in which identity consolidation is observed to be facilitated through the participation in self-defining activities that are platforms to optimal experience. In sum, the present investigation makes a cohesive case for the relationship between subjective experiences of flow and sense of self-identification. Finally, further and ongoing research directions are outlined.

Y. Mao (✉)
Dipartimento di Psicologia dei Processi di Sviluppo e Socializzazione, Sapienza Università di Roma, Rome, Italy

Department of Early Childhood Education, Alexander Technological Educational Institute of Thessaloniki, Thessaloniki, Greece
e-mail: yanhui.mao@uniroma1.it

S. Roberts
Department of Psychology, Claremont Graduate University, Claremont, CA, USA
e-mail: scott.roberts@cgu.edu

M. Bonaiuto
Dipartimento di Psicologia dei Processi di Sviluppo e Socializzazione, Sapienza Università di Roma, Rome, Italy

Centro Interuniversitario di Ricerca in Psicologia Ambientale (CIRPA), Sapienza Università di Roma, Rome, Italy
e-mail: marino.bonaiuto@uniroma1.it

L. Harmat et al. (eds.), *Flow Experience*, DOI 10.1007/978-3-319-28634-1_18

18.1 Introduction

18.1.1 Eudaimonistic Identity Theory

Eudaimonistic identity theory (Waterman 1990a, 1992, 1993a) is grounded in both Aristotle's philosophy of eudaimonia and Erikson's theories of identity (Erikson 1968, 1980). Eudaimonia is a word of Greek origin which can be traced to Aristotle's works *Nicomachean Ethics* (Aristotle IV c. B.C.), as comprised of the words "*eu*" ("good") and "*daimōn*" ("spirit"), and has been interpreted in different ways as relating to "well-being" (Ross 1949), or "flourishing" (Cooper 1999), an intrinsically good state or activity constitutive of the good life (Fraser 2014), seeking to use and develop the best in oneself (Huta 2012), the various realization of one's potential (Irwin 1985), and the highest human good that arises from activities achievable by human action (Ryff and Singer 2008). Based upon *Nicomachean Ethics*, Norton (1976) remarks in his book *Personal Destinies* that eudaimonism as an ethical theory calls individuals to recognize and live with their daimon or "true self".

According to Aristotle, eudaimonia actually requires activity – action – so that it is not sufficient for a person to possess an unpotentiated ability or disposition. Aristotle's philosophy on eudaimonia has provided philosophically grounding influence upon psychological researchers across the study of different constructs regarding personal growth and fulfillment, i.e., flow (Csikszentmihalyi 1975, 1988), personal expressiveness (Waterman 1990a, b, 1992, 1993a, 2004), intrinsic motivation (Deci and Ryan 1985, 1987, 1991, 2002; Waterman 1993a, 2004), well-being (Diener and Lucas 2000; Ryff and Singer 2006), self-determination (Deci and Ryan 1985, 2002; Ryan and Deci 2000, 2001), as well as parenting (Huta 2012). As a subjective state, eudaimonia refers to the feelings present when one is moving toward self-realization in terms of developing one's unique individual potentials and furthering one's purpose in living (Waterman et al. 2008).

Erikson's theories of identity provide the other stream of literature underpinning Eudaimonistic identity theory, and indicate that an optimally developed identity emerges from the discovery of the critical elements of one's self which result in a sense of feeling at home with who one is and what one is doing in life. A eudaimonistic identity framework focuses specifically on personally salient identity-related activities (or termed also as self-defining activities), since they help to discover and to recognize one's "daimon" or true self by allowing interests, talents and abilities to flourish (Waterman 1984, 1990a, 1992, 1993a, 2004; Coatsworth et al. 2005; Sharp et al. 2007). Overall, the eudaimonistic identity perspective provides a link for understanding the connection between identity experiences through the experience of a range of self-defining activities.

18.1.2 Self-Defining Activities

Self-defining activities are those activities that are representative of who a person is or would like to become (Coatsworth et al. 2005, 2006; Waterman 2004). They are distinct from other daily activities in that they are identified by an individual as being important to who he or she fundamentally is as a person (Sharp et al. 2007). Self-defining activities have been termed personally salient (identity-related) activities (Coatsworth et al. 2005, 2006; Sharp et al. 2007; Schwartz and Waterman 2006; Waterman 2004), or personally expressive activities (Waterman 2004). This is conveyed through a process of exploration within identity-related activities through which a person forms the basis for building a coherent personal identity. Such identity-related activities are identified by an individual as being important of who he/she is as a person. They are essential for identity consolidation particularly during adolescence and emerging adulthood in providing for example a broad sense of social identity (e.g., activities of jocks vs. brains; Eccles and Barber 1999) that suggests appropriate behaviors and how one fits into the social milieu (Coatsworth et al. 2005; Sharp et al. 2007). As Maslow (1970) expressed, activities that are important for identity development, are those that provide the impetus towards self-actualization or a full use and exploration of talents, capacities, and potentials. According to Erikson (1968, 1980), an optimally developed identity emerges from the discovery of those critical elements of one's self that result in the understanding of who one is and what one is pursuing in life. Recent research on identity development has provided evidence that self-defining activities may assist adults' exploration of sense of a more meaningful and coherent identity, facilitating identity work necessary for identity integration, and providing a unique context for the exploration of their interests and talents (Barber et al. 2001; Fredricks et al. 2002; Hansen et al. 2003; Sharp et al. 2007). The above mentioned literature has expanded the sense in which identity development is associated with action in the context of activity and is further informative for understanding which specific features of various activities may promote identity strength. Flow, being a salient category among the various possible kinds of activity-related experiences, could potentially be among the most influential, though it has yet to be systematically analyzed for its impact upon a person's identity consolidation. In general, there could be a range of activity-related features that are potentially relevant for identity development. However, several aspects of the flow experience (e.g., the balance between a person's skills and the challenges of the context, perceived control, etc.) pertain to an individual's perception of and emotional reactions to her/his relation with the situation. This could potentially contribute to making the activity (whatever the activity is) important for self-perception and self-assessment. Flow therefore is closely related to the eudaimonia concept of the crucial link between what one does and one's own experience of it (Waterman 1990b), with the psychological impact of all this on one's own self-concept.

Some activities could be more favorable for, or more frequently associated with this purpose; complementary, one may argue that some entertainment activities could be identity irrelevant, or that, on the contrary, trivial activities might end up in having personal impact in the long run. However, these kinds of question still need to be empirically tested too. For this purpose, on the basis of previous categorizations for self-defining activities (Coatsworth et al. 2005; Sharp et al. 2007; Waterman 2004, 2005; Delle Fave and Massimini 2005), participants' self-defining activities reported in the present work are clustered into six categories: productive and compulsory activities (e.g., study, writing a paper, teaching in school, working as an employee); social activities (e.g., talking with family via Skype, dating); structured leisure activities (sports/hobby: e.g., playing chess, music and dance, rock climbing); relaxed leisure (e.g. watching TV, eating, sexual relations, window shopping); performing/fine arts/music (e.g., drama, choir, band, sculpting); and finally religious/altruistic (church attendance, volunteer work).

18.1.3 Flow, an Activity Experience as Eudaimonia

Flow is defined as the mental state in which a person performing an activity is fully immersed in a task with complete involvement, intense enjoyment and intrinsic interest (Csikszentmihalyi 1977, 1990). Seligman (2002) has suggested that the good life, in alignment with Aristotle's eudaimonia, is in part a life of engagement that is characterized as one in which flow is pursued as a means towards happiness (Seligman 2002; Peterson et al. 2005). And such a good life is characterised by complete absorption in what one does (Nakamura and Csikszentmihalyi 2002). Flow may emerge in any situation when there is an ongoing activity (Csikszentmihalyi 1997), and when such activity is characterized by clear goals, immediate and unambiguious feedback, and an appropriate balance of sufficient challenges with requisite skills (Csikszentmihalyi and Csikszentmihalyi 1988; Csikszentmihalyi 1990; Nakamura and Csikszentmihalyi 2002): such flow characteristics have been interpreted alternatively as flow antecedents (Chen et al. 1999) or flow conditions (Novak et al. 2000). When these conditions are met, flow is characterized by intense concentration, merged action and awareness, perceived temporal distortion (e.g., time acceleration), unselfconsciousness, perceived control, and intrinsically rewarding action (Csikszentmihalyi 1997; Nakamura and Csikszentmihalyi 2002).

The flow experience is hedonic (pleasurable) and intrinsically enjoyable (Waterman 1993a; Seligman 2002). At the same time, however, flow's features have a eudaimonic component since they link an individual's activity with her/his own experience and feelings of that activity, as well as with the experience's impact on the subject conception of her/himself in relation to the pursuit of an activity in a certain challenging situation. The enjoyment from flow is retrospectively assessed and thus distinct (Peterson et al. 2005). Flow is seen to be inherently growth producing by making full use of an individual's skills and abilities while also leading to one's own progressive development (Nakamura and Csikszentmihalyi 2002; Waterman 2007).

18.1.4 Feelings of Personal Expressiveness, an Activity Experience Equivalent to Eudaimonia

Another activity experience – "personal expressiveness" (Waterman 1990a, 1993b) – pertains to the subjective experiences associated with intrinsically motivated, personally salient identity-related activities (Schwartz and Waterman 2006). Such an experience occurs when there is a feeling: (a) of being really alive, (b) that this is who one really is, (c) of more intense involvement than when engaged in most other activities, (d) that this is what the person was meant to do, (e) of being more complete or fulfilled than when engaged in other activities, and (f) of experiencing a special fit or meshing when engaged in the activity (Waterman 1990a, 1993b). According to Waterman, personal expressiveness seems conceptually linked with flow based on the eudaimonist perspective, as personal expressiveness is experienced in connection with furtherance of an individual's skills and talents, and such experience arises in the process of self-realization when an individual's skills meet the challenges afforded by an activity. Activities giving rise to personal expressiveness have been considered as means to identify one's optimal potential, and may serve as a basis for identifying an individual's goals in life (Schwartz and Waterman 2006; Waterman 1993b, 2004; Waterman et al. 2003).

18.1.5 Psychological and Bio-cultural Selection of Activity

Human beings are exposed to a large number of activities regularly on their daily basis, and they would preferentially select, replicate, and transform some of them that are associated with optimal experience (Delle Fave and Massimini 2005). Flow is not only an end in itself in being among the most enjoyable of human experiences. It also carries impact as being a producer of both complexity of the self as well as selection of bio-cultural information that contributes to cultural evolution (Csikszentmihalyi and Csikszentmihalyi 1988, 2006; Csikszentmihalyi and Massimini 1985; Massimini and Delle Fave 2000; Delle Fave et al. 2011). This process of preferentially selecting attentional foci that promote the cultivation of one's talents and skills is known as "psychological selection", and this orientation leads to a trajectory of skill development and cultivation of the activities that provide platforms for personal growth (Csikszentmihalyi and Massimini 1985). Because of the inherently enjoyable and beneficial qualities of flow, experiencing flow could be one reason for engagement in an activity by the individual. At the group level, if many people experience certain activities as flow promoting, they may be more likely to become established within a cultural repertoire (Massimini and Delle Fave 2000). From the individual perspective, the cultivation of optimal experiences is seen to be advantageous to personal development.

18.1.6 State of Literature

Flow itself has been widely referenced across a variety of fields (Csikszentmihalyi 1990), and has been well researched extensively over the past 40 years since the concept was first coined (Csikszentmihalyi 1975). A few recent links between flow and personal identity are traced within a limited number of research works. These include quantitative studies showing that flow is significantly and positively correlated with ego identity (Schwartz 2006), with personal expressiveness (Coatsworth et al. 2005; Schwartz and Waterman 2006; Waterman et al. 2003), and with intrinsic motivation and self-determination (Schwartz and Waterman 2006). Additionally, there are a few qualitative studies indicating that flow is associated with a person's identity (Coatsworth et al. 2006; Sharp et al. 2007; Tietze 2008; Waterman 2005).

In flow-identity literature, few studies on the relations among flow and personal identity's proxies have been carried out in the last two decades. More specifically, Coatsworth et al. (2005) explored adolescent's self-defining leisure activities and identity experiences across different countries, and they found that flow, as well as personal expressiveness, occurred across a wide variety of group, solitary, structured, and unstructured activities (Csikszentmihalyi 1990, 1996; Waterman 2004). Findings indicated that most adolescents reported high levels of identity experiences within self-defining activities: flow was moderately correlated with personal expressiveness ($r = .55$).

Coatsworth et al. (2006) examined the relations among activity participation, expressive identity, and wellness through the self-defining activities on a sample of 115 high school students, and found that most adolescents identify several activities as self-defining. Expressive identity (within which both flow and personal expressiveness were comprised) mediated the relations between self-defining activities and wellness. However the associations between flow and personal expressiveness were not tested.

Schwartz and Waterman (2006) in a three-timepoint longitudinal study drawing on theories of intrinsic motivation, investigated relations between three subjective indices of intrinsic motivation (interest, flow, and personal expressiveness) and three theoretically derived predictor variables (self-determination, the balance of challenges and skills, and self-realization values). Findings indicated that the increases or decreases in the predictor variables were associated with corresponding increases or decreases in the subjective experience indices; the correlation of flow with personal expressiveness in each timepoint was reported as .56, .49, and .48, respectively.

Schwartz (2006) ascertained the extent to which three alternative perspectives on identity development (self-construction, eudemonistic self-discovery, and agentic personality) relate to various indices of identity consolidation drawn from Erikson (identity status, and identity capital). Schwartz's focus was in particular on personal identity. The results showed that eudaimonistic self-discovery, within which flow was included together with other constructs, correlated $r = .25$ with ego identity.

The results suggested that strategies like eudaimonistic self-discovery could be used to develop an individual's sense of identity.

Drawing on Eudaimonistic identity theory, Sharp et al. (2007) examined three subjective identity-related experiences: personal expressiveness, flow, and goal-directed behavior (which are considered as the indicators of identity development). Findings indicated that both genders had similar identity-related experiences (i.e., flow), however, the relation of flow to identity was not tested.

Another qualitative study by Tietze (2008) applied the case study approach to assess the process of learning through students' response to a course of jazz music. Many of the described scenarios indicate that when engaging in the study of jazz music, the individual did not just experience flow, but he/she also experienced a creation and development of his/her unique self-identity. However, the association of flow with such a unique personal identity was not measured, neither qualitatively, nor quantitatively.

Waterman (2005) studied college students' intrinsic motivation, distinguishing between two philosophical conceptions of happiness: hedonism and eudaimonism. The results indicated that High Effort – High Enjoyment activities, compared to Low Effort – High Enjoyment activities, were associated with greater reported subjective experience of flow and personal expressiveness, greater perceived competence and higher scores for both self-realization values and importance. It was suggested that self-defining activities provided a context that facilitates not only flow, but also personal expressiveness (which could be considered as a proxy for personal identity); however, the correlations between these two constructs were not measured.

Waterman et al. (2003) conducted a research on U.S. university students' intrinsic motivation. Three predictors for the subjective experience of intrinsic motivation (interest, flow, and personal expressiveness) were measured, and flow was positively correlated with personal expressiveness in two sub-studies ($r = .50$ and $r = .66$).

More generally, it should be noted that null results are not reported in the literature. In summary, prior literature suggests a relationship between the degree of flow experience and the strength of personal identity resulting from that activity, yet previous tests of such a relationship were either conducted solely qualitatively (Tietze 2008); or they measured with alternative variables (i.e., personal expressiveness, ego identity) but did not test their direct link (Coatsworth et al. 2006; Waterman 2005; Sharp et al. 2007); or otherwise they tested their link but still using their operationalization in terms of proxy variables such as personal expressiveness (Coatsworth et al. 2005; Schwartz and Waterman 2006; Waterman et al. 2003), or ego identity (Schwartz 2006). Studies applying alternate variables were either partially convergent, activity specific, or employed a proxy of features fundamental to the activity itself (e.g., personal expressiveness within the activity). Optimal experience could be a feature of a person's experience in the context of engagement within a self-defining activity, which in turn develops the self-identity of the actor. Nevertheless, until now almost no literature deals explicitly with a direct quantitative test of the relationship between flow and personal identity. The one exception is a study carried out by our team (Mao et al. 2016) but with reference to a person's identity at the social level. Thus, to bridge this gap, the present investigation aims to use standard and specific measures to test such a link, using different tools from our previous study (Mao et al. 2015). The current study is guided by one aim (*A1*) and two hypotheses (*H1*, *H2*):

A1: To find out what kinds of activities participants reported as self-defining.
H1: There is a main effect of activity type (*Activity 1, 2, 3, 4*) on the subjective experience of flow and personal expressiveness (manipulation check for the four activity types).
H2: Subjects' experience of flow and sense of personal identity from their reported self-defining activities are positively correlated.

18.2 Methods

18.2.1 Participants[1]

A total number of 400 potential participants were contacted, and 290 of them responded (response rate was 72.5 %). After excluding those individuals who were either inattentive or non-discriminating (i.e., the same score was provided for almost all items), or for whom there was missing data on crucial study variables, or for whom their English proficiency were reported as poor, 109 participants (completion rate was 27.3 %) remained. Among these 109 respondents, 48.6 % were males and 51.4 % were females, and their age was in a range between 21 and 39 ($Mean=28.6$, $SD=4.37$): 21–25 (28.4 %), 26–30 (48.6 %), 31–35 (12.8 %), and 36–39 (10.1 %). Concerning their educational background, 2.8 % held a High school diploma, 21.1 % had a Bachelor's degree, 44 % held a Master's degree, while 32.1 % had a doctoral degree. In terms of their nationality, 11.9 % were from U.S.A., 12.8 % were Australian, 14.7 % were Canadian, 9.2 % were Chinese, 11 % were French, 10.1 % were German, 13 % were Italian, 6.4 % were Dutch, 6.4 % were Polish and 8.3 % were Spanish. 79.8 % of the participants were from urban and 20.2 % were from sub-urban settings.

[1] We conducted preliminary analyses to investigate possible age or gender difference on the subjective experience of both flow and personal expressiveness. Results obtained from Independent sample t test did not find any significant gender difference on flow (male: $M=2.87$, $S=.96$ vs. female: $M=2.67$ $SD=.81$), $t(107)=1.16$, $p>.05$), or on personal expressiveness (male: $M=2.81$, $SD=1.09$ vs. female: $M=2.42$ $SD=.91$), $t(107)=2.03$, $p>.05$). Results from univariate ANOVAs indicated that age does not affect either flow ($M=2.77$, $SD=.89$, $F=.67$, $p>.05$), or personal expressiveness ($M=2.61$, $SD=1.01$, $F=.49$, $p>.05$). Thus both gender and age groups were combined for further manipulation check and correlational tests.

18.2.2 Instruments

All tools were administered in English. Answers to all questionnaire items (flow, personal expressiveness, personal identity) were given on a 5-point Likert-type scale ranging from "*not at all characteristic of me*" to "*completely characteristic of me*" when respondents were required to decide how much each statement was characteristic of them by asking "*When engaging in this activity___* (name of *Activity 1*, or *2*, or *3*, or *4*).

18.2.2.1 Flow Experience

Flow was measured using a nine-item scale by Nielsen and Cleal (2010, e.g., *Do you feel in control of the situation? Were you able to concentrate?*). However, those items were modified into statements as "*I feel in control of the situation*; *I feel I am highly concentrated*" in the current investigation. To confirm that the scale displayed good psychometric properties in the current sample, item level results were subjected to multi-level confirmatory factor analysis (CFA[2]) using LISREL 8.80. An acceptable fit was found with one first-order factor model where nine items loaded on a single latent variable: $\chi^2/df = 2.88$, $p < .001$, root mean square error of approximation (RMSEA) = .02. Cronbach's alpha revealed an internal reliability of .88 in the current sample.

18.2.2.2 Personal Expressiveness

The Feelings of Personal Expressiveness Scale (FPES: Waterman 1990a, 1993b; Waterman et al. 2003) was designed to assess subjective experience associated with engagement in various activities (Waterman 1993a, 2005), reflecting one's core sense of being. It is applied in the current study, as with flow, to test individual's subjective experience when engaged in intrinsically motivated, personally salient, and identity-related activities, and it serves as a convergent tool with subjective flow experience in line with eudaimonia philosophy (Waterman 1990a, 1993b). From a eudaemonist perspective, when there are feelings of personal expressiveness in connection with particular identity elements, whether involving vocational goals, ideological values, or beliefs in an interpersonal context, these feelings can be taken as signifying that the individual is acting on her/his eudaimonistic potentials (1993a), i.e., the action is doing is associated to a clearer or stronger sense and

[2] A set of indices for CFA data analytic technique used in present investigation (and relative cut-off values for acceptable fit) has been considered (see Hu and Bentler 1999). Such indices are: the significance value with a cut off value of .05, the root mean square error of approximation (RMSEA) with a cut-off value of .08 (see Browne and Cudeck 1993), and finally the chi-square/*df* ratio falling below 3 (Carmine and McIver 1981).

perception of one's own personal idendity, and/or of his or her own sense of personal identity's development. The scale contains six items, e.g., *When I engage in this activity I feel more intensely involved than I do in most other activities*; *When I engage in this activity I feel that this is what I was meant to do*. A CFA of a one-factor model of the item data showed very good fit indices: $\chi^2/df=2.32$, $p<.001$, RMSEA=.05. Cronbach's alpha coefficient was .91 in the present sample.

18.2.2.3 Personal Identity

Personal identity was measured by the five functions of identity scale (FIS: Adams and Marshall 1996; Serafini and Adams 2002) that theoretically align with Erikson's concept of optimal identity (Erikson 1968). However, a shortened version with 15 items was applied (Serafini et al. 2006), It was used in the current study in order to determine to what extent "optimal identity" is associated with optimal experience (flow), as hypothesized. The FIS is designed to assess the extent to which identity provides individuals with a sense of structure for a better understanding of self-relevant information. Such structure is apparent in a sense of harmony between chosen values, beliefs and commitments, as well as in the alignment of goals within a context of achieving a sense of congruence with present and future conceptions of self. A sense of personal control, free will or agency are also conceived characteristics of this optimal identity, as is the relevant processing of life experience in a manner which enables active self-regulation in the process of goal setting and achievement. The scale has 15 items, e.g., *My values and beliefs reflect who I am*; *I have constructed my own personal goals for myself*. Each item was rated with a 5-point Likert-type scale (*1- not at all characteristic of me* to *5 – completely characteristic of me*): respondents were asked to rate how much each statement was characteristic of them by initially asking "*When engaging in this activity_* (name of *Activity 1*, or *2*, or *3*, or *4*),"; then as item completions for this scale the 15 items were presented to be rated. A CFA of five first-order factor model of the item data indicated satisfying fit indices: $\chi^2/df=2.51$, $p<.001$, RMSEA=.012. The internal consistency reliability estimates for scores on each of five factors in the present sample was .81 for structure, .85 for harmony, .82 for goals, .78 for future, and .74 for personal control.

18.2.3 Procedure

The questionnaire was conducted online for consenting participants within a Google Documents environment, in which subjects' responses were recorded and collected by voluntary participation in the survey through the administration of hyperlinks. A pool of potential young adult research participants from ten nations available through Sapienza University of Rome was contacted via E-mail, Facebook, and Skype. Participants were asked to complete the first section by listing five to ten personally salient activities and choosing four activities according to the criteria of effort (*low* vs. *high*) by enjoyment (*low* vs. *high*) combination: i.e., *Activity 1* (low effort low enjoyment – corresponding to *Apathy* in the flow model), *Activity 2* (high effort low enjoyment corresponding to *Anxiety*), *Activity 3* (low effort high enjoyment – corresponding to *Relaxation*), *Activity 4* (high effort high enjoyment – *Flow*). Responses to the second section concerning each of the four activities were filled in on separate web pages, one page per activity. Participants were then asked to respond their social demographic background in the third section. Data were gathered regarding participants' answers to above three-section self-report questionnaire from June to August in 2013, and were coded for statistical analysis with the SPSS Statistics 20.0 and LISREL 8.80 computer software program.

18.2.4 Data Analysis

We addressed the questions of the *A1* using cross-tabulation comparisons with chi-square statistics, utilized one-way analysis of variance for testing *H1*, and adopted Bravais-Pearson Bivariate correlation to examine our main hypothesis *H2*. All these analyses were conducted in SPSS 20.0.

18.3 Results

18.3.1 Results for A1

Table 18.1 presents both frequencies and percentages within the full sample that listed a self-defining activity in each of six self-defining activity categories. As indicated, the highest rates of self-defining activities for the combined sample are found in the category of structured leisure and social activities, with substantially fewer reporting productive and compulsory activities. The lowest rates are found in the category of religious and altruistic activities. The highest rate for self-defining activities in *Activity 1* is the relaxed leisure categories, while the highest rate in *Activity 2*, *Activity 3* and *Activity* 4 are consistently found in the category of structured leisure. The calculated Chi-square statistic ($\chi^2 = 45.04$, $df = 15$, $p < .001$) indicates that the six self-defining activity categories are distributed significantly differently within the four types of activities. The follow-up analyses are conducted separately for each activity type to locate significant differences: in terms of relaxed leisure category, there is significant differences comparing *Activity 1* to *Activity 2* ($\chi^2 = 20.05$, $df = 5$, $p < .001$), and comparing *Activity 1* to *Activity 4* ($\chi^2 = 28.20$, $df = 5$, $p < .001$); in terms of Performing/fine arts/music, there is significant difference comparing *Activity 2* to *Activity 3* ($\chi^2 = 11.83$, $df = 5$, $p < .05$); in terms of productive and compulsory activities, significant difference is located between *Activity 3* and *Activity 4* ($\chi^2 = 11.78$, $df = 5$, $p < .05$).

Table 18.1 Frequencies and percentage of self-defining activities within six categories by each activity

Categories of activity	Activity 1	Activity 2	Activity 3	Activity 4	Total
Productive and compulsory	N=15 (13.76 %)	N=30 (27.14 %)	N=16 (14.68 %)	N=25 (22.94 %)	N=86 (19.72 %)
Social	N=25 (22.94 %)	N=23 (21.43 %)	N=25 (22.94 %)	N=21 (19.27 %)	N=94 (21.56 %)
Structured leisure	N=26 (23.86 %)	N=38 (35 %)	N=36 (33.03 %)	N=41 (37.61 %)	N=141 (32.34 %)
Relaxed leisure	N=31 (28.44 %)	N=12 (11.43 %)	N=20 (18.35 %)	N=8 (7.34 %)	N=71 (16.28 %)
Performing/fine arts/ music	N=6 (5.5 %)	N=5 (4.29 %)	N=9 (8.26 %)	N=10 (9.17 %)	N=30 (6.88 %)
Religious/altruistic	N=6 (5.5 %)	N=1 (.71 %)	N=3 (2.75 %)	N=4 (3.67 %)	N=14 (3.21 %)
Total	N=109	N=109	N=109	N=109	N=436

18.3.2 Results for H1

One-way Analysis of Variance (ANOVA) on the flow means revealed that, as expected, significant differences among four activity types (M=3.32, SD=.86, F=44.51, p<.001) were detected. For each activity type (*Activity 1, 2, 3, 4*), the mean value for the flow experience was: 2.77 for *Apathy*; 3.14 for *Anxiety*; 3.48 for *Relaxation*; and 3.90 for *Flow*. Post-hoc analysis using Turkey-HSD approach indicated the following varying trends: $Flow_1 < Flow_2$ (p<.005), $Flow_1 < Flow_3$ (p<.001), $Flow_1 < Flow_4$ (p<.001), $Flow_2 < Flow_3$ (p<.05), $Flow_2 < Flow_4$ (p<.001), $Flow_3 < Flow_4$ (p<.005) (Table 18.2). This manifested that flow is best achieved when both effort and enjoyment are high (i.e., when engaging in *Activity 4*). Importantly, high enjoyment high effort activity is associated with greater reported level of flow than high enjoyment low effort activity. On the whole, these results support the case that the four-activity types are relatively different in terms of flow degree. On the basis of the previous study by Waterman et al. (2003), it is known the varying degrees of flow relate to correspondingly varying degrees of both effort and enjoyment. A similar trend also applied to personal expressiveness (M=3.35, SD=1.00, F=58.66, p<.001) across four types of activities that went from *Apathy* (2.61), to *Anxiety* (3.11), to *Relaxation* (3.62), and up to *Flow* (4.05). Post-hoc analysis by Turkey-HSD technique located specific significant differences among four activity types ($PE_1 < PE_2$, p<.001; $PE_1 < PE_3$, p<.001; $PE_1 < PE_4$, p<.001; $PE_2 < PE_3$, p<.001; $PE_2 < PE_4$, p<.001; $PE_3 < PE_4$, p<.005), such varying trends once again proved that the manipulation check serves to validate that the categories are indeed composed of four activities with differing characteristics.

Table 18.2 Multiple comparisons among activities on flow and personal expressiveness (N=109)

Dependent variable	(I) Activity type	(J) Activity type	Mean difference (I–J)	Std. error	Sig.
FLOW	1 (Apathy)	2	−.38*	.10	.001
		3	−.72*	.10	.000
		4	−1.14*	.10	.000
	2 (Anxiety)	1	.38*	.10	.001
		3	−.34*	.10	.006
		4	−.76*	.10	.000
	3 (Relaxation)	1	.72*	.10	.000
		2	.34*	.10	.006
		4	−.42*	.10	.000
	4 (Flow)	1	1.14*	.10	.000
		2	.76*	.10	.000
		3	.42*	.10	.000
PE	1 (Apathy)	2	−.50*	.11	.000
		3	−1.01*	.11	.000
		4	−1.43*	.11	.000
	2 (Anxiety)	1	.50*	.11	.000
		3	−.51*	.11	.000
		4	−.93*	.11	.000
	3 (Relaxation)	1	1.01*	.11	.000
		2	.51*	.11	.000
		4	−.42*	.11	.001
	4 (Flow)	1	1.43*	.11	.000
		2	.93*	.11	.000
		3	.42*	.11	.001

*The mean difference is significant at the 0.05 level

18.3.3 Results for H2

Correlations between flow and personal identity (See Table 18.3) were calculated on the activity level (concerning 4 different activity types) and at the individual level across all the activity types. Specifically, when engaging in *Activity 1* – the "*low effort – low enjoyment*" combination in the *Apathy* activity type, as it would be expected, the individual's reported flow was significantly, strongly correlated with feelings of personal expressiveness ($r=.81$, $p<.001$), with each of the five FIS (r's ranged from .66 to .72, all p's$<.001$), and overall sense of FIS ($r=.80$, $p<.001$). When engaging in *Activity 2* – the "*high effort – low enjoyment*" combination as in the *Anxiety* activity type, the correlations of flow to personal expressiveness ($r=.74$, $p<.001$), and personal identity (r's ranged from .65 to .84, all p's$<.001$) were all significant and positive as hypothesized. When engaging in *Activity 3* – the "*low effort – high enjoyment*" combination as in the *Relaxation* activity type, the correlations of flow to personal expressiveness ($r=.75$, $p<.001$), and to the five functions

Table 18.3 Correlations of flow to personal expressiveness and personal identity (N = 109)

Correlation	Flow				
	Activity level				
	Activity1 (*apathy*)	Activity2 (*anxiety*)	Activity 3 (*relaxation*)	Activity4 (*flow*)	Individual level
PE	.81**	.74**	.75**	.78**	.83**
FIS_control	.71**	.65**	.68**	.80**	.76**
FIS_future	.66**	.67**	.53**	.43**	.64**
FIS_goals	.72**	.79**	.72**	.62**	.75**
FIS_harmony	.71**	.78**	.65**	.68**	.72**
FIS_structure	.72**	.73**	.60**	.71**	.73**
FIS	.80**	.84**	.75**	.73**	.82**

**Correlation is significant at the 0.01 level (two-tailed)

of identity (r's ranged from .53 to .75, $p<.001$) were significant and positive. Finally when engaging in *Activity 4* – the "*high effort – high enjoyment*" combination in the *Flow* activity type, the various indices of flow were significantly positively correlated with personal expressiveness ($r=.78$, $p<.001$), and personal identity (r's ranged from .43 to .80, $p<.001$). Since both flow and personal expressiveness are subjective experiences, and personal identity per se is a personal level variable too, thus, an additional correlation was calculated at the individual level. Similarly as for the previous four correlational situations, flow at the individual level was significantly correlated with personal expressiveness ($r=.83$, $p<.001$), with each of five functions of identity (r's ranged from .64 to .76, $p<.001$), and with overall sense of FIS ($r=.82$, $p<.001$).

18.4 Discussion

The present work draws upon theoretical underpinnings of Eudaimonistic identity theory, flow, and personal expressiveness, while incorporating personal identity theory and the theory of psychological selection, in order to quantitatively support the potential associations between flow and personal identity, within a systematic approach. Support is found for the primary hypothesis, and it is seen that the individuals report higher levels of personal identification through self-defining activities that they see comprised of a balance of higher effort and also more enjoyment.

The self-defining activities that participants selected from their daily domain and placed respectively in each of the four activity types according to the flow channel (*Apathy*, *Anxiety*, *Relaxation*, *Flow*), have been categorized and coded into six primary categories. Such categories allow for the investigation of the activities with respect to optimal experience, as well as other psychological states based on the flow channel (i.e., Apathy, Relaxation, Anxiety). Specifically, the structured leisure activity category, within which sports and hobbies are mostly reported, is found to be associated with flow, and this finding confirms prior works (Coatsworth et al. 2005; Csikszentmihalyi 1990; Delle Fave and Massimini 2005; Mao et al. 2015; Sharp et al. 2007). Next is the category of productive and compulsory, which is seen to provide less flow than active leisure, yet is seen to significantly relate to flow overall. This is as might be expected since it is study or work that comprised the majority of daily activities for the young adults (Delle Fave and Massimini 2005). In sum, these two activity categories associated with more flow, reaffirm the findings from a cross-cultural study by Delle Fave (2007), in which the categories of both productive and structured leisure activities were reported as prominent opportunities for optimal experience.

The category of passive leisure activities, within which watching TV is broadly reported, is most frequently reported in Activity 1 (Apathy), and such a finding is also in alignment with previous research (Bassi and Delle Fave 2004; Csikszentmihalyi 1990; Delle Fave and Bassi 2003; Kubey and Csikszentmihalyi 1990), and it shows that low effort and low enjoyment apathy activities are rarely associated with optimal experience. Though in certain conditions it may temporarily reduce loneliness, transiently mask or abate negative affect (Kubey and Csikszentmihalyi 2002), and offer behavioral and identity models (Larson 1995), or even may provide stimuli to attract attention thus facilitating passive involvement; but it does not require any skills to conquer any challenges, and thus it unlikely leads to personal growth feelings (Delle Fave et al. 1993). Such a finding may well explain why watching TV has kept its leading position among leisure activities. Such a finding has also been confirmed by the manipulation check in the present work, as the lowest mean score for flow is located in Activity 1, irrespective of its relation to personal identity. In conclusion, the structured leisure activity, the compulsory and productive activity are typical activity categories associated with flow experiences as reported by present sample, since they have something in common: providing a sense of discovery and feelings of transporting the individuals into a new reality, while pushing them to higher levels of performance in a manner which can lead to personal growth. As flow activities are freely chosen, and are more intimately related to the source of what is ultimately meaningful, they are perhaps more precise indicators of who one is (Csikszentmihalyi 1990).

The results of the manipulation check on flow have served to validate the flow channel proposed by Csikszentmihalyi (1975, 1990) that the four different types are indeed composed of activities with differing characteristics (*Apathy*, *Anxiety*, *Relaxation*, *Flow*); and that flow experience is prominently reported in Activity 4. The different combinations of effort by enjoyment within four different activity types result in both different levels of reported flow ($p < .001$), and also different levels of reported personal expressiveness ($p < .001$). These empirical results are also in alignment with the inherently enjoyable quality that is retrospectively associated with the flow state (Csikszentmihalyi 1977, 1982, 1990). In regards to the reported experience of flow across different activity types that is increasingly produced from *Activity 1* up to *Activity 4*, this confirms that flow involves the combination of effort and enjoyment, and it is best achieved when enjoyment and effort are each high and in balance. When an activity has a component of enjoyment, which stays at the same high level, the balanced high effort-enjoyment activity is associated with greater reported level of flow than the low effort activity. This finding confirms the research by Waterman (2005) that the category of high effort-enjoyment activities is more associated with reports of flow than the low effort-enjoyed activities.

Finally, significant positive correlations of flow to personal identity, on both of the activity level and individual level are observed. These relationships confirm previous qualitative works (Coatsworth et al. 2006; Sharp et al. 2007; Waterman 2005; Tietze 2008), and the effects are observed greater than in previous quantitative findings obtained using convergent constructs (Coatsworth et al. 2005; Schwartz 2006; Schwartz and Waterman 2006; Waterman et al. 2003). Such flow-personal identity correlations indicate that through participating in self-defining activities, whenever there is both an increased level of effort as well as enjoyment, when participants experience an increased level of flow, they report an increased degree of personal identity solidification. The fact that the positive correlations among degree of flow and five functions of identity are detected on both the activity level and the individual level, shows how flow experience and solidification of the identity covariate at any level of flow. That is to say, even when the flow degree is at a minimum (i.e., when engaging in *Activity 1-Apathy*), it still plays a positive role in promoting feelings of personal identification. Thus, the positive relation holds true within any type of activity (*Activity1*, or *2*, or *3*, or *4*), from *Apathy* to *Anxiety* up to *Relaxation* and finally to *Flow*: any achieved further flow degree may be seen as a useful step in promoting one's own personal identity. Of course the strongest effects are observed comparing the highest flow to lack of flow degrees, but even activities that elicit during *Apathy* or *Anxiety* – as long as people manage to experience small flow degree variations – are still useful ways to promote corresponding small positive variations in the perceived personal identity strength. In sum, the findings reported here demonstrate that when people experience flow in self-defining activities, they undergo the self-defining consolidation of personal identity to a greater extent. In other words, whenever the individuals enjoy the greatest likelihood of personal identity development (Coatsworth et al. 2005; Sharp et al. 2007; Waterman 2004), their flow experience is seen integral to the process of identity formation (Waterman 2004). This finding supports the Eudaimonistic identity perspective: it is through a process of exploration within self-defining activities, individuals discover identity elements, develop motivation, and find self-direction, which in turn facilitate the consolidation of a coherent personal identity (Waterman 1993b).

In conclusion, the present investigation provides support for the main hypothesis and is in line with previous literature. Given the correlational nature of the present research design, no claims can be made about the origins of causality, and it is possible that activities that the individuals identify with are more likely to be productive of flow, or vice versa. It is also possible that the relationship between the two considered variables, personal identity and flow experience, is spurious in nature: that is, they both relate to a third variable (e.g., genetics, personality, etc.) which is actually the hidden cause behind their co-variation. Further research needs to explore those alternative explanations using experimental and multi-factorial research designs. Still, the findings reported here demonstrate that when flow is experienced within a self-defining activity, the sense of personal identity is significantly stronger than when the activity is less conducive to the flow state, thus providing further evidence supporting a link between flow and identity. The basic link between optimal experience and personal identity has been supported within the present investigation, and the underpinnings of Eudaimonistic identity theory (Waterman 1990a, 1992, 1993a, 2005; Waterman et al. 2008) as well as psychological selection (Delle Fave et al. 2011) provide platforms for future work seeking to nuance the topic, and/or directionality of the findings.

These results are also convergent with those obtained using different tools and instruments, but a similar conceptual apparatus and methodological procedure (Mao et al. 2016). Ongoing investigations that are currently in the final stages allow for examining the associations between flow and a variety of distinct facets of identity, i.e., cultural identity, and place identity. When engaged in an activity that requires effort, and yet in which the experience is enjoyable, young persons may discover their strengths and, by overcoming the challenges, they may build more complex identities in this process. Further, this process of flourishing through an individual's talents and abilities may promote the selection of bio-cultural information (Csikszentmihalyi and Massimini 1985; Della Fave et al. 2011), in a way that promotes identification with and development of a culture in turn. In sum, a mutually supportive relationship between flow and identity may be an important addition to our understanding of personal growth.

References

Adams, G. R., & Marshall, S. (1996). A developmental social psychology of identity: Understanding the person in context. *Journal of Adolescence, 19*, 429–442.

Aristotle. (IV c. B.C.). *The Nicomachean ethics* (D. Ross, Trans., 1925). New York: Oxford University Press.

Barber, B. L., Eccles, J. S., & Stone, M. R. (2001). Whatever happened to the jock, the brain, and the princes? Young adult pathways linked to adolescent activity involvement and social identity. *Journal of Adolescent Research, 16*, 429–455.

Bassi, M., & Delle Fave, A. (2004). Adolescence and the changing context of optimal experience in time: Italy 1986–2000. *Journal of Happiness Studies, 5*, 155–179.

Browne, M. W., & Cudeck, R. (1993). Alternative ways of assessing model fit. In K. A. Bollen & J. S. Long (Eds.), *Testing structural equation models* (pp. 136–162). Newbury Park: Sage.

Carmines, E., & McIver, J. (1981). Analysing models with unobserved variables: Analysis of covariance structures. In G. Bhornstedt & E. Borgatta (Eds.), *Social measurement* (pp. 65–115). Beverly Hills: Sage.

Chen, H., Wigand, R. T., & Nilan, M. S. (1999). Optimal experience of web activities. *Computers in Human Behavior, 15*, 585–608.

Coatsworth, J. D., Sharp, E. H., Palen, L., Darling, N., Cumsille, P., & Marta, E. (2005). Exploring adolescent self-defining leisure activities and identity experiences across three countries. *International Journal of Behavioral Development, 29*, 361–370.

Coatsworth, J. D., Palen, L., & Sharp, E. H. (2006). Self-defining activities, expressive identity, and adolescent wellness. *Applied Developmental Science, 10*(3), 157–170.

Cooper, J. M. (1999). The psychology of justice in Plato. In J. M. Cooper (Ed.), *Reason and emotion. Essays on ancient moral psychology and ethical theory* (pp. 138–149). Princeton: Princeton University Press.

Csikszentmihalyi, M. (1975). *Beyond boredom and anxiety*. San Francisco: Jossey-Bass.

Csikszentmihalyi, M. (1977). *Beyond boredom and anxiety, second printing*. San Francisco: Jossey-Bass.

Csikszentmihalyi, M. (1982). Towards a psychology of optimal experience. In L. Wheeler (Ed.), *Annual review of personality and social psychology* (Vol. 3, pp. 13–36). Beverly Hills: Sage.

Csikszentmihalyi, M. (1988). The flow experience and its significance for human psychology. In M. Csikszentmihalyi (Ed.), *Optimal experience: Psychological studies of flow in consciousness* (pp. 15–35). Cambridge: Cambridge University Press.

Csikszentmihalyi, M. (1990). *Flow: The psychology of optimal experience*. New York: Harper & Row.

Csikszentmihalyi, M. (1996). *Flow: The psychology of discovery and invention*. New York: Harper Perennial.

Csikszentmihalyi, M. (1997). *Finding flow: The psychology of engagement with everyday life*. New York: Basic Books.

Csikszentmihalyi, M., & Csikszentmihalyi, I. (Eds.). (1988). *Optimal experience*. Cambridge: Cambridge University Press.

Csikszentmihalyi, M., & Csikzsentmihalyi, I. (Eds.). (2006). *A life worth living: Contributions to positive psychology* (Series in positive psychology). Oxford University Press: New York.

Csikszentmihalyi, M., & Massimini, F. (1985). On the psychological selection of bio-cultural information. *New Ideas in Psychology, 3*, 115–138.

Deci, E. L., & Ryan, R. M. (1985). *Intrinsic motivation and self-determination in human behavior*. New York: Plenum Press.

Deci, E. L., & Ryan, R. M. (1987). The support of autonomy and the control of behavior. *Journal of Personality and Social Psychology, 53*(6), 1024–1037.

Deci, E. L., & Ryan, R. M. (1991). A motivational approach to self: Integration in personality. In R. Dienstbier (Ed.), *Nebraska symposium on motivation: Perspectives on motivation* (Vol. 38, pp. 237–288). Lincoln: University of Nebraska Press.

Deci, E. L., & Ryan, R. M. (2002). An overview of self-determination theory: An organismic dialectical perspective. In E. L. Deci & R. M. Ryan (Eds.), *Handbook of self-determination research* (pp. 3–33). Rochester: Univeristy of Rochester Press.

Delle Fave, A. (2007). Individual development and community empowerment: Suggestions from studies on optimal experience. In J. Haworth & G. Hart (Eds.), *Well-being: Individual, community, and societal perspectives* (pp. 41–56). London: Palgrave McMillan.

Delle Fave, A., & Bassi, M. (2003). Italian adolescents and leisure: The role of engagement and optimal experience. In S. Verma & R. Larson (Eds.), *Examining adolescent leisure time across cultures: Developmental opportunities and risks. New directions in child and adolescent development* (pp. 79–93). San Francisco: Jossey Bass.

Delle Fave, A., & Massimini, F. (2005). The investigation of optimal experience and apathy. *European Psychologist, 10*, 264–274.

Delle Fave, A., Massimini, F., & Borri Gaspardin, M. (1993). Televisione e qualita' dell'esperienza quotidiana [Television and daily quality of experience]. *Ikon, 26*, 81–109.

Delle Fave, A., Massimini, F., & Bassi, M. (2011). Acculturation and optimal experience. In *Psychological selection and optimal experience across cultures* (pp. 273–293). Dordrecht: Springer.

Diener, E., & Lucas, R. E. (2000). Explaining differences in societal levels of happiness: Relative standards, need fulfillment, culture, and evaluation theory. *Journal of Happiness Studies, 1*, 41–78.

Eccles, J. S., & Barber, B. L. (1999). Student council, volunteering, basketball, or marching band: What kind of extracurricular involvement matters? *Journal of Adolescent Research, 14*, 10–43.

Erikson, E. H. (1968). *Identity: Youth and crisis*. New York: Norton.

Erikson, E. H. (1980). *Identity and the life cycle*. New York: Norton.
Fraser, C. (2014). Wandering the way: A eudaimonistic approach to the Zhuāngzǐ. *Dao: A Journal of Comparative Philosophy, 13*, 541–565.
Fredricks, J. A., Alfeld-Liro, C. J., Hruda, L. Z., Eccles, J. S., Patrick, H., & Ryan, A. M. (2002). A qualitative exploration of adolescents' commitments to athletics and the arts. *Journal of Adolescent Research, 17*(1), 68–97.
Hansen, D. M., Larson, R. W., & Dworkin, J. B. (2003). What adolescents learn in organized youth activities: A survey of self-reported developmental experiences. *Journal of Research on Adolescence, 13*, 25–55.
Hu, L., & Bentler, P. M. (1999). Cutoff criteria for fit indexes in covariance structure analysis: Conventional criteria versus new alternatives. *Structural Equation Modeling, 6*, 1–55.
Huta, V. (2012). Linking peoples' pursuit of eudaimonia and hedonia with characteristics of their parents: Parenting styles, verbally endorsed values, and role modeling. *Journal of Happiness Studies, 13*, 47–61.
Irwin, H. (1985). *Flight of mind: A psychological study of the out-of-body experience*. Metuche: Scarecrow Press.
Kubey, R. W., & Csikszentmihalyi, M. (1990). *Television and the quality of life*. New Jersey: Erlbaum.
Kubey, R. W., & Csikszentmihalyi, M. (2002). Television addiction is no mere metaphor. *Scientific American, 286*, 62–68.
Larson, R. (1995). Secrets in the bedroom: Adolescents' private use of media. *Journal of Youth and Adolescence, 24*, 535–550.
Mao, Y., Robert, S., Pagliaro, S., Csikszentmihalyi, M., & Bonaiuto, M. (2016). Optimal experience and optimal identity: A multinational study of the associations between flow and social identity. *Frontiers in Psychology, 7*:67. doi: 10.3389/fpsyg.2016.00067
Maslow, A. H. (1970). *Religions, value, and peak experiences*. New York: Harper & Row.
Massimini, F., & Delle Fave, A. (2000). Individual development in a bio-cultural perspective. *American Psychologist, 55*, 24–33.
Nakamura, J., & Csikszentmihalyi, M. (2002). The concept of flow. In C. R. Snyder & S. J. Lopez (Eds.), *Handbook of positive psychology* (pp. 89–105). Oxford: Oxford University Press.
Nielsen, K., & Cleal, B. (2010). Predicting flow at work: Investigating the activities and job characteristics that predict flow states at work. *Journal of Occupational Health Psychology, 15*(2), 180–190.
Norton, D. L. (1976). *Personal destinies*. Princeton: Princeton University Press.
Novak, T. P., Hoffman, D. L., & Yung, Y. (2000). Measuring the flow construct in online environments: A structural modeling approach. *Marketing Science, 19*, 22–44.
Peterson, C., Park, N., & Seligman, M. E. (2005). Orientations to happiness and life satisfaction: The full life versus the empty life. *Journal of Happiness Studies, 6*(1), 25–41.
Ross, W. D. (1949). *Aristotle* (5th ed.). London: Methuen.
Ryan, R. M., & Deci, E. L. (2000). Self-determination theory and the facilitation of intrinsic motivation, social development, and well-being. *American Psychologist, 55*, 68–78.
Ryan, R. M., & Deci, E. L. (2001). On happiness and human potentials: A review of research on hedonic and eudaimonic well-being. *Annual Review of Psychology, 52*, 141–166.
Ryff, C. D., & Singer, B. H. (2006). Best news yet on the six-factor model of well-being. *Social Science Research, 35*, 1103–1119.
Ryff, C. D., & Singer, B. H. (2008). Know thyself and become what you are: A eudaimonic approach to psychological well-being. *Journal of Happiness Studies, 9*, 13–39.
Serafini, T. E., & Adams, G. R. (2002). Functions of identity: Scale construction and validation. *Identity, 2*(4), 361–389
Schwartz, S. J. (2006). Predicting identity consolidation from self-construction, eudaimonistic self-discovery, and agentic personality. *Journal of Adolescence, 29*, 777–793.
Schwartz, S. J., & Waterman, A. S. (2006). Changing interests: A longitudinal study of intrinsic motivation for personally salient activities. *Journal of Research in Personality, 40*, 1119–1136.

Seligman, M. E. (2002). *Authentic happiness: Using the new positive psychology to realize your potential for lasting fulfillment*. New York: Free Press.

Serafini, T. E., Maitland, S. B., & Adams, G. R. (2006, March). *The functions of identity scale: revisions, validation and model testing*. Poster presented at the Biennial Meeting of the Society for Research on Adolescence, San Francisco, California.

Sharp, E. H., Coatsworth, J. D., Darling, N., Cumsille, P., & Ranieri, S. (2007). Gender difference in the self-defining activities and identity experiences of adolescents and emerging adults. *Journal of Adolescence, 30*, 251–269.

Tietze, R. L. (2008). Jazz and American identity: Case study of a college course. *Psychology of Aesthetics, Creativity, and the Arts, 2*, 245–255.

Waterman, A. S. (1984). Identity formation: Discovery or creation? *Journal of Early Adolescence, 4*, 329–341.

Waterman, A. S. (1990a). Personal expressiveness: Philosophical and psychological foundations. *Journal of Mind and Behavior, 11*, 47–74.

Waterman, A. S. (1990b). The relevance of Aristotle's conception of eudaimonia for the psychological study of happiness. *Theoretical and Philosophical Psychology, 10*, 39–44.

Waterman, A. S. (1992). Identity as an aspect of optimal psychological functioning. In G. R. Adams, T. P. Gullotta, & R. Montemayor (Eds.), *Adolescent identity formation: Advances in adolescent development* (pp. 50–72). Newbury Park: Sage.

Waterman, A. S. (1993a). Finding something to do or someone to be: A Eudaimonist perspective on identity formation. In J. Kroger (Ed.), *Discussions of ego identity* (pp. 147–167). Hillsdale: Lawrence Erlbaum & Associates.

Waterman, A. S. (1993b). Two conceptions of happiness: Contrasts of personal expressiveness (eudaimonia) and hedonic enjoyment. *Journal of Personality and Social Psychology, 64*, 678–691.

Waterman, A. S. (2004). Finding someone to be: Studies on the role of intrinsic motivation in identity formation. *Identity, 4*, 209–228.

Waterman, A. S. (2005). When effort is enjoyed: Two studies of intrinsic motivation for personally salient activities. *Motivation and Emotion, 29*, 165–188.

Waterman, A. S. (2007). On the importance of distinguishing hedonia and eudaimonia when contemplating the hedonic treadmill. *American Psychologist, 62*, 612–613.

Waterman, A. S., Schwartz, S. J., Goldbacher, E., Green, H., Miller, C., & Philip, S. (2003). Predicting the subjective experience of intrinsic motivation: The roles of self-determination, the balance of challenges and skills, and self-realization values. *Personality and Social Psychology Bulletin, 29*, 1447–1458.

Waterman, A. S., Schwartz, S. J., & Conti, R. (2008). The implications of two concept of happiness for the understanding of intrinsic motivation. *Journal of Happiness Studies, 9*, 41–79.

Chapter 19
The Flow Experience in Clinical Settings: Applications in Psychotherapy and Mental Health Rehabilitation

Eleonora Riva, Teresa Freire, and Marta Bassi

Abstract In mental health care settings, the positive psychology approach has been widely incorporated in traditional cognitive-behavioral therapy aiming to foster change in individuals' behavior and approach to life. The aim of this chapter is to integrate findings stemming from three lines of research focusing on the use of flow in psychotherapy and mental health rehabilitation. We will present studies in which the ability to find flow in everyday life was connected with individuals' well-being and reduced symptomatology. Results also suggested a relationship between flow and psychotherapeutic intervention: finding flow fosters positive and meaningful changes both inside and outside the therapeutic and rehabilitation processes. Finally, we will present a new psychotherapeutic model in which flow is part and parcel in facing daily life challenges and in promoting clients' integration and active involvement in society.

E. Riva (✉)
Department of Cultural Heritage and Environment, University of Milan, Milan, Italy
e-mail: eleonora.riva@unimi.it

T. Freire
School of Psychology, University of Minho, Braga, Portugal
e-mail: tfreire@psi.uminho.pt

M. Bassi
Department of Biomedical and Clinical Sciences "Luigi Sacco", University of Milan, Milan, Italy
e-mail: marta.bassi@unimi.it

L. Harmat et al. (eds.), *Flow Experience*, DOI 10.1007/978-3-319-28634-1_19

19.1 Positive Psychology and Health: From Theory to Applications

Since the 1980s the researchers who later became the founders of positive psychology have embraced a vision of the human being as a complex, proactive and intentional entity (Csikszentmihalyi 1975/2000, 1990, 1993; Csikszentmihalyi and Csikszentmihalyi 2006; Seligman 2002a; Peterson and Seligman 2004; Fredrickson 2001). From their perspective, psychological well-being should be considered as much more than a lack of distress or sufferance (Delle Fave et al. 2010, 2011; Ryff 1989; Ryff and Keyes 1995); mental health is to be regarded as more than absence of pathology (Seligman 2008); and the positive psychological experience is to be considered more complex than the ephemeral emotion of joy or happiness (Inghilleri 1999; Freire 2013). This view is consistent with definition of mental health of the WHO (1946, 2004 – p. 59): "Mental health is a state of well-being in which the individual realizes his or her own abilities, can cope with the normal stresses of life, can work productively and fruitfully, and is able to make a contribution to his or her community". This definition includes terms such as well-being, abilities, coping, work performance, and social contribution that are widely used in Positive Psychology research (Delle Fave and Fava 2011).

Ryff and Singer (1996) remarked that, historically, mental health research is dramatically weighted on the side of psychological dysfunction and that health is equated with the absence of illness rather than the presence of wellness. They suggested that the absence of well-being creates conditions of vulnerability to possible future adversities and that the route to enduring recovery lies not exclusively in eliminating symptoms and sufferance, but in promoting positive skills. The authors (Ryff et al. 1998) propose that, from a clinical perspective, there are major advantages in applying a conceptualization of health viewed not simply as the absence of disease but as the presence of wellness in a biopsychosocial perspective. Keyes (2002) demonstrated empirically that mental health and mental illness are not opposite ends of a single measurement continuum. Measures of the symptoms of mental illness correlate negatively and modestly with measures of mental health. In Keyes' conceptualization (2007), mental health is best viewed as a complete state consisting in the presence of mental health and the absence of mental illness Individuals with complete mental health are flourishing in life, while persons with an incomplete mental health are languishing (Fredrickson 2001, 2002; Keyes 2002). Developing the *Broad-and-Build Theory* (2001, 2002, 2013), From a similar perspective, Fredrickson proposes a new approach for evaluating human experience, promoting the concept of "*flourishing*" as a measure of overall life well-being, which is considered to be the subjective capability to live within an optimal range of human functioning including components like goodness, generativity,[1] growth,

---

[1] Generativity in essence refers to the ability to create, generate, or produce new content unique to the social or cultural system. In Developmental Psychology generativity is a struggle against stagnation that ascends during adulthood. In a wider, psychosocial sense it refers to the concern for

and resilience (Fredrickson 2006, p. 57; Fredrickson and Losada 2005, p. 678; Riva et al. 2014). From this viewpoint, full mental health thus means to be filled with positive emotion and to be functioning well psychologically and socially (Fava and Tomba 2009). Moreover, we have to take into consideration that the condition of languishing is neither pathological per se, nor is it recognized by therapists, but can have important negative effects on daily functioning just like mental illnesses, and sometimes can become a precondition for the development of pathology.

In 2004 Seligman and Peterson proposed a new model of the human mental structure, and published a manual of psychological *Virtues and Strength*, also called *VIA (Values In Action) model*. In this wide and detailed definition of human mental abilities they lay the foundations for the development of clinical and educational tools (Park et al. 2006; Peterson 2006; Peterson and Seligman 2004; Peterson et al. 2007). According to these authors, mental health depends first on the promotion and development of subjective psychological skills, and only at a later level on the elimination of symptoms. Following this vision, the authors proposed to use the *VIA* model for clinical and therapeutic goals (Peterson 2006), and developed a positive psychology approach for psychotherapists and health professionals, in order to make their therapeutic methods more complex and qualified (Seligman 2006, 2008). Seligman and Peterson developed positive psychology's theories and methods for mental health care and psychotherapy, within the frame of cognitive-behavioral therapeutic approach (Seligman 2002b, 2006; Seligman and Peterson 2003; Seligman et al. 2005, 2006). Joseph and Linley also elaborated a similar reflection; they defined the characteristics of *Positive Therapy*, an approach to psychological clinical practice and psychotherapy in which positive psychology is used as a meta-theory (Joseph and Linley 2004, 2006; Linley and Joseph 2004). Other practical approaches have been developed in this direction, such as Frisch's *Quality of Life Therapy* (2006, 2009a, b) or Fava's *Well-Being Therapy* (Fava 2012; Fava and Tomba 2009; Ruini and Fava 2008; Ruini et al. 2007). The strategy of these psychotherapeutic models is to focus on the development of psychological well-being subjectively perceived by the client, which becomes the core of a short-term therapeutic process. In this way the therapy, oriented toward the reinforcement of the client's subjective abilities, will obtain both the result of eliminating or diminishing the symptoms, and reinforcing the client's personality in order to prevent future relapse (Fava and Tomba 2009; Frisch 2006; Goldwum et al. 2007; Goldwum and Colombo 2010; Seligman 2002b; Seligman and Peterson 2003).

Following this perspective, we will now try to highlight the features of a model of optimal experience that is related to the operation of psychodynamic processes of individuals. Then we will evaluate the possible implications of the model in mental health care. Evidence showed a relationship between flow and well-being (Asakawa 2010; Bassi et al. 2014; Delle Fave et al. 2011; Fullagar and Kelloway 2009; Steele and Fullagar 2009). Between the 1980s and 1990s Mihaly Csikszentmihalyi analyzed and defined *Optimal Experience* as an experience of temporary subjective

establishing and guiding the next generation having as a starting point a sense of optimism about humanity (Erikson 1950; Slater 2003).

psychological well-being, strictly connected to the involvement in a specific activity which corresponds to the characteristics of the individual's personality (1975/2000, 1982; Csikszentmihalyi and Csikszentmihalyi 1988). He also defined the specific characteristics of Optimal Experience, also called *Flow of Consciousness* (1990, 1997) which is a psychological optimal state from three points of view: from the cognitive perspective, as there is the possibility of comprehension; from the emotional perspective, as there is the possibility of positive emotions; from the motivational perspective, as there is the possibility of engagement. This theory could also be considered from a cultural transmission perspective, as it highlights the close relationship between the past life of the individual, their motivations, cognitions, current emotions and the development of material culture and ideas (Inghilleri 2014). Csikszentmihalyi and colleagues demonstrated that the repeated experience of flow is associated with the development of an autotelic[2] personality (Baumann 2012; Csikszentmihalyi 1989, 1996; Leontiev 2006; Gardner 1993a, b, 2007; Nakamura and Csikszentmihalyi 2002) and with the construction of a more complex and resilient self (Csikszentmihalyi 1993; Csikszentmihalyi and Rathunde 1993; Csikszentmihalyi et al. 1993; Inghilleri 1999). In the health care setting, Delle Fave and her colleagues found that occasions for optimal experience can be retrieved also in suboptimal physical conditions – such as the case of people with chronic motor and sensory disabilities – and can facilitate adjustment to illness as well as personal growth (Delle Fave 2006, 2010; Delle Fave and Massimini 1992; Delle Fave et al. 2003, 2011). In addition, studies among individuals undergoing physical rehabilitation (Sartori et al. 2014) and among women with eating disorders attending a hospital programme for obesity (Preziosa et al. 2008) showed that flow played a crucial role in treatment adherence, supporting treatment outcomes and improved functioning in daily life.

In our work we have developed the frame of application of flow in mental health care settings and in psychotherapy, following three different lines of research. The first one was developed at the Medical School of the University of Milano and focuses on the association of flow with rehabilitation activities as a means to promote treatment adherence, skill development, and ultimately community integration. The second one, developed at the School of Psychology of the University of Minho, suggests a model of psychotherapy intervention for adolescents in which flow is used as an assessment tool of the subjective experience of patients and as a framework to promote the development of skills and positive evolution of a richer and more flexible personality.[3] The third one was developed at the Department of

[2] Csikszentmihalyi and Gardner defined autotelic personality for the first time in their research on optimal experiences and creativity (Csikszentmihalyi 1996; Gardner 1993a, b). It is a quality that characterizes a person who is receptive, active and open to detecting new challenges adapted to promoting their own experience of flow. An autotelic person is a person with the ability to understand and extract the intrinsic characteristics of the activities connected to flow, starting from self-experience, and investigate their presence in other activities of daily experience, in order to maximize the opportunities to find flow and satisfaction in life.

[3] The development of a more flexible personality would result in a reinforcement of the self, that will be richer and more complex, and thus better able to deal with problematic situations and to

Human and Environmental Studies of the University of Milano and proposes a definition of Flow Therapy: this is the first model of psychotherapeutic treatment with a psychodynamic approach that is completely centered on concepts and practices derived from positive psychology. These three interconnected lines of application allow us to see the impact that positive psychology could have on mental health care, both in terms of better understanding of the patients' experience, and in terms of a more rapid and more effective promotion of their resources and skills.

19.2 Flow and Mental Health: From Rehabilitation Programs to Everyday Life

Psychologists and psychiatrists working in clinical settings are traditionally trained to identify signs and symptoms of disorders, neglecting for the most part those aspects of individuals' lives and experiences that are "healthy" per se and do not apparently deserve therapeutic intervention. In a series of studies conducted by our research group at the Medical School of the University of Milano, we have challenged this narrow focus of analysis and have explored the potential of optimal experience as a tool for intervention in the mental health domain. Specifically, in line with the concept of positive mental health described in the introduction, we investigated the overall ability of individuals with mental disorders to find flow in their daily lives irrespective of their mental health condition, as well as the possibility of associating flow with rehabilitation practices as a means to support treatment adherence and social integration.

Three assessment instruments were applied in our studies. One is the Experience Sampling Method (Csikszentmihalyi et al. 1977), the procedure described in chapter of Bassi and Delle Fave that provides repeated real-time information on the participant's time-budget (activity, social context, location) and the associated quality of experience during the unfolding of daily events and situations. This procedure proved effective in monitoring the fluctuation of experience and pathological symptoms in relation to various daily activities and social contexts, and can be applied to evaluate and predict treatment progress (Ebner-Priemer and Trull 2009; Massimini et al. 1987). The other two are self-report single-administration questionnaires measuring optimal experience (*Flow Questionnaire*; Csikszentmihalyi 1975/2000; Csikszentmihalyi and Csikszentmihalyi 1988; Delle Fave and Massimini 1988) and individuals' life themes (*Life Theme Questionnaire*; Delle Fave 2004). Through open-ended questions and Likert-type scales, participants were asked to identify and describe the activities and situations they associated with optimal experience – if any – and to provide additional information on the conditions that facilitate flow onset and continuation over time. They were also asked to report on specific aspects

find practical solutions (Csikszentmihalyi 1993; Csikszentmihalyi et al. 1993; Inghilleri 1999), without elapse in development of disease.

of one's life theme such as positive and negative life influences, current challenges, and future goals (for a detailed description: Delle Fave et al. 2011).

In line with our research objectives, the administration of these instruments to individuals with various mental disorders allowed us to gather empirical data on the role of flow in clinical settings. Results showed that individuals with mental disorders can experience flow in their daily lives and, particularly, that rehabilitation activities (RA) can be sources of optimal experience. This was testified in a study with 54 schizophrenic participants undergoing pharmacological treatment who were involved in a psychiatric rehabilitation program based on mountain-therapy (Lanfranchi et al. 2011). Mountain therapy is an original therapeutic approach based on the bio-psycho-social paradigm that aims to enhance individuals' growth potentials in the mountain environment. Intervention includes mountain activities performed in small groups, such as trekking, excursions and walks, which are coordinated and supervised by therapists and alpine guides. Participants in this research study were administered Flow Questionnaire and a shorter version of the Life Theme Questionnaire. All but two participants identified sources of flow in their lives, and primarily named structured leisure activities (76 %) as their most intense optimal experience compared to activities such as socialization with friends (8 %) or work (6 %). Among reported leisure activities, 80 % of the answers referred to mountain-therapy (e.g. trekking, mountain walks). Similar results were obtained in an ESM study conducted at the Psychiatric Rehabilitation Center of a University Hospital in Milano with a group of 27 residential and semi-residential patients diagnosed with psychoses, mood disorders, and personality disorders (Bassi et al. 2012). These participants associated flow more frequently with RA such as workshops on photography, cooking, gardening and art therapy (21.2 %) than with free-time activities, namely activities at the center they could choose to engage in that were not part of their rehabilitation program (10.1 %; $t(25)=2.64$, $p<.015$).

Findings from these two studies suggest the importance for people involved in rehabilitation programs to engage in challenging tasks, favoring both the onset of positive and complex experiences and skill development. In particular, they raise two crucial issues health professionals should take into account when devising intervention protocols. The first one concerns *personalized intervention*: participants should be actively involved in all the stages of the rehabilitation program, above all in choosing activities within the gamut of available opportunities based on personal interests and goals. Moreover, professionals should evaluate individuals' proficiency levels in different activities so as to calibrate levels of activity complexity (challenge) and favor the onset of optimal experiences, instead of situations generating anxiety – in which perceived challenges are higher than perceived skills – or generating apathy – in which both challenges and skills are perceived as low (see Chap. 12 by Bassi and Delle Fave, in this volume). The second issue concerns what we may call the *generalization of flow*, that is the individuals' ability to understand, recognize and promote the factors leading to flow. The participants in our research rarely found occasions of optimal experience outside their rehabilitation activities. Intervention should therefore aim to help individuals export into their daily lives the competences they acquired during the rehabilitation process and also encourage the autonomous search for opportunities for action in other daily activities, thus fostering higher levels of well-being and integration in the community.

In this respect, research findings indicated that flow could be conceived as both a means to counteract mental illness symptoms and as a target of intervention by itself. Among groups of adolescents and university students, finding flow was shown to contribute to individuals' well-being, while the lack thereof was associated with reduced well-being (Asakawa 2010; Bassi et al. 2014; Fullagar and Kelloway 2009; Steele and Fullagar 2009). In the clinical setting, we performed a longitudinal case study involving a woman diagnosed with panic disorder and agoraphobia (Delle Fave and Massimini 1992). Besides adopting a cognitive-behavioral approach to tackle dysfunctional symptoms and thoughts, the psychotherapy program included strategies to promote optimal experiences, goal setting and meaning development in the client's living environment (Delle Fave and Fava 2011; Fava and Tomba 2009). The therapy lasted one and half years, during which the woman completed nine ESM sessions to assess her daily quality of experience. A comparison of the findings obtained in the first and in the last session showed that the frequency of optimal experiences substantially increased during the psychotherapy process from 15 to 51 % of the ESM forms: The participant progressively devoted more time to complex and structured activities such as volunteering, reading, socializing, and less time to activities associated with apathy and disengagement, like watching TV. At the same time, by the end of the therapy, the participant's panic attacks as well as unease of being alone and need for social support had greatly reduced, leading her to go to public places and walk in the streets mostly unattended.

19.3 Positive Interventions and Optimal Functioning of Adolescents

In the scope of positive interventions, children and adolescents have been a major target for applying new strategies that make the promotion of well-being possible while individuals are *in* development. This approach brings up the concept of positive development associated to normative processes as well as psychopathology or its onset. The emphasis on the positive side of individuals' experiences has shed light on a new comprehension about developmental healthy trajectories by integrating self-enhancement and external opportunities or adversities, mainly in adolescence. In fact, the concept of positive clinical psychology has emerged stating that "the understanding and treatment of clinical levels of distress is based on a balanced and equally weighted focus on the positive and negative aspects of life" (Wood and Tarrier 2010, pp. 820). Following this conceptual framework, the aim of interventions is not to achieve positive functioning only; instead, they need to embrace a broader perspective based on optimal functioning that improves individuals' lives contextualized in their daily cultural environment (Leong and Wong 2003). Following this perspective, a series of studies have been conducted by our group at the School of Psychology (The Research Group on Optimal Functioning), aimed at studying optimal functioning of children and adolescents and related forms of psychological interventions. For the purposes of this chapter we will present two intervention programs designed for the promotion of a positive youth development and optimal functioning of adolescents, namely: *Desafio: Ser⁺* (Challenge: to be⁺; Lima et al. unpublished manual); and *Optimal Functioning Therapy for Adolescents* (OFTA; Teixeira and Freire unpublished manual). While the former is a group intervention for normative adolescent populations, the second consists of an individual intervention following a psychotherapeutic process for clinical adolescent populations, more specifically, depressed adolescents. Both interventions address the concept of flow, promoting the identification of activities that produce flow, encouraging adolescents to use and optimize them in their daily routines. The importance of engaging in flow activities and the benefits for adolescents' positive development and optimal functioning are also discussed, by working on adolescents' involvement and initiative behaviors.

The group intervention program, *Challenge: to be⁺*, was developed based on the scientific knowledge and empirical evidence in the field of positive psychology from the last years, and it is aimed at the promotion of a positive youth development (Freire et al. 2012). More specifically, this program aims to help youth to increase positive emotions and positive experiences in their daily life and to identify, use and optimize their personal strengths and resources in order to make adolescents active agents in promoting their own development and psychological well-being. This intervention program includes a total of eight sessions of 90 min each (one session per week) and it is structured into three modules: (1) emotions and positive life experiences; (2) positive individual characteristics and engagement; (3) flow/optimal experiences and positive development. It was developed especially for ninth grade adolescents (Freire et al. 2012). For the evaluation of this program, a quasi-experimental design was used with pre and post-test evaluations considering two groups, the experimental one (program implemented) and the comparison group (program not implemented). Both quantitative (assessment of positive dimensions, such as self-esteem, self-concept, psychological well-being and life satisfaction) and qualitative (general appreciation of adolescents with respect to each session and the entire program, preferred activities, accomplished learnings and importance of the program for their lives) measures were used to assess the intervention program. A total of 104 students in the ninth grade year (mean age = 14.36, DP=0.68) were involved in the quasi-experimental design, with 78 students participating in the experimental group and 26 in the comparison group (class-based distribution). Quantitative results showed a main effect for the moment (pre and post-test), for all variables: self-esteem (F (1, 97) = 12.51, p < .001), self-concept (F (1,97) = 18.58, p < .001), psychological well-being (F (1,97) = 18.37, p < .001) and life satisfaction (F (1,97) = 6.02, p = .02) at post-test, (Freire et al. 2012); but not a group main effect (experimental versus comparison groups). Only for satisfaction with life was a marginally significant interaction effect (group × moment) obtained, with adolescents from the experimental group showing higher values of satisfaction with life than their counterparts in the comparison group, after the participation in the program (F (1, 97) = 3.19, p = .08). These results suggest a tendency for a positive impact of the program in these positive development-related variables, with a particular emphasis on satisfaction with life. However, future implementations of the program need to overcome limited quasi-experimental designs by the implementation of experimental designs, where causal-effect analyses are possible in terms of the impact of the program. Qualitative results indicated that the participants made a positive appraisal of the intervention program, valuing what they had learned, the attainment of major personal changes in thinking, feeling and acting, the acquisition of personal knowledge and the role of flow experiences, and the sharing of their positive experiences and strengths with the group (Freire et al. 2012). Furthermore, ongoing studies using a total of 43 adolescents from 8th (n = 26; mean age = 13.81, DP = 0.80) and 11th (n = 17; mean age = 15.26, DP = 1.97) grade have shown that, although both groups increased the levels of self-esteem, self-concept, psychological well-being and life satisfaction at the end of the intervention, an analysis of the group main effects showed that eighth grade students seemed to benefit more from the implementation of the program, suggesting that the program is more suitable for younger adolescents. This program is still at a validation phase, but it aims to be an effective intervention program for the promotion of a positive development by means of the achievement of daily flow experiences.

As concerns individual intervention, our team is developing the OFTA manual for the treatment of depression in adolescents. This intervention aims to reduce and/or eliminate depressive symptoms through the use of cognitive-behavioral strategies, and to promote optimal functioning through the use of positive psychotherapy strategies like enhancing positive experiences in everyday life; identifying and optimizing personal resources; promoting flow/optimal experiences; and constructing meaning and purpose in life (Freire et al. 2014). The novelty of this therapy is the integration of techniques from cognitive-behavioral therapy and positive psychology interventions that were adapted for the purpose of this specific intervention (Freire and Teixeira 2014). OFTA consists of a total of 14 group therapy sessions, one per week, and is structured into three modules: (1) promotion of positive emotions, by increasing positive life experiences and positive ways of thinking; (2) identification and optimization of adolescents' strengths and personal resources in order to solve problems; (3) promotion of flow/optimal experience, hope and optimism and development of a life project for the future (Freire et al. 2014). At present, this therapy is being validated for the treatment of depression in adolescents from 14 to 17 years old. The assessment of this therapy effectiveness includes four different moments of the therapeutic process (pre-intervention; middle-intervention; post-intervention; and follow-up), using retrospective instruments and real time measures, namely the Experience Sampling Method. This last measure is being used to assess the impact of the therapy, understanding related changes in the daily lives of adolescents in terms of life contexts (activities, social interactions, places), psychological variables (affective, cognitive and motivational), and the occurrence of flow experiences in daily life. Results from an in-course clinical case study with a 17-year-old adolescent diagnosed with Major Depression Disorder have shown significant decreases in depressive symptoms and increases in well-being in parallel with flow experiences, that were maintained until follow-up. Although in a validation phase, this therapy has already shown promising results with regard to the reduction of depressive symptoms and increased well-being, with significant results in terms of the occurrence of flow experiences, which contributes to optimal functioning of adolescents.

The results of these two types of intervention (group and individual) mirror a continuum of developmental processes from normative to psychopathology, and underline some of the main issues that can be associated to the enhancement of healthy life trajectories, buffering the onset of psychopathology and providing individual strengths and resources in relation to daily contexts. In both cases the results show that the participants could learn about the flow experience, identify it during the course of their life; more importantly, adolescents realized how to become more proactive in managing or producing the occurrence of flow experiences across their lived contexts (e.g., school, leisure, family or friendship), were made aware of the importance of taking the initiative and of their involvement in tasks and activities of the milieu.

Clinical professionals themselves must be aware of the potentialities of the therapies as effective structures in giving support and promoting changes, either through individual or in group interventions, to enable adolescents to realize their potential, and how the flow experience is an important ingredient in creating positive interventions for adolescents. In both group and individual interventions flow experience has a significant role, as an intervention tool and as an experience to be promoted inside and outside therapy, enhancing an intentional *equilibrium* or balance between challenges and skills into self-complexity of adolescents.

19.4 Flow Therapy: A Psychodynamic Model

To develop a clinical approach that uses flow as an instrument in therapeutic processes, it is necessary to define a theoretical and methodological framework based on the connection of selected models from both positive psychology and psychodynamic psychotherapies. Most of the modern approaches in psychodynamic psychotherapies (e.g. Gislon 2000; Stern 2004, 2010; Winston and Winston 2002) have a major focus on the patient's daily experience in order to accompany the latter in a gradual process of change which can give, right from the start, a contribution to the improvement of the client's quality of life. In this direction positive psychology provides a clear, comprehensive, exhaustive and dynamic definition of the psychological state of *subjective daily experience* (Inghilleri 1999) that can be used as a frame for the psychotherapeutic setting. The author defines *SDE* as a perception of the concrete events of everyday life that produces feelings, emotions and a psychological state that orientates the individual towards a subjective selection of the experiences and cultural objects that will be looked for or avoided in the future. In the context within which we introduce the Flow concept in psychotherapy *Subjective Experience* is interconnected with other three theories originating from positive psychology: *Optimal Experience* (Csikszentmihalyi 1982, 1990; Csikszentmihalyi and Rathunde 1993), *Creativity Theory* (Gardner 1993a, b, 2007) and *Subjective Experience* (Inghilleri 1999). These three models share two common focuses: the first focuses on the importance of the relationship between concrete, situated, daily experiences and intrapsychic dynamics; the second refers to the centrality of the subjective capacity to select situations able to promote psychological well-being (i.e. autotelic personality). In Csikszentmihalyi's theory, flow emerges from a situation or activity in which the psychological features and skills of the individual are maximally potentiated; according to Gardner, creativity develops when a person encounters a specific activity or discipline of study that fuels his or her ability to interpret reality in an unconventional and personal way. According to the author creative skills are closely linked to a specific domain, or field of action, and to concrete activities. Creative skills grow from micro-conflicts that the subject perceives within or between three "nodes" of experience (i.e. idiosyncratic characteristics, social forces and cultural context). These conflicts, rather than producing a state of illness or disease, trigger "fruitful asynchronies" in the subject's psyche that are the basis of the construction of creative skills. Inghilleri argues that the way in which daily experience is subjectively perceived, together with psychological states and emotions that derive from it, are the central point for the development of a complex and flexible self. The autotelic person is considered as able to identify and select new activities that promote flow experiences, states of well-being and self-satisfaction. Following this vision in which flow, creativity and subjective experience are closely related in a relationship of reciprocal causality, the three characteristics of flow that are most noteworthy for psychotherapeutic purposes setting are: *self-determination, intrinsic motivation* and *balance between challenges and skills*, as subjectively perceived by the person.

19.4.1 Flow Therapy

Flow, as a universal experience of mankind, can be considered a feature of every individual psychodynamic. In this sense it has to be considered not only as an instrument to evaluate the evolution of therapy, but also as a mental process on which to work. In this sense, *should flow be seen as a therapeutic experience or as an object of investigation?* The answer is both. The therapist may examine the occurrence of flow in the present and previous daily life of the client, in order to promote new opportunities of flow; at the same time the experience of psychotherapy per se can be a fruitful situation in which to live the flow experience.

19.4.1.1 The Therapy Session as an Experience of Flow

Psychotherapy is a continuous transition between the inner (the session) and the outer (the daily life). This constant movement is not only cognitive but also affective, and fosters the development of a close personal relation between client and therapist. This particular emotional and relational situation may be generative of flow experiences. Flow can be considered a shared experience when it is developed in more than one partner simultaneously, thanks to the relational characteristics of an activity or a situation (Aubè et al. 2014; Delle Fave and Bassi 2009). In the case of psychotherapeutic setting, both the interacting persons are deeply involved in the therapeutic relationship. The communication with the counterpart and the development of mutual understanding and empathy focus the attention and the energy of both patient and therapist; both of them are involved in an activity of great interest, and they share the intense emotions derived from the intimate contact with another human being. In some phases of therapy, these conditions may lead to experiencing shared moments of flow, which allow the therapeutic relationship to make a significant leap forward and enable the patient to feel both more accepted by the therapist and closer to the acquisition of their own autonomy. A simple indicator of these situations is to be traced in the perception of time, which is often slowed down, in contrast with the need to measure and define the times of the encounters that is characteristic of this profession. The therapeutic sessions become a protected place in which clients can find flow for the first time, or rediscover it after many years in which they have been depressed, emotionally deprived and unhappy.

19.4.1.2 Flow as an Object of the Therapy

The process of psychodynamic psychotherapy is a path of personal growth and change that can last from several months to several years, with the aim of leading the person to a more positive, strong and complex way of being. In this journey all the experiences of life that may have contributed to the actual situation of illness, and the ways in which the patient perceives and reacts to daily situations are taken into consideration. In the same way in which they examine the structuring and pathogenic experiences of the client's past and present life, therapists can consider the occurrence of flow in the present and previous daily life of the client, quantify it and identify its idiosyncratic characteristics, in order to promote new opportunities of flow in present and future experience.

The first step is *to identify the flow experience*. The therapist can use different instruments to help the client in this detection and characterization process: the first place is in the clinical interview, which can be combined with the use of diaries (including virtual ones – e.g. Bassi et al. 2012; de Cordova et al. 2010), questionnaires (e.g. Boffi et al. 2012; Jackson et al. 2008) or other similar instruments. The therapist can also ask the patient to bring cultural artifacts such as photographs, drawings or objects related to past experiences of flow. The patient has to be given a clear and detailed definition of optimal experience, so that they can be able to identify any connected situation even in the distant past. First of all the patient has to describe the presence of flow in their remote and recent past life, in order of quantity, quality and subjective perception. In a following step the patient is required to define, in a narrative way, the most recurrent situations or activities promoting flow, the tasks proposed by the environment and the skills brought into play by the patient themselves.

Once the raw data is collected, the therapist must use the clinical interview, through the interpretation of the events shared by the patient, in order to obtain a *characterization of the experience of flow* for that specific person. This means first of all, the description of the trend of flow experience in the patient's history (in order of quantity and quality) and the identification of the moments in the patient's life which have marked an evolution or involution of this trend, or a change in the activities promoting flow. Then the therapist has to extrapolate the characteristics that define such situations promoting flow. These are to be intended both as general characteristics of the experiences connected to flow, and as the personality and psychological features elicited in the subject by the situation. A person may be more inclined to develop a state of flow in individual situations rather than in social ones, in physical or in mental activities, in experiences with a high or low degree of risk.

Then a *Flow Profile* of the patient has to be compiled: it defines the client's experience of flow in a unique way, by relating the characteristics of their personality with their daily experience and with the cultural opportunities provided by the environment. The information provided by the profile can be used to stimulate an increase in the flow-promoting situation in the everyday life of the patient.

The *promotion of flow* can follow different strategies. Firstly, it has to recover or redefine a space for activities and situations already known as triggers of flow, in order to increase the frequency and quality of well-being experience present in the subject or potentially available to clients. It is just like recovering space for self-care, for sport and leisure activity, for social relations, for natural environment frequentation. At a second level, the therapist can use the Flow Profile to detect other kinds of situations or activities that possess similar characteristics or elicit the same area of skills in the client. This is a way of stimulating the development of some form of *autotelic skills*. Besides working on flow, the therapist can work on the enhancement and strengthening of other subjective strengths (Peterson 2006; Peterson and Seligman 2004; Ryff and Singer 2008), to reinforce the psychological structure of the patient and increase their predisposition to perceive and detect flow. A restoration of self-esteem, for example, can return a more accurate perception of the balance between challenges and skills and decrease the level of anxiety, making it easier to achieve the state of flow. A recovery of a broader social network can facilitate the contact with richer and more varied activities within which it is possible for the person to identify new and unexpected sources of flow.

Finally, the transfer of the experience of *Flow in Therapy* to situations of life "outside the sessions" can support the regeneration of social relations, supporting the social reintegration of the patient and their perception of a better quality of relational experience.

References

Asakawa, K. (2010). Flow experience, culture, and well-being: How do autotelic Japanese college students feel, behave, and think in their daily lives? *Journal of Happiness Studies, 11*, 205–223.

Aubè, C., Brunelle, E., & Rousseau, V. (2014). Flow experience and team performance: The role of team goal commitment and information exchange. *Motivation & Emotion, 38*, 120–130. doi:10.1007/s11031-013-9365-2.

Bassi, M., Ferrario, N., Ba, G., Delle Fave, A., & Viganò, C. (2012). Quality of experience during psychosocial rehabilitation: A real-time investigation with experience sampling method. *Psychiatric Rehabilitation Journal, 35*, 447–453.

Bassi, M., Steca, P., Monzani, D., Greco, A., & Delle Fave, A. (2014). Personality and optimal experience in adolescence: Implications for well-being and development. *Journal of Happiness Studies, 15*, 829–843.

Baumann, N. (2012). Autotelic personality. In S. Engeser (Ed.), *Advances in flow research*. Dordrecht: Springer.

Boffi, M., Diana, B., Riva, E., Inghilleri, P., Argenton, L., Villani, D., Muzio, M., & Riva, G. (2012). L'adattamento italiano della *Dispositional Flow Scale* IIDFS-2. In M. Muzio, G. Riva, & L. Argenton (Eds.), *Flow, benessere e prestazione eccellente. Dai modelli teorici alle applicazioni nello sport e in azienda*. Milano: Franco Angeli.

Csikszentmihalyi, M. (1975/2000). *Beyond boredom and anxiety*. S. Francisco: Jossey Bass.

Csikszentmihalyi, M. (1982). Towards a psychology of optimal experience. In L. Wheeler (Ed.), *Review of personality and social psychology* (Vol. 2). Beverly Hills: Sage.

Csikszentmihalyi, M. (1989). *Research on motivation in education, vol. 3, goals and cognitions*. New York: Academic.

Csikszentmihalyi, M. (1990). *Flow: The psychology of optimal experience*. New York: Harper & Row.

Csikszentmihalyi, M. (1993). *The evolving self: A psychology for a third millennium*. New York: HarperCollins.

Csikszentmihalyi, M. (1996). *Creativity. Flow and the psychology of discovery and invention*. New York: Harper Perennial.

Csikszentmihalyi, M. (1997). *Finding flow. The psychology of engagement with everyday life*. New York: Basic Books.

Csikszentmihalyi, M., & Csikszentmihalyi, I. (Eds.). (1988). *Optimal experience. Psychological studies of flow in consciousness*. New York: Cambridge University Press.

Csikszentmihalyi, M., & Csikszentmihalyi, I. (2006). *A life worth living: Contributions to positive psychology* (pp. 165–181). New York: Oxford University Press.

Csikszentmihalyi, M., & Rathunde, K. (1993). *The measurement of flow in everyday life. Toward a theory of emergent motivation*. In Nebraska symposium of motivation (Vol. 40). Lincoln: University of Nebraska Press.

Csikszentmihalyi, M., Larson, R. W., & Prescott, S. (1977). The ecology of adolescent activity and experience. *Journal of Youth and Adolescence, 6*, 281–294.

Csikszentmihalyi, M., Rathunde, K., & Whalen, S. (1993). *Talented teenagers: A longitudinal study of their development*. New York: Cambridge University Press.

de Cordova, F., Riva, E., & Vittadini, N. (2010) Emerging communication practices and how they affect immigrant adolescents in their developmental process. In Billias, N. (Ed.) *Proceedings of the 5. Global conference of cybercultures*, Interdisciplinary Net.

Delle Fave, A. (2004). A feeling of wellbeing in learning and teaching. In M. Tokoro & L. Steels (Eds.), *A learning zone of one's own* (pp. 97–110). Amsterdam: Ios Press.

Delle Fave, A. (2006). The impact of subjective experience on the quality of life. A central issue for health professionals. In M. Csikszentmihalyi & I. Csikszentmihalyi (Eds.), *A life worth living: Contributions to positive psychology* (pp. 165–181). New York: Oxford University Press.

Delle Fave, A. (2010). Development through disability. The unfolding and sharing of psychological resources. In G. W. Burns (Ed.), *Happiness, healing, enhancement. Your casebook collection for applying positive psychology in the therapy* (pp. 88–99). Hoboken: Wiley.
Delle Fave, A., & Bassi, M. (2009). Sharing optimal experiences and promoting good community life in a multicultural society. *Journal of Positive Psychology, 4*, 280–289.
Delle Fave, A., & Fava, G. A. (2011). Positive psychotherapy and social change. In R. Biswas-Diener (Ed.), *Positive psychology as social change* (pp. 267–291). Dordrecht: Springer.
Delle Fave, A., & Massimini, F. (1988). Modernization and the changing contexts of flow in work and leisure. In M. Csikszentmihalyi & I. Csikszentmihalyi (Eds.), *Optimal experience. Psychological studies of flow in consciousness* (pp. 193–213). New York: Cambridge University Press.
Delle Fave, A., & Massimini, F. (1992). The ESM and the measurement of clinical change: A case of anxiety disorder. In M. W. deVries (Ed.), *The experience of psychopathology: Investigating mental disorders in their natural settings* (pp. 280–289). New York: Cambridge.
Delle Fave, A., Lombardi, M., & Massimini, F. (2003). Disability and development: Individual and cultural issues. In L. Loewenstein, D. Trent, & R. Roth (Eds.), *Catching the future: Women and men in global psychology* (pp. 104–113). Lengerich: Pabst Science Publishers.
Delle Fave, A., Brdar, I., Freire, T., Vella-Brodrick, D. A., & Wissing, M. P. (2010). The investigation of eudaimonic happiness: Qualitative and quantitative findings. *Social Indicators Research, 100*, 185–207. doi:10.1007/s11205-010-9632-5.
Delle Fave, A., Massimini, F., & Bassi, M. (2011). *Psychological selection and optimal experience across cultures: Social empowerment through personal growth*. Dordrecht: Springer.
Ebner-Priemer, U. W., & Trull, T. J. (2009). Ecological momentary assessment of mood disorders and mood dysregulation. *Psychological Assessment, 21*, 463–475.
Erikson, E. H. (1950). *Childhood and society*. New York: Norton.
Fava, G. A. (2012). The clinical role of psychological well-being. *World Psychiatry, 2012*(11), 102–103.
Fava, G. A., & Tomba, E. (2009). Increasing psychological well-being and resilience by psychotherapeutic methods. *Journal of Personality, 77*, 1–32.
Fredrickson, B. L. (2001). The role of positive emotions in positive psychology: The broaden-and-build theory of positive emotions. *American Psychologist, 56*, 218–226.
Fredrickson, B. L. (2002). Positive emotions. In C. R. Snyder & S. J. Lopez (Eds.), *Handbook of positive psychology* (pp. 120–134). New York: Oxford University Press.
Fredrickson, B. L. (2006). Un packing positive emotions: Investigating the seeds of human flourishing. *The Journal of Positive Psychology, 1*(2), 55–57.
Fredrickson, B. L. (2013). Positive emotions broaden and build. In E. Ashby Plant & P. G. Devine (Eds.), *Advances on experimental social psychology* (Vol. 47, pp. 1–53). Burlington: Academic.
Fredrickson, B. L., & Losada, M. (2005). Positive affect and the complex dynamics of human flourishing. *American Psychologist, 60*(7), 678–686.
Freire, T. (2013). *Positive leisure science: From subjective experience to social context*. Dordrecht: Springer. doi:10.1007/978-94-007-5058-6_1.
Freire, T., & Teixeira, A. (2014). Terapia cognitivo-comportamental: da psicopatologia ao funcionamento ótimo de crianças e adolescentes. In P. Monteiro (Ed.), *Psicologia e Psiquiatria da Infância e da Adolescência* (pp. 475–494). Lisboa: Lidel.
Freire, T., Araújo, M., Teixeira, A., & Lima, I. (2012). Implementação e avaliação de um programa de intervenção em grupo para o desenvolvimento positivo de adolescentes: Desafio: ser+. *Psicologia Educação e Cultura, XVI*(1), 231–255.
Freire, T., Teixeira, A., Silva, E., & Matias, G. (2014). Interventions for youth depression: From symptom reduction to well-being and optimal functioning. *Journal of Behavior, Health & Social Issues, 6*(2), 9–19.
Frisch, M. B. (2006). *Quality of life therapy: Applying a life satisfaction approach to positive psychology and cognitive therapy*. Hoboken: Wiley.

Frisch, M. B. (2009a). Quality of life therapy and coaching (QOLTC). In S. J. Lopez (Ed.), *Encyclopedia of positive psychology* (pp. 824–826). New York: Wiley-Blackwell.
Frisch, M. B. (2009b). *The quality of life inventory (QOLI') handbook: A practical guide for laypersons, clients, and coaches*. Minneapolis: Pearson Assessments.
Fullagar, C. J., & Kelloway, E. K. (2009). 'Flow' at work: An experience sampling approach. *Journal of Occupational Health Psychology, 82*, 595–615.
Gardner, H. (1993a). *Multiple intelligences: The theory in practice*. New York: Basic Books.
Gardner, H. (1993b). *Creating minds. An anatomy of creativity seen thorough the lives of Freud, Einstein, Picasso, Stravinsky, Eliot, Graham and Ghandi*. New York: Basic Books.
Gardner, H. (2007). *Five minds for the future*. Boston: Harvard Business School Press.
Gislon, M. C. (2000). *Trattato di psicoterapia breve integrata*. Dialogos: Bassano del Grappa.
Goldwum, G., & Colombo, F. (2010). *Psicologia Positiva: Applicazioni per il benessere*. Trento: Erickson.
Goldwum, G., Baruffi, M., Bielli, D., Colombo, F., Corsale, B., & Marchi, S. (2007). Training Applicativi in Psicologia Positiva. In A. Delle Fave (Ed.), *La Condivisione del Benessere. Il Contributo della Psicologia Positiva*. Milano: Franco Angeli.
Inghilleri, P. (1999). *From subjective experience to cultural change*. Cambridge: Cambridge University Press.
Inghilleri, P. (2014). Phenomenology of positive change: Social growth. In P. Inghilleri, G. Riva, & E. Riva (Eds.), *Enabling positive change. Flow and complexity in daily experience* (pp. 105–122). Warsaw: De Gruyter.
Jackson, S. A., Martin, A. J., & Eklund, R. C. (2008). Long and short measures of flow: The construct validity of the FSS-2, DFS-2, and new brief counterparts. *Journal of Sport and Exercise Psychology, 30*(5), 561–587.
Joseph, S., & Linley, P. A. (2004). Positive therapy: A positive psychological theory of therapeutic practice. In P. A. Linley & S. Joseph (Eds.), *Positive psychology in practice*. Hoboken: Wiley.
Joseph, S., & Linley, P. A. (2006). *Positive therapy: A meta-theory for positive psychological practice*. London: Taylor & Francis.
Keyes, C. L. M. (2002). The mental health continuum: From languishing to flourishing in life. *Journal of Health and Social Research, 43*, 207–222.
Keyes, C. L. M. (2007). Promoting and protecting mental health as flourishing: A complementary strategy for improving national mental health. *American Psychologist, 62*(2), 95–108.
Lanfranchi, F., Frecchiami, A., & Delle Fave, A. (2011). Interventi riabilitativi nel contesto montano [Rehabilitation interventions in the mountain context]. *Psichiatria di Comunità, 10*, 95–102.
Leong, F. T. L., & Wong, P. T. P. (2003). Optimal functioning from cross-cultural perspectives. In B. Walsh (Ed.), *Counseling psychology and optimal human functioning* (pp. 123–150). Mahwah: Lawrence.
Leontiev, D. (2006). Positive personality development: Approaching personal autonomy. In M. Csikszentmihalyi & I. Csikszentmihalyi (Eds.), *A life worth living. Contribution to positive psychology*. Oxford: Oxford University Press.
Linley, P. A., & Joseph, S. (2004). *Positive psychology in practice*. Hoboken: Wiley.
Massimini, F., Csikszentmihalyi, M., & Carli, M. (1987). The monitoring of optimal experience. A tool for psychiatric rehabilitation. *Journal of Nervous and Mental Disease, 175*, 545–549.
Nakamura, J., & Csikszentmihalyi, M. (2002). The concept of flow. In C. R. Snyder & S. J. Lopez (Eds.), *Handbook of positive psychology* (pp. 89–105). New York: Oxford University Press.
Park, N., Peterson, C., & Seligman, M. E. P. (2006). Character strengths in fifty-four nations and in the fifty US states. *The Journal of Positive Psychology, 1*(3), 118–129.
Peterson, C. (2006). The values in action (VIA) classification of strengths. In M. Csikszentmihalyi & I. Csikszentmihalyi (Eds.), *A life worth living. Contribution to positive psychology*. Oxford: Oxford University Press.
Peterson, C., & Seligman, M. E. P. (2004). *Character strengths and virtues a handbook and classification*. Washington, DC: APA Press/Oxford University Press.

Peterson, C., Ruch, W., Beermann, U., Park, N., & Seligman, M. P. E. (2007). Strengths of character, orientations to happiness, and life satisfaction. *The Journal of Positive Psychology, 2*(3), 149–156.
Preziosa, A., Riva, G., & Delle Fave, A. (2008). L'esperienza soggettiva dell'obesità: implicazioni diagnostico-terapeutiche [The subjective experience of obesity: Therapeutical and diagnostical implications]. *Psicologia della Salute, I*, 39–55.
Riva, E., Rainisio, N., & Boffi, M. (2014). Positive change in clinics: Flow experience in psychodynamic therapies. In P. Inghilleri, G. Riva, & E. Riva (Eds.), *Enabling positive change. Flow and complexity in daily experience* (pp. 105–122). Warsaw: De Gruyter.
Ruini, C., & Fava, G. A. (2008). New psychotherapeutic technique for preventing relapse: Well-being therapy. *Journal of Affective Disorders, 107*, S98–S99.
Ruini, C., Tomba, E., & Fava, G. A. (2007). Well-Being Therapy (WBT): una strategia psicoterapica per la promozione del benessere psicologico. In A. Delle Fave (Ed.), *La Condivisione del Benessere. Il Contributo della Psicologia Positiva* (pp. 113–128). Milano: Franco Angeli.
Ryff, C. D. (1989). Happiness is everything, or is it? Explorations on the meaning of psychological well-being. *Journal of Personality and Social Psychology, 57*, 1069–1081.
Ryff, C., & Keyes, C. (1995). The structure of psychological well-being revisited. *Journal of Personality and Social Psychology, 69*, 719–727.
Ryff, C. D., & Singer, B. (1996). Psychological well-being: Meaning, measurement, and implications for psychotherapy research. *Psychotherapy and Psychosomatics, 65*, 14–23.
Ryff, C. D., & Singer, B. H. (2008). Know thyself and become what you are: A eudaimonic approach to psychological well-being. *Journal of Happiness Studies, 9*, 13–39.
Ryff, C. D., Singer, B., Dienberg Love, G., & Essex, M. J. (1998). Resilience in adulthood and later life. In J. Lomranz (Ed.), *Handbook of aging and mental health* (pp. 69–96). New York: Plenum.
Sartori, R. D. G., Marelli, M., Garavaglia, P., Castelli, L., Busin, S., & Delle Fave, A. (2014). The assessment of patients' quality of experience: Autonomy level and perceived challenges. *Rehabilitation Psychology, 59*, 266–277.
Seligman, M. E. P. (2002a). *Authentic happiness: Using the new positive psychology to realize your potential for lasting fulfillment*. New York: Free Press.
Seligman, M. E. P. (2002b). Positive psychology, positive prevention and positive therapy. In C. R. Snyder & S. Lopez (Eds.), *Handbook of positive psychology*. Oxford: Oxford University Press.
Seligman, M. E. P. (2006). Afterward: Breaking the 65 percent barrier. In M. Csikszentmihalyi & I. Csikszentmihalyi Selega (Eds.), *A life worth living. Contribution to positive psychology*. Oxford: Oxford University Press.
Seligman, M. E. P. (2008). Positive health. *Applied Psychology: An International Review, 57*, 3–18.
Seligman, M. E. P., & Peterson, C. (2003). Positive clinical psychology. In L. G. Aspinwall & U. M. Staudinger (Eds.), *A psychology of human strengths: Fundamental questions and future directions for a positive psychology*. Washington, DC: APA Books.
Seligman, M. E. P., Park, N., & Peterson, C. (2005). Positive psychology progress. Empirical validation for intervention. *American Psychologist, 60*(5), 410–421.
Seligman, M. E. P., Rashid, T., & Park, A. C. (2006). Positive psychotherapy. *American Psychologist, 61*, 774–788.
Slater, C. L. (2003). Generativity versus stagnation: An elaboration of Erikson's adult stage of human development. *Journal of Adult Development, 10*, 53–65.
Steele, J. P., & Fullagar, C. J. (2009). Facilitators and outcome of student engagement in a college setting. *Journal of Psychology, 143*, 5–27.
Stern, D. N. (2004). *The present moment in psychotherapy and everyday life*. New York: Norton.
Stern, D. N. (2010). *Forms of vitality: Exploring dynamic experience in psychology and the arts*. Oxford: Oxford University Press.

Winston, A., & Winston, B. (2002). *Handbook of integrated short-term psychotherapy*. Washington, DC: American Psychiatric Publishing.
Wood, A. M., & Tarrier, N. (2010). Positive clinical psychology: A new vision and strategy for integrated research and practice. *Clinical Psychology Review, 30*, 819–829.
World Health Organization (1946, June 19–22). Preamble to the constitution of the World Health Organization as adopted by the International Health Conference, New York; signed on 22 July 1946 by the representatives of 61 States (Official Records of the World Health Organization, no. 2, p. 100) and entered into force on 7 April 1948.
World Health Organization. (2004). *Promoting mental health: Concepts, emerging evidence, practice (summary report)*. Geneva: World Health Organization.

Part VIII
Physiological Correlates of the Flow Experience

Chapter 20
Experimental Paradigms to Investigate Flow-Experience and Its Psychophysiology: Inspired from Stress Theory and Research

Tahmine Tozman and Corinna Peifer

Abstract In this chapter, we present new psychological and physiological research paradigms to assess and investigate flow-experience. We compare flow theory and research with concepts of challenge and threat, as well as with mental effort. By taking a closer look at physiological processes during challenge and threat and during mental effort, we outline physiological measures that might relate to flow-experience but have not yet been considered by flow-research yet. Also, we describe research paradigms from the research-traditions of challenge and threat and mental effort and discuss applications for flow-research. Within this chapter, we aim at stimulating experimental research on flow-experience for a better understanding of its psychological and physiological mechanisms.

20.1 Introduction

Flow-theory has been linked to stress-theory (e.g., Csikszentmihalyi 1990; Peifer 2012), particularly to Lazarus' Transactional Stress Model (Lazarus and Folkman 1984). It was empirically shown that flow occurs at a state of moderate physiological arousal, whereas low and high arousal corresponds to relaxation or stress (Peifer et al. 2014). Psychological stress theories and research offer paradigms that might be of great use for flow-research – both with respect to its psychological and psychophysiological processes. In the following, we will thus discuss the biopsychosocial (BPS) model of challenge and threat and the concept of mental effort. Based on the link between flow and stress, we will transfer psychological as well as psychophysiological research methods and paradigms from stress-research to flow-research. In each section, we will first present a short description of the theory

T. Tozman (✉)
Institute of Psychology, Goethe University Frankfurt, Frankfurt, Germany
e-mail: t.tozman@psych.uni-frankfurt.de

C. Peifer
Department of Applied Psychology in Health, Work and Development, Ruhr University Bochum, Bochum, Germany
e-mail: corinna.peifer@rub.de

L. Harmat et al. (eds.), *Flow Experience*, DOI 10.1007/978-3-319-28634-1_20

including its psychological and physiological findings and discuss its similarities and differences with flow. Then we will present the experimental designs used in the tradition of the presented theory and discuss how flow research could adapt these paradigms for future studies.

20.1.1 The Biopsychosocial Model of Challenge and Threat

In the social motivation literature, the BPS model of challenge and threat (Blascovich 2008; Blascovich and Mendes 2010; Tomaka et al. 1993, 1997) is a well-established model, which integrates biological, psychological and social psychological approaches to explain stress and motivated performance. Psychologically, it is based on the transactional stress model (Lazarus and Folkman 1984) and postulates that a situation leads to an experience of challenge or threat as a consequence of the subjective evaluation of situational demands (e.g., required effort, controllability of a task, novelty etc.; see Blascovich 2008) compared to the personal resources to cope with them (e.g., abilities, skills, knowledge, support etc.). Challenge and threat only occur in situations that are self-relevant and relevant to reach personal goals – called motivated performance situations (see Blascovich 2008). Such motivated performance situations are, for example, exams and sport competitions. When individuals are confronted with motivated performance situations, they either consciously or automatically (Blascovich 2008) evaluate their resources to cope with the demands of the task. An experience of threat results when individuals evaluate their resources as insufficient to cope; an experience of challenge results when individuals evaluate their resources as meeting the demands of the task. Blascovich (2008) determines a state of challenge as a "positive, hedonically toned motivational state". Thus, it appears that the motivational state of challenge in terms of Blascovich resembles the state of flow-experience, as a positively toned state of high task engagement. As challenge in the BPS model, flow results when the skills of a person are meeting the demands of a situation (i.e., challenge-skill-balance, compare flow-channel model, Csikszentmihalyi 1975). Consequently, challenge can be regarded as a precondition for flow experience (Fig. 20.1). A similar theoretical integration has already been conducted with flow and stress within Lazarus' transactional stress model (compare Peifer 2012; Peifer et al. 2014, 2015).

20.1.2 The Psychophysiology of Challenge and Threat

However, a clear strength of the BPS model beyond the transactional stress model is that it integrates assumptions with regard to the psychophysiology of challenge and threat, which can be applied to achieve new insights into possible physiological mechanisms of flow. Based on assumptions of the theory of physiological toughness (Dienstbier 1989), Blascovich and colleagues found in their research that challenge

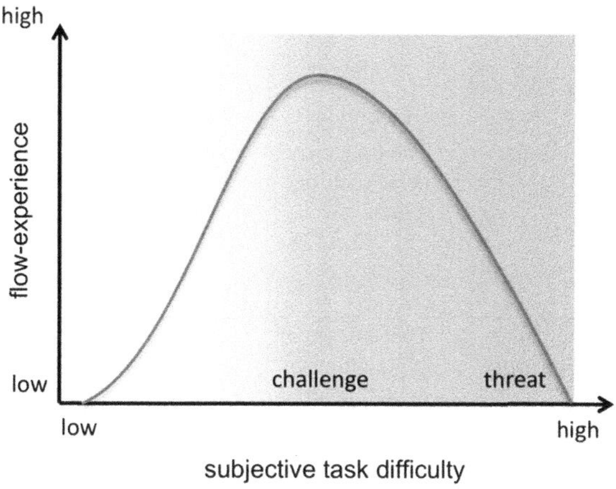

Fig. 20.1 Relation of flow experience with challenge and threat

causes an increase of sympathetic activation, as measured through increased heart rate, ventricular contractility (the strength of contractions of the left ventricle of the heart), cardiac output (the amount of blood pumped by the heart), the release of epinephrine, and a decrease in total peripheral resistance (Blascovich 2008; Obrist 1981; Seery 2011).

The physiological pattern that Blascovich and colleagues identified for the state of threat is also characterized by sympathetic activation, but, additionally, by activation of the hypothalamic pituitary adrenal (HPA) axis. Accordingly, threat – like challenge – is also marked by increased heart rate and ventricular contractility, but – in opposite to challenge – by increased cortisol, decreased cardiac output and an increased total peripheral resistance (Seery 2011). These indicators have been well validated in the literature (Blascovich 2008) (Table 20.1).

Based on the past 5 years of flow-research, we have first evidence that flow is related to moderately increased sympathetic activation (Peifer et al. 2014; De Manzano et al. 2010) and moderate HPA axis activation (Keller et al. 2011a; Peifer et al. 2014; Tozman et al. 2014). These findings show that – on top of the theoretical similarities of the states flow and challenge – the physiological pattern of flow has similarities to both, the physiology of challenge and the physiology of threat, as it involves (at least moderate) increases in sympathetic activation and also (at least moderate) HPA axis activation. Still, the physiological pattern for the flow-state is yet less consistent than the patterns observed for challenge and threat and different physiological indicators have been used to investigate the concepts. Thus, (psychophysiological) flow-research could profit from applying research paradigms from the tradition of the BPS model. As a first step, it seems to be necessary to empirically test the postulated relatedness of the concepts of challenge and flow succeeded by systematical investigation of the physiology of flow with respective research methods. In the following, we will present research paradigms used to investigate challenge and threat and discuss their applicability and value for flow research. Subsequently, we will propose physiological parameters that could be used in future investigations of the physiology of flow.

Table 20.1 Physiological measures in relation to challenge and threat and to flow-experience

Physiological measure	Description	Relation to threat	Relation to challenge	Relation to flow-experience
Heart rate	The frequency of heart beats per minute	Increase (Tomaka et al. 1993, 1997)	Increase (Tomaka et al. 1993, 1997)	Decrease in heart period (inverse of heart rate) (de Manzano et al. 2010)
Ventricular contractility	The strength of contractions of the left ventricle of the heart	Increase (Tomaka et al. 1993, 1997)	Increase (Tomaka et al. 1993, 1997)	Research gap
Cardiac output	The volume of blood pumped by the heart in one minute	Decrease (Tomaka et al. 1993, 1997)	Increase (Tomaka et al. 1993, 1997)	Decrease (measured as decreased heart period and increased blood pressure; de Manzano et al. 2010)
Total peripheral resistance	The total resistance to blood flow in the systemic circuit	Increase (Tomaka et al. 1993, 1997)	Decrease (Tomaka et al. 1993, 1997)	Research gap
Epinephrine	Hormone released by the sympathetic nervous system in response to stress	Increase (Blascovich et al. 2004; Henry 1993)	Increase (Blascovich et al. 2004; Henry 1993)	Research gap
Cortisol	Hormone released by the hypothalamic-pituitary-adrenal axis in response to stress	Increase (Dickerson and Kemeney 2004; Frankenhaeuser and Lundberg 1985)	Unrelated (Dickerson and Kemeney 2004; Frankenhaeuser and Lundberg 1985)	Inverted-u shaped relationship (Peifer et al. 2014; Tozman et al. 2016); increase of cortisol in a demand-skill balance-condition (Keller et al. 2011a)

20.1.3 Experimental Designs from the Tradition of the BPS Model

Despite similarities between flow theory and the BPS model, there are several differences in experimental designs that have been applied so far. In the tradition of the BPS model, researchers make use of experimental methods such as framing – in order to influence the cognitive appraisal towards a task (Tomaka et al. 1997), or social evaluation – in order to manipulate the self relevance of a task (Blascovich et al. 1999), to investigate the different patterns of challenge and threat. In the following, we present selected experimental paradigms in order to demonstrate how challenge and threat are investigated in the laboratory and discuss how these methods can complement psychological and psychophysiological flow research.

20.1.3.1 Framing: Cognitive Appraisal of a Challenge-Skill Balance

Besides theoretical and physiological similarities between flow and challenge, there are also striking similarities with respect to their assessment. As mentioned above, an important precondition for challenge and flow to occur is the cognitive appraisal of one's own skills in meeting the demands of a given task (Blascovich and Tomaka 1996; Csikszentmihalyi 1975). Almost identical to early measures of flow (e.g., the Experience Sampling Form, Csikszentmihalyi and Larson 1987), Blascovich and Tomaka (1996) have assessed challenge by two items: (1) "How threatening do you expect the upcoming task to be?" And (2) "How able are you to cope with the upcoming task?" They assumed a state of challenge if the subjective ability of coping (item 2) was higher than the subjective threat of the task (item 1) – and they assumed a state of threat in case of the opposite pattern. Building upon this operationalization of challenge, Blascovich and Tomaka (1996) have developed experimental paradigms to manipulate challenge and threat appraisals to measure their distinct psychophysiological pattern. The manipulation was realized using a framing technique: To induce challenge, participants were informed that the upcoming task would be challenging and they were encouraged to "think of themselves as someone capable of meeting that challenge" (Tomaka et al. 1997, p. 65); to induce threat, participants were informed that the upcoming task would be mandatory, and they were told to complete the task "as quickly and accurately as possible" (Tomaka et al. 1997, p. 65) and that their task performance was assessed. By means of this manipulation, Tomaka and colleagues (1997) were able to find distinct physiological patterns for challenge and threat as reported earlier in this chapter.

In flow research, framing-paradigms have so far not been used in laboratory experiments. Considering the conceptual similarities between challenge and threat with flow-experience, using framing paradigms in flow-research can bring new insights into the concept of flow. Building on the just described paradigm of Tomaka and colleagues (1997), psychophysiological flow research could apply the framing technique to test whether individuals in the challenge-frame experience more flow than individuals in the threat-frame.

As physiological measures in their experiment, Tomaka and colleagues (1997) analyzed heart rate, preejection period, cardiac output and total peripheral resistance. In flow-research, first findings exist with respect to heart rate and indicators of cardiac output (decreased heart period and increased blood pressure) – although based on a very different experimental design (De Manzano et al. 2010): De Manzano and colleagues (2010) compared a flow-condition to a baseline but not to a threat-condition. In order to distinguish states of flow or challenge with states of threat, future studies should look at these physiological measures using the described framing paradigm. Furthermore, preejection period and peripheral resistance have not yet been investigated in the context of flow but were shown to distinguish challenge from threat. Recently, it was found that flow is associated with moderate sympathetic activation as assessed by low-frequency heart rate variability (Peifer et al. 2014) – a measure that was criticized for being an insufficient indicator of sympathetic activation. As preejection period is a reliable indicator for sympathetic activation, it would be able to complement and clarify those recent findings.

Another scope of application for framing paradigms relates to the concept of self-relevance: The BPS model postulates that challenge and threat only occur in motivated performance situations, i.e. in those situations that are self-relevant and relevant to achieve personal goals (e.g., Blascovich 2008; Blascovich and Mendes 2010; Blascovich and Tomaka 1996). Based on the conceptual similarities between flow and challenge outlined above, we postulate that self-relevance of a situation is facilitating flow, accordingly. This means that if the demands of a situation meet the skills of a person, flow is more likely to occur, if the situation is self-relevant and relevant to achieve personal goals. Thus, flow-experience should more likely occur if a situation is framed as a self-relevant task. In other words, if a comparatively boring task (e.g., a simple d2-Test) is framed as a task that has predictive value for later job success, this should increase the probability to experience flow during that task. Also, tasks where demands exceed the skills of a person will not cause threat, unless the task is evaluated as self-relevant.

In line with these assumptions, cortisol was not increased in an overload condition of the computer game Tetris compared to a demand-skill-fit condition (Keller et al. 2011a). By increasing self-relevance of Tetris using framing (e.g., by telling participants that Tetris would be an indicator for intelligence), an overload condition might cause a state of threat and, in consequence, an increase in cortisol compared to a fit condition. First evidence supporting this assumption can be found in a study of Tozman and colleagues (2016). They investigated professional chess players for whom chess is highly self-relevant. In contrast to results from the Tetris study, their results indicated that cortisol increased in the overload condition of a chess-simulation compared to a fit condition. Accordingly, future studies on flow-experience should take the self-relevance of tasks into account and complement existing paradigms to manipulate flow experience. One paradigm, which has successfully been applied to investigate flow-experience, was developed by Keller and colleagues (e.g., Keller and Bless 2008; Keller et al. 2011b) and operationalized flow by realizing an objective demand-skill balance. They have modified the computer game Tetris and invented a version, in which task difficulty (i.e. speed) automatically adapts to the skills of the person. While subjective flow-ratings were found to be highest in the demand-skill-fit condition, a major critique of this paradigm is that an *objective* demand-skill fit does not sufficiently meet the subjective nature of flow-experience. As the described framing paradigm of Tomaka and colleagues (1997) uses the manipulation of *subjective* appraisal of the demand-skill-ratio, possibly a combination of both paradigms – realizing an objective demand-skill-fit and framing the task as a challenge – would come closer to a genuine experimental manipulation of flow-experience.

20.1.3.2 Social Evaluation as a Means to Enhance Self-Relevance

The presence of others has been a central topic of interest in social psychology since Triplett (1898) observed that bikers were faster in the presence of coactors. In many following studies, it was found that the presence of others (coactors or an audience) has strong effects on task performance (compare Bond and Titus 1983): simple or well-trained tasks were improved (social facilitation), while complex, unlearned tasks were impaired (social inhibition). Two processes seem to mediate the effect of others on task performance: increased arousal through the presence of others (Zajonc 1968), and evaluation apprehension (Cotrell et al. 1968). According to Seta and Seta (1992), social observation "increases the value of task performance"; performing well is related to "praise and recognition" and, in contrast, poor performance is related to "shame and embarrassment" (Seta and Seta 1992, p. 97). Building upon the literature on audience effects, Blascovich and colleagues (1999) took a closer look at the influence of social observation on cardiovascular response during challenge or threat. Participants had to perform either a well-learned or an unlearned task (number categorization task or pattern recognition task), either alone or with the presence of an audience. Cardiovascular responses were recorded using an impedance cardiograph and a blood pressure monitor. The no-observation condition caused no cardiovascular reaction – neither in learned nor in unlearned tasks. Under social observation, however, the cardiovascular response during a learned task showed a pattern as characteristic for challenge; and during an unlearned task a pattern as typical for threat. As self-relevance is a condition for challenge and threat (and their physiological patterns) to occur, the presence of an audience must have caused an increase in self-relevance. In line with these insights, established stress-protocols for stress manipulations in the laboratory involve social evaluation, e.g., the Trier Social Stress Test (TSST, Kirschbaum et al. 1993) and the Socially Evaluated Cold Pressure Test (Schwabe et al. 2008).

In order to investigate the relationship of stress and flow-experience, Peifer and colleagues (2014) made use of the described effects of social evaluation by confronting participants with the TSST (Kirschbaum et al. 1993) before participants performed a computer task under social observation. Framing the task as having predictive value for later job success further increased the goal relevance of the computer task. The results showed that high sympathetic and HPA-axis activation (as typical for threat) during the computer game following the TSST were associated with low flow values, while moderate sympathetic and HPA-axis-activation (similar to a challenge pattern) was associated with high flow-values. Thus, retrospectively, this pattern is indeed in line with expectations of the BPS model. However, Peifer and colleagues (2014) did not use a full experimental design, but treated the whole sample with the TSST. Future research should thus compare social-evaluative conditions with control conditions in order to unravel the exact effects of social evaluation on flow-experience. Presumably, not only the increase of self-relevance, but also the increase in physiological arousal mediated the effects. The answer to these research questions is highly applicable to the practice: many of the activities that have been named with respect to flow are performed in social contexts and in front of an audience, such as sports competitions, music or actor performance, teaching and many more.

20.1.4 Summary: What Can We Learn from the BPS Model for Flow-Research?

The high similarity between the concepts flow and challenge enables hypotheses on physiological flow indicators, which have not yet been considered in flow-research, such as preejection period, epinephrine, ventricular contractility, and total peripheral resistance. Also, the differentiation between challenge and threat according to the BPS model is a reminder of the differentiation between flow and stress according to Peifer and colleagues (2014) and reveals further hypotheses on a distinct physiological pattern of those states that should be tested in future studies.

With respect to experimental designs, we would like to highlight two approaches of challenge and threat studies, which are of high interest to flow research: (1) Framing and (2) Social evaluation. Through framing, it is possible to experimentally manipulate the cognitive appraisal of a demand-skill-fit (e.g., in terms of challenge or threat), as well as of the self-relevance of a task. Through social evaluation, it is possible to increase the self-relevance of a task, as well as physiological arousal during a task. Both approaches will complement actual flow research and help to better understand its (pre)conditions.

20.2 Mental Effort

Mental effort is defined as the amount of resources that are mobilized to cope with cognitive tasks and mental demands (Gaillard and Kramer 2001; see also Kahneman 1973). According to Kahneman (1973), mental effort, and – at the same time – physiological arousal vary with task difficulty. Building upon Kahneman's model, the Compensatory Control model (Hockey 1993, 1997) described an increase of mental effort as a compensatory strategy to protect performance in the presence of increased task demands – but under the expense of physiological costs. Until today, many studies have confirmed that mental effort is accompanied by physiological arousal (Blascovic and Tomaka 1996; Wright 1996; Obrist 1976, 1981). As a consequence, physiological indicators to measure mental effort have been established.

Adding to the approaches of Kahneman (1973) and Hockey (1993, 1997), motivational intensity theory (Brehm and Self 1989) offers a close look at the role of task-difficulty on mental effort: It postulates that the amount of effort spent in accomplishing a task is predicted to increase proportionally with the level of perceived difficulty. When a task is perceived as very difficult, more effort will be invested in the task *as long as success is possible and justified.* However, disengagement occurs when task difficulty is experienced as impossible to cope. This assumption was supported by many psychophysiological studies: effort-related physiological activation was found to be more evident and persistent under moderately difficult conditions than under easy or impossible conditions (Aasman et al. 1987; Gendolla and Krüsken 2001; Light and Obrist 1983; Wright and Lockard 2006). In line with these findings, Obrist's (1981) active coping theory postulates that cardiovascular reactivity is related to resource mobilization during activities in which individuals have control over their performance outcomes.

According to the flow-channel-model, individuals experience flow when they evaluate a task or situation as challenging, but accomplishable by means of their own skills (challenge-skill balance) (Csikszentmihalyi 1975). A challenging task is the result of an evaluation of current demands and the resources of the individual to cope with them (Rheinberg 2010). According to the definitions of flow experience and mental effort, both concepts show some similarities: both are high, if the task is challenging but not impossible. The effects of task difficulty on flow-experience were first studied by Rheinberg and Vollmeyer (2003) using two different video game tasks (Roboguard and Pacman). Their results supported the assumption that flow is highest during conditions of a demand-skill fit. Following studies (Engeser and Rheinberg 2008; Keller and Bless 2008; Moller et al. 2007) supported their findings. Thus, flow and mental effort both depend on task difficulty in relation to the personal skill level. For example, regarding a chess player during a tournament, we can assume that playing against an equally skilled opponent will likely lead to flow experience. In contrast, if the opponent is superior, flow experience is less likely (Abuhamdeh and Csikszentmihalyi 2009; Tozman et al. 2014). However, with regard to mental effort, the chess player has to mobilize resources to protect his performance in both scenarios – with an equal or superior opponent. This means, both, flow and mental effort increase with increased task difficulty compared to low task difficulty. However, when task difficulty increases beyond a challenge-skill balance, flow will decrease, while mental effort still increases. Mental effort stops as soon as task difficulty is evaluated as impossible to cope (Fig. 20.2).

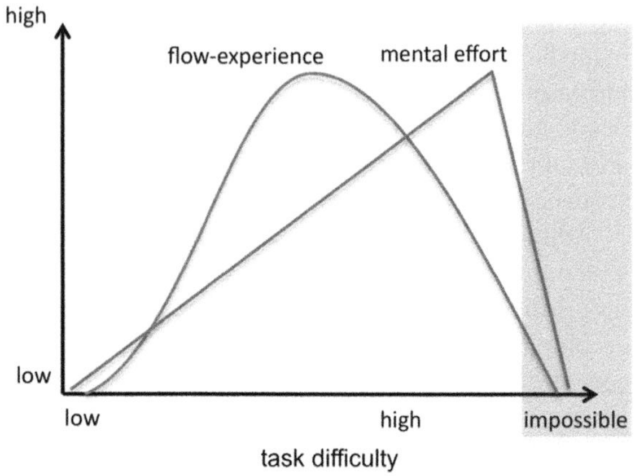

Fig. 20.2 Relation of task difficulty with mental effort and flow-experience

20.2.1 The Physiology of Mental Effort

Integrating motivational intensity theory (Brehm and Self 1989) and active coping theory (Obrist 1981), Wright (1996) postulated that cardiovascular adjustments during mental effort are driven by sympathetic activation (i.e., sympathetic discharge). Based on this assumption, systolic blood pressure, diastolic blood pressure, heart rate and preejection period (e.g., Richter and Gendolla 2009) have been assessed in relation to mental effort (see Table 20.2). Furthermore, findings demonstrate associations between mental effort and skin conductance (Gendolla and Richter 2005; Richter et al. 2008), pupil dilation (Kahneman and Beatty 1966) as well as salivary cortisol (Peters et al. 1998) and blood glucose (Fairclough and Houston 2004; Scholey et al. 2006) (see Table 20.2). The relationship of mental effort with these physiological indicators will now be outlined.

Systolic blood pressure has been considered to be a highly sensitive measure of mental effort (Smith et al. 1990). The intensity of the heart muscle pump causes the difference in the systolic blood pressure and is related to beta-adrenergic discharge of the sympathetic nervous system and the mobilization of resources. In contrast, sympathetic arousal affects diastolic blood pressure unsystematically. Recent studies show that systolic blood pressure is related to objective task difficulty as long as success is likely and justified (Bongard 1995; Light 1981; Lovallo et al. 1985; Sherwood et al. 1990). Heart rate, which is affected by both, sympathetic and parasympathetic arousal, was only found to be sensitive to energy mobilization when sympathetic influence dominates (Berntson et al. 1993). In a study conducted by Richter and colleagues (2008), the preejection period proves to be an even more sensitive measure of mental effort. Preejection period was highest in a condition of high task difficulty compared to two easier conditions and, importantly, compared to an impossible task condition. Preejection period is mainly influenced by beta-adrenergic activity (e.g., Schächinger et al. 2001), and is a very good indicator of

Table 20.2 Physiological measures in relation to mental effort and flow-experience

Physiological measure	Description	Relation to mental effort	Relation to flow-experience
Systolic blood pressure	The maximum arterial pressure during contraction of the heart	Increase (e.g., Bongard 1995; Gendolla and Richter 2005; Light 1981; Lovallo et al. 1985; Sherwood et al. 1990; Wright 1996; Obrist 1981)	Decreased (de Manzano et al. 2010)
Diastolic blood pressure	The pressure in the vessels between two heart beats when the heart rests	Less consistent findings (e.g., Gendolla and Richter 2005; Obrist 1981; Schwerdtfeger 2004; Storey et al. 1996; Wright 1996)	Increased (de Manzano et al. 2010)
Heart rate	The frequency of heart beats per minute	Increase, when sympathetic influence dominates (e.g., Berntson et al. 1993; Gendolla and Richter 2005; Obrist 1981; Schwerdtfeger 2004; Wright 1996)	Decrease in heart period (inverse of heart rate) (de Manzano et al. 2010)
Preejection period	The force of myocardial contraction	Increase (e.g., Richter and Gendolla 2009; Richter et al. 2008)	Research gap
Pupil dilation	Dilation of the pupil	Increased dilation during activity (e.g., Kahneman and Beatty 1966)	Research gap
Low-frequency heart rate variability	Spectral component of HRV 0·04–0·15 Hz	Less consistent findings (e.g., Bernardi et al. 2000; Blitz et al. 1970; Hjortskov et al. 2004)	Inverted-u shaped relationship (Peifer et al. 2014; during stressful activities: Tozman et al. 2015); negative linear relation (Harmat et al. 2015; Tozman et al. 2015)
High-frequency heart rate variability	Spectral component of HRV 0·15–0·4 Hz	Decrease (e.g., Bernardi et al. 2000; Blitz et al. 1970; Hjortskov et al. 2004)	**Inconsistent findings** negative linear relation (de Manzano et al. 2010); positive linear relation during stress (Peifer et al. 2014); curvilinear relation during stress (Tozman et al. 2015)
RMSSD	HRV parameter, highly related to high-frequency HRV		Decrease (Keller et al. 2011a)

(continued)

Table 20.2 (continued)

Physiological measure	Description	Relation to mental effort	Relation to flow-experience
Blood glucose	Measure of energy mobilization	Decrease during activity (e.g., Fairclough and Houston 2004; Scholey et al. 2006)	Research gap
Skin conductance	Physiological measure of autonomic and psychological arousal	Increase in unspecific skin conductance responses (e.g., Dawson et al. 2000; Gendolla and Richter 2005)	**Inconsistent findings** positive relationship (Nacke and Lindley 2009) no relationship (Kivikangas 2006)
Salivary cortisol	Hormone released by the hypothalamic-pituitary-adrenal axis in response to stress	Increase under uncontrollable conditions (e.g., Peters et al. 1998)	Inverted-u shaped relationship (Peifer et al. 2014; Tozman et al. 2016); increase of cortisol in a demand-skill balance-condition (Keller et al. 2011a); no relation (Brom et al. 2014)

sympathetic activation. These results give, thus, further support to Wright's (1996) assumptions regarding the role of sympathetic activation during mental effort.

Similarly, research on the psychophysiology of flow also suggested an association with sympathetic activity with flow (de Manzano et al. 2010; Peifer et al. 2014), however, evidence is still scarce and inconsistent. Peifer and colleagues (2014) have used low-frequency HRV as an indicator for sympathetic activation and found an inverted u-shaped relationship with flow in a stress-relevant situation. Recently, Harmat and colleagues (2015) found a negative relationship of low-frequency HRV with subjective flow as measured in three different difficulty conditions (easy, optimal, difficult). De Manzano and colleagues assumed a relationship between flow and sympathetic activation based on the ratio of high-frequency and low-frequency HRV and on heart period (the inverse of heart rate). While heart period represents both, sympathetic and parasympathetic influence, low-frequency HRV as well as the ratio of low-frequency and high frequency have been critically discussed in their relation to sympathetic activation. The inconsistencies of these findings could thus partly trace back to the imprecise measures of sympathetic activation that have been used so far. Thus, flow-research could profit from the research tradition of mental effort and integrate measures such as preejection period to clarify the role of sympathetic activation for flow-experience.

Heart rate variability (HRV) has also been shown to be sensitive to changes in mental effort (Aasman et al. 1987; Jorna 1992; Mulder and Mulder 1981; Veltman and Gaillard 1993) and, accordingly, to be a reliable measure of mental effort (Mukherjee et al. 2011). Thayer and colleagues (2009) have explained this relationship in their network model: The prefrontal cortex plays an active role in

HRV-regulation. During mental load, the capacities of the prefrontal cortex are fully used by cognitive functions, and, as a consequence, HRV decreases (Thayer et al. 2009). Many studies support the postulated suppression of HRV with increasing cognitive load, particularly for tasks that require central executive functions (e.g., Di Bernadi et al. 2009; Kalsbeek and Ettema 1964; Redondo and Del Valle-Inclán 1992). Particularly the high-frequency-band of the HRV was found to be a stable indicator for mental effort, whereas inconsistent results exist for the low-frequency-band (Bernardi et al. 2000; Blitz et al. 1970; Hjortskov et al. 2004). Additionally, high-frequency HRV is a reliable indicator for parasympathetic activation (Task Force of the European Society of Cardiology and the North American Society of Pacing and Electrophysiology 1996). With respect to flow-experience, Keller and colleagues (2011a) found a decrease in HRV (RMSSD) in a demand-skill-fit (or "flow") condition, compared to an easy and an overload condition, and suggested that flow has physiological parallels to mental effort. However, Keller and colleagues (2011a) found that although the demand-skill-fit condition had a negative effect on HRV, this effect did not reflect self-reported flow-experience. Consequently, they suggested that the decrease in HRV (RMSSD) in the fit-condition could also indicate mental effort. Future studies need to disentangle what is manipulated in a skills-demand-fit-condition: flow-experience or mental effort or both?

In a very different design, Peifer and colleagues (2014) found that self-reported flow-experience under stressful conditions was positively associated with high-frequency HRV. This finding speaks for a parasympathetic modulation of sympathetic activation, and for decreased mental effort during flow in the context of stressful situations. In an experimental study conducted with a driving simulator Tozman and colleagues (2015) found a negative linear relation between low-frequency HRV and flow when participants were faced with a balanced skill-demand level task. However, faced with a stressful task, flow and low-frequency as well as high-frequency HRV showed a curvilinear relation. In their study, Tozman and colleagues used low-frequency HRV as an indicator for baroreflex modulation of the cardiovascular activity. The baroreflex is one of the elementary mechanisms through which acute changes in the heart rate and blood pressure is controlled (Guyton 1980) and has also been associated with several cognitive functions (e.g., mental stress, del Paso et al. 1996). In an experimental study Yasumasu and colleagues (2006) showed that decrease in baroreflex activity was associated with increase in mental effort.

Furthermore, blood glucose - an explicit measure of energy mobilization – has been found to be a sensitive physiological indicator of mental effort. Increase of energy mobilization was associated with reduced glucose levels in blood (Fairclough and Houston 2004; Scholey et al. 2006). Glucose provides the required energy to the metabolism to cope with a task or an activity. Especially, cognitive functions (Taylor and Rachman 1988) such as attentional control (Gailliot et al. 2007) and memory (Manning et al. 1990) are associated with increased consumption of glucose in blood. Under conditions of high task difficulty (high effort) and low controllability (e.g., noise), an increase in salivary cortisol causes an increase of glucose levels in blood to mobilize energy resources to address current task demands. Whereas glucose levels have not yet been investigated in flow research, cortisol was: Findings reveal that moderately elevated cortisol-levels (as compared to baseline) are related to flow-experience (Keller et al. 2011a; Peifer et al. 2014; Tozman et al. 2016) and indicate an inverted-u shaped relationship between flow and cortisol in stress-relevant situations (Peifer et al. 2014; Tozman et al. 2014). However, Brom and colleagues (2014) found no relationship of cortisol and flow in serious games. Thus, further studies should address the flow-cortisol link to clarify results. Measures of blood glucose could complement the picture.

One of the earliest measures of mental effort is pupil dilation (Hess and Polt 1964). Pupil dilation was found to be increased in response to increases in task demands and difficulty – and the effects were confirmed in many contexts, from mental arithmetic (Bradshaw 1968; Payne et al. 1968) to short-term memory tasks (Kahneman and Beatty 1966; compare also Kahneman 1973). To our knowledge, no research has yet investigated the relationship of pupil dilation with flow-experience, although this could be an interesting real-time measure of flow, which could complement psychophysiological flow-research.

20.2.2 Experimental Designs to Investigate Mental Effort

In the following, we will present experimental paradigms from the tradition of mental effort and discuss them with respect to their relevance for flow-research. We will address paradigms manipulating task difficulty, as well as paradigms manipulating ego-involvement.

20.2.2.1 Task Difficulty

Different types of tasks were used to investigate mental effort, such as mental arithmetic (Bradshaw 1968; Payne et al. 1968), short-term memory tasks (Kahneman and Beatty 1966), Stroop tasks (e.g., Fairclough and Houston 2004), pitch discrimination tasks (Kahneman and Beatty 1967), concentration tests (d2, Brickenkamp 1981), sentence comprehension tasks (Ahern and Beatty 1979), or imagery tasks (Eysenck 1979). Those tasks were usually presented at varying difficulty levels in order to investigate different levels of mental effort. A clear strength of designs in the tradition of mental effort is the rigorous experimental approach to create objective conditions. Probably because flow-experience is characterized a subjective evaluation of challenges and skills, clear experimental paradigms are scarce until now. However, the transfer of methods from the tradition of mental effort to flow research has one important challenge: many of the tasks are not applicable for flow-research, as flow requires tasks to be skill-related, with clear goals and direct feedback (Csikszentmihalyi 1975). Considering this claim, one task paradigm from mental effort research that is applicable to flow is mental arithmetic (Bradshaw

1968; Payne et al. 1968). Indeed, mental arithmetic has already been used successfully in flow-research: Ulrich and colleagues (2014) have applied a mental arithmetic paradigm in a neuropsychological study on flow. Similar to the Tetris paradigm described in Sect. 20.1.3.1, they developed one task condition, in which math tasks were adapted to the skills of the participant and compared this condition to a very easy and an overload condition.

Other experimental paradigms to investigate the role of task difficulty during flow-experience (and that fulfill the challenge of being interesting and to create objective experimental conditions at the same time), are computer games or work simulations. Using two types of computer games (Roboguard and Pacman) Rheinberg and Vollmeyer (2003) developed a successful experimental paradigm. As a first step, they tested the skills of their participants in the respective video game. In the experimental phase, they assigned participants to their optimal difficulty level that was in balance with their personal skills as assessed in the test phase. Optimal difficulty levels were then played alternating with low and high difficulty levels. Their results showed that self-reported flow is highest during a medium (optimal) level of task difficulty. Results from subsequent studies (Engeser and Rheinberg 2008; Keller and Bless 2008; Moller et al. 2007) supported their findings. At this point, we need to recall the paradigm of Keller and colleagues (2008; see 2.1.1), which can be seen as an advancement of the paradigm of Rheinberg and Vollmeyer (2003). Keller and colleagues (2008) adapted the computer game Tetris to achieve three different difficulty levels, one easy, one optimal and one overload condition. Inspired by the concept of challenge-skill-balance as a precondition of flow-experience (e.g., Csikszentmihalyi 1975), the optimal condition was realized by a constant adaptation of task demands (i.e. speed) to the skills of the participant. However, one big challenge for flow-research using different difficulty levels to manipulate flow, is to distinguish if findings reflect flow or probably mental effort. As a consequence, subjective flow measures should always be taken into account in experimental flow-studies.

20.2.2.2 Ego Involvement

It has been shown that the effects of task difficulty and of value of success have a combined influence on the cardiovascular system during motivated performance activities. Gendolla and Richter (2005) pointed out that in addition to the incentive of success, there are motivational implications of a task with consequences for the subject's ego. That means, there are tasks which are more important for oneself than other tasks. Similar to Blascovich's (2008) self-relevant situations, Gendolla and Richter (2005) refer to ego involvement as task and performance conditions important for an individual's self-esteem such as prestige and academic standing (e.g., student participants). For example, for the grandmaster a chess game at a tournament is highly ego-involving, as is dancing for dancers, playing basketball for basketball players, and so on. To investigate the effect of ego-involvement on mental effort, Gendolla and Richter (2005) conducted an adapted version of the d2 attention and concentration task (Brickenkamp 1981) at two levels of difficulty: in the unfixed condition ('do your best'), different letters were presented on a computer screen and participants had to decide to press a button (in case of a 'd') or not (in case of any other letter) as quickly and correctly as possible. In the easy condition, each letter was presented for 3 s, before participants could press the button. Furthermore, Gendolla and Richter (2005) manipulated ego involvement by means of the instructions: In the high ego involvement condition, the task was presented as a concentration and achievement test for students (Gendolla and Richter 2005, p. 597) and participants were told that the result of the test could predict their study success. In the no ego involvement condition, the d2 test was presented as a fill-in task. Results indicated that high ego involvement increased performance-related cardiovascular reactivity, systolic blood pressure, diastolic blood pressure and heart rate as well as skin conductance when task difficulty was unfixed (do your best) but not when the task was easy. In the easy condition, ego involvement did not have an impact on cardiovascular reactivity.

Accordingly, when comparing flow and stress in terms of task difficulty, increasing the importance of a task using framing paradigms in combination with optimal or high task difficulty seems to be a promising approach. These recommendations based on mental effort research are, thus, in line with recommendations based on the BPS model, making them even more promising for future investigations. Instead of framing paradigms to manipulate task importance, one could alternatively work with homogenous samples and use a task that is highly relevant for the sample, e.g., playing chess with a sample of professional chess players or playing poker with professional poker players (Tozman et al. 2014).

One more research question evolving from the described paradigm to investigate mental effort, is how the fixation of difficulty and subjective importance interact. In case of the relatively monotone d2 attention task, it could be that flow is particularly high if the task difficulty is unfixed *and* the task is framed as highly important.

20.2.3 Summary: What Can We Learn from Mental Effort Studies for Flow Research?

The concepts of flow and mental effort show some parallels, as both concepts depend on task difficulty and self-relevance. Based on these similarities, we extracted physiological measures, which have not yet been considered in flow-research, beyond them pupil dilation, blood glucose and preejection period.

With respect to research paradigms used in mental effort research, flow-research can profit from the rigorous experimental approach with objective conditions of task difficulty – and there are already first studies applying those kind of experimental designs. Another important finding from mental effort research is that mental effort decreases when the task is evaluated as impossible. This aspect is nicely applicable to flow-research and should be considered in any experimental study design. Furthermore, and similar to the research for the BPS model, mental effort research also outlines the importance of ego involvement. By adding framing of importance in order to increase ego-involvement, the existing experimental paradigms to induce flow could be progressed.

20.3 General Conclusion

Although recently, there has been an increasing body of research addressing the psychophysiology of flow-experience, there are still many research gaps to close. Within this chapter, we have outlined similarities and differences to theories and research of challenge and threat and of mental effort. From these research traditions, new ideas for physiological flow measures were derived in order to stimulate future flow-research.

Furthermore, we have outlined that there is only relatively little experimental work on flow. And despite some already very good approaches to experimentally investigate flow-experience in the laboratory, further rigorous paradigms are needed to complement actual psychological and psychophysiological knowledge on flow-experience. By means of enhancing self-relevance (see Sect. 20.2.2.2), it might be possible to further enhance the probability of flow in a demand-skill-fit condition. However, the subjective measurement of flow-experience – at least as a control variable – will probably always be necessary. It will be a challenge for future flow-research to focus more on experimental designs to investigate flow-experience, thereby maintaining the balance between objective conditions and measures – including physiological measures - and self-reports to assess flow.

References

Aasman, J., Mulder, G., & Mulder, L. J. (1987). Operator effort and the measurement of heart-rate variability. *Human Factors: The Journal of the Human Factors and Ergonomics Society, 29*(2), 161–170.

Abuhamdeh, S., & Csikszentmihalyi, M. (2009). Intrinsic and extrinsic motivational orientations in the competitive context: An examination of person–situation interactions. *Journal of Personality, 77*(5), 1615–1635.

Ahern, S. K., & Beatty, J. (1979). Physiological signs of information processing vary with intelligence. *Science, 205*, 1289–1292.

Bernardi, L., Wdowczyk-Szulc, J., Valenti, C., Castoldi, S., Passino, C., Spadacini, G., & Sleight, P. (2000). Effects of controlled breathing, mental activity and mental stress with or without verbalization on heart rate variability. *Journal of the American College of Cardiology, 35*(6), 1462–1469.

Berntson, G. G., Cacioppo, J. T., & Quigley, K. S. (1993). Cardiac psychophysiology and autonomic space in humans: Empirical perspectives and conceptual implications. *Psychological Bulletin, 114*, 296–322.

Blascovich, J. (2008). Challenge and threat. In A. J. Elliot (Ed.), *Handbook of approach and avoidance motivation* (pp. 431–446). New York: Psychology Press.

Blascovich, J., & Mendes, W. B. (2010). Social psychophysiology and embodiment. In S. T. Fiske, D. T. Gilbert, & G. Lindzey (Eds.), *The handbook of social psychology* (5th ed., pp. 194–227). New York: Wiley.

Blascovich, J., & Tomaka, J. (1996). The biopsychosocial model of arousal regulation. *Advances in Experimental Social Psychology, 28*, 1–51.

Blascovich, J., Mendes, W. B., Hunter, S. B., & Salomon, K. (1999). Social "facilitation" as challenge and threat. *Journal of Personality and Social Psychology, 77*(1), 68–77.

Blitz, P. S., Hoogstraten, J., & Mulder, G. (1970). Mental load, heart rate and heart rate variability. *Psychologische Forschung, 33*, 277–288.

Bond, C. F., & Titus, L. J. (1983). Social facilitation: A meta-analysis of 241 studies. *Psychological Bulletin, 94*(2), 265.

Bongard, S. (1995). Mental effort during active and passive coping: A dual task analysis. *Psychophysiology, 32*, 242–248.

Bradshaw, J. L. (1968). Pupil size and problem solving. *The Quarterly Journal of Experimental Psychology, 20*(2), 116–122.

Brehm, J. W., & Self, E. A. (1989). The intensity of motivation. *Annual Review of Psychology, 40*(1), 109–131.

Brickenkamp, R. (1981). *Test d2. Aufmerksamkeits-Belastungs-Test*. Göttingen: Verlag für Psychologie J. Hogrefe.

Brom, C., Buchtová, M., Šisler, V., Děchtěrenko, F., Palme, R., & Glenk, L. M. (2014). Flow, social interaction anxiety and salivary cortisol responses in serious games: A quasi-experimental study. *Computers & Education, 79*, 69–100.

Cottrell, N. B., Wack, D. L., Sekevak, G. J., & Rittle, R. H. (1968). Social facilitation of dominant responses by the presence of an audience and the mere presence of others. *Journal of Personality and Social Psychology, 9*, 245–250.

Csikszentmihalyi, M. (1975). *Beyond boredom and anxiety* (The Jossey-Bass behavioral science series 1st ed.). San Francisco: Jossey-Bass Publishers.

Csikszentmihalyi, M., & Larson, R. (1987). Validity and reliability of the experience-sampling method. *The Journal of Nervous and Mental Disease, 175*(9), 526–536.

Csikszentmihalyi, M. (1990). *Flow: The psychology of optimal experience*. New York: Harper & Row.

Dawson, M. E., Schell, A. M., Hazlett, E. A., Nuechterlein, K. H., & Filion, D. L. (2000). On the clinical and cognitive meaning of impaired sensorimotor gating in schizophrenia. *Psychiatry Research, 96*(3), 187–197.

de Manzano, Ö., Theorell, T., Harmat, L., & Ullén, F. (2010). The psychophysiology of flow during piano playing. *Emotion, 10*(3), 301–311.

del Paso, G. A. R., Langewitz, W., Robles, H., & Pérez, N. (1996). A between-subjects comparison of respiratory sinus arrhythmia and baroreceptor cardiac reflex sensitivity as non-invasive measures of tonic parasympathetic cardiac control. *International Journal of Psychophysiology, 22*(3), 163–171.

Di Bernadi, L. C., Takase, E., & Darby, D. (2009). Heart rate variability and cognitive function: Effects of physical effort. *Biological Psychology, 82*, 186–191.

Dickerson, S. S., & Kemeny, M. E. (2004). Acute stressors and cortisol responses: A theoretical integration and synthesis of laboratory research. *Psychological Bulletin, 130*(3), 355.

Dienstbier, R. A. (1989). Arousal and physiological toughness: Implications for mental and physical health. *Psychological Review, 96*(1), 84.

Engeser, S., & Rheinberg, F. (2008). Flow, performance and moderators of challenge-skill balance. *Motivation and Emotion, 32*(3), 158–172. doi:10.1007/s11031-008-9102-.

Eysenck, M. W. (1979). Anxiety, learning, and memory: A reconceptualization. *Journal of Research in Personality, 13*(4), 363–385.

Fairclough, S. H., & Houston, K. (2004). A metabolic measure of mental effort. *Biological Psychology, 66*(2), 177–190.

Frankenhaeuser, M., & Lundberg, U. (1985). Sympathetic-adrenal and pituitary-adrenal response to challenge. In *Biological psychiatry, higher nervous activity* (pp. 699–704). New York: Springer US.

Gaillard, A. W. K., & Kramer, A. F. (2001). Theoretical and methodological issues in psychophysiological research. In R. W. Backs & W. Boucsein (Eds.), *Engineering psychophysiology* (pp. 31–58). Mahwah: Erlbaum.

Gailliot, M. T., Baumeister, R. F., DeWall, C. N., Maner, J. K., Plant, E. A., Tice, D. M., ... & Schmeichel, B. J. (2007). Self-control relies on glucose as a limited energy source: Willpower is more than a metaphor. *Journal of Personality and Social Psychology, 92*(2), 325–336.

Gendolla, G. H., & Krüsken, J. (2001). The joint impact of mood state and task difficulty on cardiovascular and electrodermal reactivity in active coping. *Psychophysiology, 38*(03), 548–556.

Gendolla, G. H., & Richter, M. (2005). Ego involvement and effort: Cardiovascular, electrodermal, and performance effects. *Psychophysiology, 42*(5), 595–603.

Guyton, A. C. (1980). *Arterial pressure and hypertension*. Philadelphia: Saunders WB Co.

Harmat, L., de Manzano, Ö., Theorell, T., Högman, L., Fischer, H., & Ullén, F. (2015). Physiological correlates of the flow experience during computer game playing. *International Journal of Psychophysiology, 97*(1), 1–7.

Henry, J. P. (1993). Biological basis of the stress response. *Physiology, 8*(2), 69–73.

Hess, K. H., & Polt, J. M. (1964). Pupil size in relation to mental activity during simple problem-solving. *Science, 143*, 1190–1192.

Hjortskov, N., Rissen, D., Blangsted, A. K., Fallentin, N., Lundberg, U., & Sogaard, K. (2004). The effect of mental stress on heart rate variability and blood pressure during computer work. *European Journal of Applied Physiology, 92*, 84–89.

Hockey, G. R. J. (1993). Cognitive-energetical control mechanisms in the management of work demands and psychological health. In A. D. Baddeley & L. Weiskrantz (Eds.), *Attention, selection, awareness and control: A tribute to Donald Broadbent* (pp. 328–345). Oxford: Oxford University Press.

Hockey, G. R. J. (1997). Compensatory control in the regulation of human performance under stress and high workload: A cognitive-energetical framework. *Biological Psychology, 45*, 73–93.

Jorna, P. G. A. M. (1992). Spectral analysis of heart rate and psychological state: A review of its validity as a workload index. *Biological Psychology, 34*(2), 237–257.

Kahneman, D. (1973). *Attention and effort*. Englewood Cliffs: Prentice-Hall.

Kahneman, D., & Beatty, J. (1966). Pupil diameter and load on memory. *Science, 154*(3756), 1583–1585.

Kahneman, D., & Beatty, J. (1967). Pupillary responses in a pitch-discrimination task. *Perception & Psychophysics, 2*(3), 101–105.

Kalsbeek, J. W. H., & Ettema, J. H. (1964). Physiological and psychological evaluation of distraction stress. In: *Proceedings of 2nd International Congress On Ergonomics* (pp. 443–447). London: Taylor and Francis.

Keller, J., & Bless, H. (2008). Flow and regulatory compatibility: An experimental approach to the flow model of intrinsic motivation. *Personality & Social Psychology Bulletin, 34*(2), 196–209.

Keller, J., Bless, H., Blomann, F., & Kleinböhl, D. (2011a). Physiological aspects of flow experiences: Skills-demand-compatibility effects on heart rate variability and salivary cortisol. *Journal of Experimental Social Psychology, 47*(4), 849–852.

Keller, J., Ringelhan, S., & Blomann, F. (2011b). Does skills–demands compatibility result in intrinsic motivation? Experimental test of a basic notion proposed in the theory of flow-experiences. *The Journal of Positive Psychology, 6*(5), 408–417.

Kirschbaum, C., Pirke, K.-M., & Hellhammer, D. H. (1993). The "Trier Social Stress Test" – A tool for investigating psychobiological stress responses in a laboratory setting. *Neuropsychobiology, 28*(1–2), 76–81.

Kivikangas, J. M. (2006). Psychophysiology of flow experience: An explorative study. Faculty of behavioural sciences, department of psychology. Master's thesis. Retrieved from http://ethesis.helsinki.fi/julkaisut/kay/psyko/pg/kivikangas

Lazarus, R. S., & Folkman, S. (1984). *Stress, appraisal, and coping*. New York: Springer.

Light, K. C. (1981). Cardiovascular responses to effortful active coping: Implications for the role of stress in hypertension development. *Psychophysiology, 18*, 216–225.

Light, K. C., & Obrist, P. A. (1983). Task difficulty, heart rate reactivity, and cardiovascular responses to an appetitive reaction time task. *Psychophysiology, 20*(3), 301–312.

Lovallo, W. R., Wilson, M. F., Pincomb, G. A., Edwards, G. L., Tompkins, P., & Brackett, D. J. (1985). Activation patterns to aversive stimulation in man: Passive exposure versus effort to control. *Psychophysiology, 22*, 283–291.

Manning, C. A., Hall, J. L., & Gold, P. E. (1990). Glucose effects on memory and other neuropsychological tests in elderly humans. *Psychological Science, 1*(5), 307–311.

Moller, A. C., Csikszentmihalyi, M., Nakamura, J., & Deci, E. I. (2007, February). *Developing an experimental induction of flow*. Poster presented at the Society for Personality and Social Psychology Conference, Memphis, TN.

Mukherjee, S., Yadav, R., Yung, I., Zajdel, D. P., & Oken, B. S. (2011). Sensitivity to mental effort and test–retest reliability of heart rate variability measures in healthy seniors. *Clinical Neurophysiology, 122*(10), 2059–2066.

Mulder, G., & Mulder, L. J. M. (1981). Information processing and cardiovascular control. *Psychophysiology, 18*(4), 392–402.

Nacke, L. E., & Lindley, C. A. (2009). Affective ludology, flow and immersion in a first-person shooter: Measurement of player experience. *Loading..., 3*(5), 1–21. doi:10.1016/j.neulet.2008.02.00.

Obrist, P. A. (1976). The cardiovascular-behavioral interaction—As it appears today. *Psychophysiology, 13*(2), 95–107.

Obrist, P. A. (1981). *Cardiovascular psychophysiology: A perspective*. New York: Plenum Press.

Payne, D. T., Parry, M. K., & Harasymin, S. J. (1968). Percentage of papillary dilation as a measure of item difficulty. *Perception and Psychophysics, 4*, 139–143.

Peifer, C. (2012). Psychophysiological correlates of flow-experience. In S. Engeser (Ed.), *Advances in flow research* (pp. 139–165). New York: Springer.

Peifer, C., Schulz, A., Schächinger, H., Baumann, N., & Antoni, C. H. (2014). The relation of flow-experience and physiological arousal under stress – Can u shape it? *Journal of Experimental Social Psychology, 53*, 62–69.

Peifer, C., Schächinger, H., Engeser, S., & Antoni, C. H. (2015). Cortisol effects on flow-experience. *Psychopharmacology, 232*(6), 1165–1173.

Peters, M. L., Godaert, G. L., Ballieux, R. E., van Vliet, M., Willemsen, J. J., Sweep, F. C., & Heijnen, C. J. (1998). Cardiovascular and endocrine responses to experimental stress: Effects of mental effort and controllability. *Psychoneuroendocrinology, 23*(1), 1–17.

Redondo, M., & Del Valle-Inclán, F. (1992). Decrements in heart rate variability during memory search. *International Journal of Psychophysiology, 13*, 29–35.

Rheinberg, F. (2010). Intrinsische Motivation und Flow-Erleben [Intrinsic motivation and flow experience]. In J. Heckhausen & H. Heckhausen (Eds.), *Motivation und Handeln* [Motivation and action] (4th ed., pp. 365–388). Berlin: Springer.

Rheinberg, F., & Vollmeyer, R. (2003). Flow-Erleben in einem Computerspiel unter experimentell variierten Bedingungen [Flow-experience in a computer game under experimentally controlled conditions]. *Zeitschrift für Psychologie, 211*, 161–170.

Richter, M., & Gendolla, G. H. (2009). The heart contracts to reward: Monetary incentives and preejection period. *Psychophysiology, 46*(3), 451–457.

Richter, M., Friedrich, A., & Gendolla, G. H. (2008). Task difficulty effects on cardiac activity. *Psychophysiology, 45*(5), 869–875.

Schächinger, H., Weinbacher, M., Kiss, A., Ritz, R., & Langewitz, W. (2001). Cardiovascular indices of peripheral and central sympathetic activation. *Psychosomatic Medicine, 63*, 788–796.

Scholey, A. B., Laing, S., & Kennedy, D. O. (2006). Blood glucose changes and memory: Effects of manipulating emotionality and mental effort. *Biological Psychology, 71*(1), 12–19.

Schwabe, L., Haddad, L., & Schachinger, H. (2008). HPA axis activation by a socially evaluated cold-pressor test. *Psychoneuroendocrinology, 33*(6), 890–895.

Schwerdtfeger, A. (2004). Predicting autonomic reactivity to public speaking: Don't get fixed on self-report data! *International Journal of Psychophysiology, 52*(3), 217–224.

Seery, M. D. (2011). Challenge or threat? Cardiovascular indexes of resilience and vulnerability to potential stress in humans. *Neuroscience & Biobehavioral Reviews, 35*(7), 1603–1610.

Seta, C. E., & Seta, J. J. (1992). Increments and decrements in mean arterial pressure as a function of audience composition: An averaging and summation analysis. *Personality and Social Psychology Bulletin, 18*(2), 173–181.

Sherwood, A., Dolan, C. A., & Light, K. C. (1990). Hemodynamics of blood pressure responses during active and passive coping. *Psychophysiology, 27*, 656–668.

Smith, T. W., Baldwin, M., & Christensen, A. J. (1990). Interpersonal influence as active coping: Effects of task difficulty on cardiovascular reactivity. *Psychophysiology, 27*, 429–437.

Storey, P. L., Wright, R. A., & Williams, B. J. (1996). Need as a moderator of the difficulty-cardiovascular response relation: The case of fluid deprivation. *Journal of Psychophysiology, 10*, 228–238.

Task Force of the European Society of Cardiology the North American Society of Pacing Electrophysiology. (1996). Heart rate variability. Standards of measurement, physiological interpretation, and clinical use. *European Heart Journal, 17*(3), 354–381.

Taylor, L. A., & Rachman, S. J. (1988). The effects of blood sugar level changes on cognitive function, affective state, and somatic symptoms. *Journal of Behavioral Medicine, 11*(3), 279–291.

Thayer, J. F., Hansen, A. L., Saus-Rose, E., & Johnsen, B. H. (2009). Heart rate variability, prefrontal neural function, and cognitive performance: The neurovisceral integration perspective on self-regulation, adaptation, and health. *Annals of Behavioral Medicine, 37*, 141–153.

Tomaka, J., Blascovich, J., Kelsey, R. M., & Leitten, C. L. (1993). Subjective, physiological, and behavioral effects of threat and challenge appraisal. *Journal of Personality and Social Psychology, 65*(2), 248.

Tomaka, J., Blascovich, J., Kibler, J., & Ernst, J. M. (1997). Cognitive and physiological antecedents of threat and challenge appraisal. *Journal of Personality and Social Psychology, 73*(1), 63.

Tozman, T., Burns, B., & Vollmeyer, R. (2014). *The biology of flow during chess and poker play*. Talk, 02.07.2014, 7th European Conference on Positive Psychology, Amsterdam.

Tozman, T., Magdas, E.S., MacDougall, H.G., Vollmeyer, R. (2015). Understanding the psychophysiology of flow: A driving simulator experiment to investigate the relationship between flow and heart rate variability. *Computers in Human Behavior, 52*, 408–418.

Tozman, T., Zhang, Y. Y., & Vollmeyer, R. (2016). Inverted U-shaped function between flow and cortisol release during chess play. *Journal of Happiness Studies* 1–22.

Triplett, N. (1898). The dynamogenic factors in pacemaking and competition. *American Journal of Psychology, 9*, 507–533.

Ulrich, M., Keller, J., Hoenig, K., Waller, C., & Grön, G. (2014). Neural correlates of experimentally induced flow experiences. *NeuroImage, 86*, 194–202. doi:10.1016/j.neuroimage.2013.08.01.

Veltman, J. A., & Gaillard, A. W. K. (1993). Indices of mental workload in a complex task environment. *Neuropsychobiology, 28*(1–2), 72–75.

Wright, R. A. (1996). Brehms theory of motivation as a model of effort and cardiovascular response. In P. M. Gollwitzer & J. A. Bargh (Eds.), *The psychology of action: Linking cognition and motivation to behavior* (pp. 424–453). New York: Guilford.

Wright, R. A., & Lockard, S. (2006). Sex, outcome expectancy, and cardiovascular response to a masculine challenge. *Psychophysiology, 43*(2), 190–196.

Yasumasu, T., del Paso, G. A. R., Takahara, K., & Nakashima, Y. (2006). Reduced baroreflex cardiac sensitivity predicts increased cognitive performance. *Psychophysiology, 43*(1), 41–45.

Zajonc, R. B. (1968). Attitudinal effects of mere exposure. *Journal of Personality and Social Psychology, 9*(2p2), 1–27.

Chapter 21
The Flow Experience Revisited: The Influence of Skills-Demands-Compatibility on Experiential and Physiological Indicators

Johannes Keller

Abstract The experience of flow is typically described as an "optimal experience". In the literature discussing the flow experience, one frequently finds the advice to maximize time in flow to enhance life-satisfaction and well-being. However, this advice seems premature because consequences of flow experiences have not been systematically assessed yet. In order to address this gap, we investigated the influence of skills-demands-compatibility (the central precondition of flow experiences) on several experiential and physiological processes in a series of experiments. The experience of (non-)flow was manipulated based on different modes of computerized tasks. Participants worked on the tasks either in one of two non-adaptive conditions ("boredom" or "overload"), or in an adaptive condition, in which the difficulty level is constantly adapted to participants' individual performance level. The results of our studies provide evidence documenting the specific nature of the state of flow – specifically regarding experiential and physiological processes.

21.1 Introduction

The experience of flow, as reflected in the deep involvement in a (skill-related) activity is typically defined with reference to three antecedents (clear goals, unambiguous and immediate feedback, skills-demands-compatibility) and five elements: (1) a modified *perception of time* (hours seem to pass like seconds; time flies), (2) a deep concentration on the activity associated with a *reduced level of reflexive self-consciousness*, (3) a strong *feeling of control*, (4) a deep *involvement* in and *enjoyment* of the activity, and (5) a high level of *intrinsic motivation* (*the exact number of elements mentioned in the definition of the state of flow can vary reflecting the fact that some authors seem to prefer a more fine-grained distinction of components whereas others seem to prefer a more reductionist perspective*). Based on these defining characteristics, the experience of flow is frequently described as an

J. Keller (✉)
Department of Psychology & Education, Ulm University, Ulm, Germany
e-mail: johannes.keller@uni-ulm.de

L. Harmat et al. (eds.), *Flow Experience*, DOI 10.1007/978-3-319-28634-1_21

"optimal experience" (Csikszentmihalyi 1990). Accordingly, in the literature discussing the flow experience, one frequently finds the advice to maximize time in flow to enhance life-satisfaction and well-being (e.g. Lyubomirsky 2008). However, this advice (to maximize time in flow) seems premature because the consequences of flow experiences have not been *systematically* assessed yet. Specifically, little is known regarding the *causal* role that the experience of flow may (or may not) have on (subjective) well-being and (mental) health. This chapter provides a condensed summary of findings obtained in our research on the state of flow based on *experimental* paradigms (involving a manipulation of the crucial boundary condition for flow to emerge – skills-demands-compatibility) regarding experiential and physiological consequences. Some of the obtained findings indicate that the proposed beneficial impact of flow experiences on (subjective) well-being and (mental) health is not as straightforward as one may expect. For instance, we did not find effects of experimental skills-demands variations on mood (as an indirect indicator of subjective well-being). Also, endocrinological results (based on salivary cortisol and its precursor ACTH [adrenocorticotropic hormone]) as well as cardiovascular patterns suggest that flow may involve an experience of straining tension. That is, our findings suggest that flow experiences can be associated with physiological stress responses. The main goal of this line of research is to contribute to our understanding of the specific nature of the state of flow. As will be discussed in the concluding section, it seems that the theoretical model as well as the conceptualization and measurement of flow experience may profit from reexamination.

21.2 Methods

In most of the empirical work summarized in a condensed form below, the studies designed to analyze the specific nature of the state of flow were *experimental* in character. That is, we tested the influence of skills-demands-compatibility (the central precondition of flow experiences) on several experiential and physiological processes. The experience of (non-)flow was manipulated based on different modes of computerized tasks. Participants worked on the tasks either in one of two non-adaptive conditions ("boredom" or "overload"), or in an adaptive condition, in which the difficulty level was constantly adapted to participants' individual performance level. In this Methods section, the experimental paradigms that we used as well as the assessment of experiential and physiological outcome variables will be described in some detail.

21.2.1 Experimental Flow Paradigms

As briefly mentioned above, participants in our experimental studies worked on tasks either in one of two non-adaptive conditions ("boredom" or "overload"), or in an adaptive condition, in which the difficulty level was constantly adapted to participants' individual performance level. That is, our experimental manipulation is essentially based on a variation of the difficulty level of the respective task such that the difficulty is either experienced as too low (boredom condition), too high (overload condition) or as largely compatible with the individual's skill level (adaptive condition). We realized this general logic in several paradigms using different types of tasks. It should be noted that the types of tasks selected for the development of the paradigms described below were intentionally restricted to tasks that do not require bodily movements (other than minor hand movements in order to move the mouse or to type in numbers on the keyboard), which may affect (or bias) psychophysiological processes.

21.2.1.1 Tetris Paradigm

In the Tetris computer game (see Fig. 21.1) the aim is to arrange "falling" objects so that they constitute completely filled lines at the bottom of the playing field. The objects move downwards from the top of the screen and can be moved to the right or left and rotated in 90° steps with assigned keys on the keyboard. The game is programmed in three specific playing modes. In the "*boredom*" *condition* the objects keep falling at a very slow rate, regardless of the player's performance, and the player has no tool available to accelerate the speed of the objects. Accordingly, it

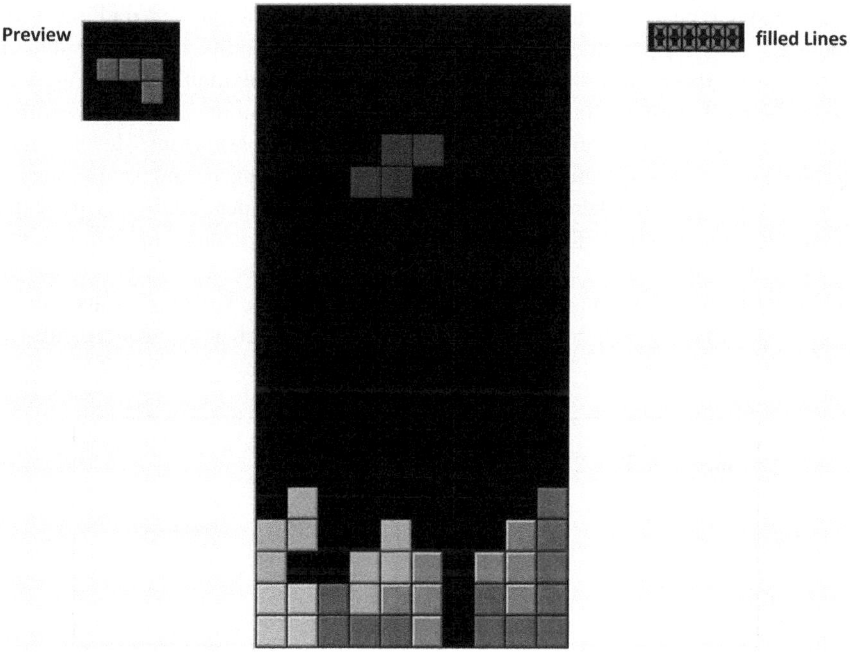

Fig. 21.1 Screen shot of the Tetris game paradigm

can be expected that persons experience a state of boredom in this playing mode condition. In the "*adaptive*" (*flow*)-*condition* the speed with which the objects keep falling is adapted to the player's performance. If the player successfully fills a predetermined number of lines (e.g., five lines or more) using a maximal number of 30 consecutive objects, the speed is automatically increased by one step. If the player accomplishes only a lower number of lines (e.g., three lines or less) using a maximal number of 30 consecutive objects, the speed is decreased by one step. Thus, the speed is adapted to the player's performance to keep the player working on the task under conditions of skills-demands-compatibility. One may reasonably anticipate that persons in this playing mode differ significantly from the other conditions regarding the intensity and quality of their experiences while playing the game. In the "*overload*" -*condition* objects initially start falling pretty fast and the speed is increased to an even higher level if the person manages to fill five lines (so that it is extremely difficult to successfully fill complete lines). Note that in this paradigm, *speed* of object movements (and accordingly the available time to react) determines difficulty level. This paradigm builds on a prototypical (old school) computer game where eye-hand-coordination and visual-spatial ability are relevant skills.

21.2.1.2 Mental Arithmetic Paradigm

In order to test the generalizability of effects based on manipulating skills-demands-compatibility, we designed additional paradigms with features substantially deviating from the typical computer game Tetris. One of these alternative paradigms is the mental arithmetic paradigm (see Fig. 21.2) where the ability to solve arithmetic problems (in this case summation of a series of single- and double-digit figures; we typically work with a maximum response time of 18 s). In the *adaptive condition*, task demands adapt automatically and continuously to participants' level of skill (which can also be estimated beforehand in a preparation phase and used as starting level for the period where participants are working under conditions of skills-demands-compatibility). The algorithm for this paradigm is designed in a way that after each set of two completed calculations the results entered by the participant are analyzed with respect to accuracy. When two out of these last two results are correct, task difficulty will be increased by one level, which is achieved using two

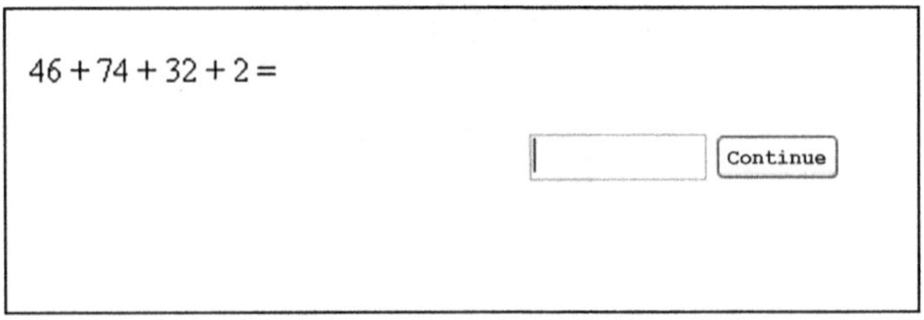

Fig. 21.2 Screen shot of the mental arithmetic paradigm (response entered via keyboard)

distinct mechanisms. In case the last summand had only one digit, the level increased by changing the last summand to a two-digit number in the upcoming calculations (e.g., Level 5: 23 + 45 + 59 + 3 changes to Level 6: 73 + 46 + 54 + 17). For a further up-level change, an additional one-digit number was added to the mathematical expression (e.g., Level 6: 89 + 38 + 65 + 15 changes to Level 7: 26 + 24 + 33 + 60 + 8). Both mechanisms are applied alternately. Analogously, when two out of the last two results are incorrect, task difficulty is decreased by one level, and this is achieved by the two mechanisms outlined above but in this case by way of deletion of a summand (or deletion of a digit). Otherwise, task demands remained unchanged.

In the *overload condition*, the starting level of task difficulty is typically set three levels higher than the starting level of the adaptive condition. A level-up adjustment occurs when at least three out of the last five results entered by the participant are correct. Task demands decreased when at least four out of five results are wrong. This algorithm is applied to make sure that task demands are always higher than participants' level of skill, thus providing participants with very ambitious problems but also minimizing the probability to permanently frustrate participants resulting in resignation. In the *boredom condition*, only two numbers have to be summed, with the first summand randomly drawn from the interval 100–109, and the second summand from the interval 1–9. Also, the result of summation was confined to numbers between 101 and 110, so that participants did not have to break up the second summand to obtain the result. As a consequence, task demands are constantly low.

Note that in this paradigm, number of figures (and digits) involved in the math problem in combination with the available time to solve the problem (18 s) determines difficulty level.

21.2.1.3 Knowledge Quiz Paradigm

In this paradigm, participants engage in a computerized knowledge task and have to answer questions in a multiple-choice format (Fig. 21.3). The questions are selected from the German version of a game based on the TV show "Who wants to be a millionaire?" (Jumbo Spiele® 2000). Each question is presented with four response

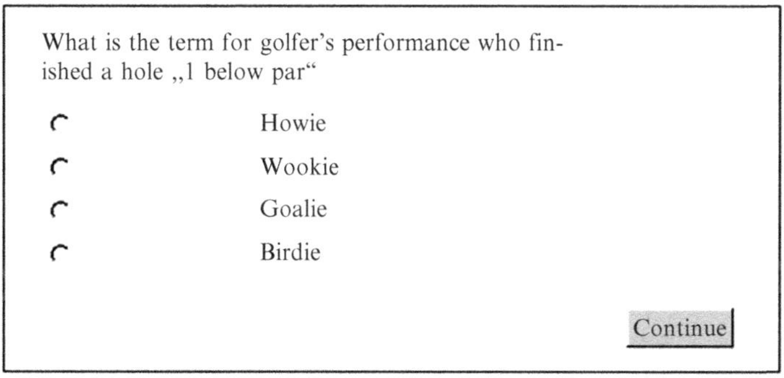

Fig. 21.3 Screen shot of the knowledge quiz paradigm

options and participants have to select one response within a limited time period (we typically work with a 15 s maximum response time; in the boredom condition the response can be submitted only after 20 s have passed so that the player has no option to increase the speed of the setting by submitting answers in a rapid fashion). We made use of the fact that the game comes with a large set of knowledge questions assigned to distinct categories reflecting levels of difficulty.

In the *boredom condition*, the difficulty level is rather low (i.e., questions from the categories where players can earn only little money in case of a correct answer in the "Who wants to be a millionaire" game) and participants have no option to increase it. In the *adaptive condition*, the difficulty level is constantly adapted to each participant's performance level. If the participant successfully answers a certain number of questions (we typically use the criterion three out of four consecutive questions correctly solved), the difficulty level is automatically increased by one step. If the participant fails a certain number of times (we typically use the criterion three out of four consecutive questions not solved), the difficulty level is decreased by one step. Thus, the difficulty level is constantly adjusted to realize a skills-demands-compatibility. In the *overload condition*, the task starts at the highest difficulty level and is decreased by one step if the participant fails a certain number of times (we typically use the criterion two out of two consecutive questions not solved). The lowest possible level is fixed (maximum decrease is six levels) so that questions are drawn from a category of questions with a relatively high level of difficulty even after a long run of wrong answers.

In this paradigm, the required *expertise* in the relevant domain in order to answer correctly determines the difficulty level. That is, questions from categories where players can earn only little money in case of a correct answer require almost no (special) expertise whereas questions from categories where players can earn a substantial amount of money in case of a correct question require expert knowledge. Given that the response has to be submitted within 15 s, this task has also a speed component (in the adaptive and overload conditions).

21.2.1.4 Chess Paradigm

This paradigm was developed with the idea in mind that analyzing effects of *extended episodes* involving flow experience (lasting for hours and not just a few minutes) should be feasible (Fig. 21.4). This requires (a) a paradigm that allows for a substantial number of trials with varying levels of difficulty (which is hardly possible when working with a knowledge question paradigm where one would need to have hundreds of pre-tested questions available) and (b) a paradigm that confronts participants with a task they are willing (and able) to engage in for an extended period of time (mental arithmetic is certainly not a good option in this respect). We opted for a chess paradigm (based on the open-source chess engine "Stockfish") because it is widely known that chess players are frequently engaging in chess

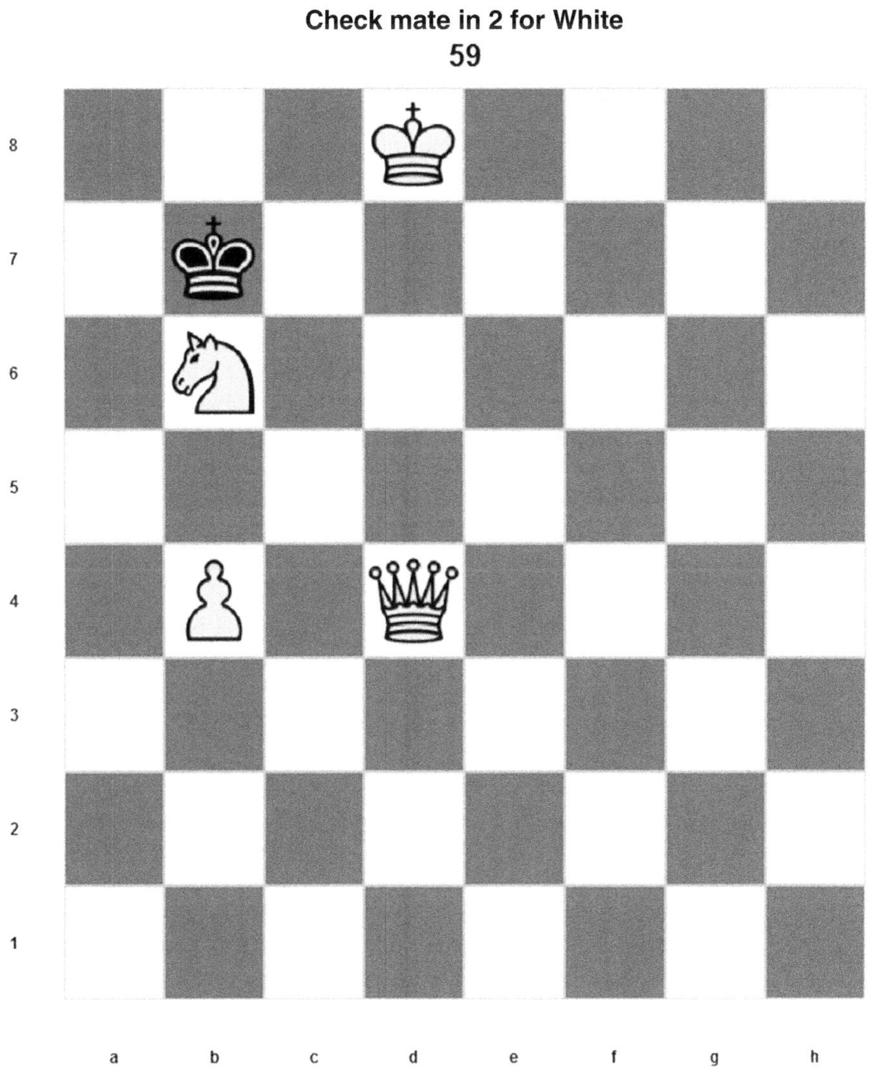

Fig. 21.4 Screen shot of the chess paradigm (checkmate-in-two)

matches or chess problem solving lasting for several hours. Also, it is possible to create an almost infinite set of problems in the domain of chess (we opted for checkmate-in-two problems), which can be modified in difficulty level by way of varying the time granted to solve the respective problem.

In the *boredom condition* of the chess paradigm, the difficulty level is rather low, that is, the time granted to solve the checkmate-in-two problem is substantial (based on pre-tests we consider a time-to-solve period of 6 min appropriate) and participants have no option to proceed to the next problem before the time assigned for each trial elapsed (one may also select specific problems with a reliably lower level of difficulty for the boredom condition, e.g. problems with compulsion to move for the king [zugzwang]). In the *adaptive condition*, the difficulty level is constantly adapted to each participant's performance level. If the participant successfully solved a certain number of chess problems (so far, we worked with a criterion of two [or more] out of four consecutive problems solved correctly), the time granted to solve the problem is automatically decreased by one step (we typically work with a reduction of 11 s). If the participant fails a certain number of times (we use a criterion of two [or less] out of four consecutive problems not solved), the time granted to solve the problem is automatically increased by one step (we typically work with an expansion of 22 s). In the *overload condition*, the time granted to solve the problem is restricted to 120 s (and checkmate-in-three problems – which are substantially more challenging – may also be used to ensure overload even for outstanding chess players). In this paradigm, the *time available* to solve the chess problem essentially determines the difficulty level of the task.

Concluding this section on the experimental paradigms, it is important to note that the specific operationalization used to vary the difficulty level of the task has implications regarding the resulting quality of experience during task engagement. Specifically, difficulty is operationalized based on the time available to solve the task (i.e., to submit a response). Accordingly, it is obvious that participants' perception of time will be particularly affected (in the sense of time passing quickly) when they are working on a task under conditions where they experience a certain level of time pressure (which is the case in the adaptive and also in the overload conditions). Also, given that in these paradigms overload is realized by relatively short time periods available to edit a response, it stands to reason that overload will result in participants responding with low estimates on measures of the subjective experience of time spent on the task (similar to participants working under adaptive conditions). It is also a sensitive issue how exactly the overload condition is operationalized. Specifically, the question has to be considered whether participants have the option to *selectively* work on some questions (in the knowledge quiz paradigm) or problems (in the Chess and mental arithmetic paradigm) while skipping many others after only a brief consideration of the question or problem (in our paradigms this is skipping option is *not* available). Furthermore, it is crucial to take into consideration that participants may just "give up" and actually not engage in the task any more after some experiences of failure. It is evident that such an overload experience reflecting resignation is fundamentally different from overload reflecting a continued struggle. In our paradigms we included measures to ensure an overload experience reflected a continued struggle (i.e., in the math, chess and knowledge quiz paradigms the algorithm is designed in a way that the difficulty level decreases down – to a still relatively ambitious level – after a certain number of consecutive failures).

21.2.2 Assessment of Experiential Processes

In line with the conceptualization of flow as a specific combination of experiential states, we included self-report measures addressing five basic elements that are mentioned in virtually every (scientific) paper addressing the conceptualization of flow. These five elements are (1) a modified *perception of time* (hours seem to pass like seconds; time flies), (2) a deep concentration on the activity associated with a *reduced level of reflexive self-consciousness*, (3) a strong *feeling of control*, (4) a deep *involvement* in and *enjoyment* of the activity, and (5) a high level of *intrinsic motivation*. In addition to these core features of the flow experience, we typically assess the degree to which participants experienced what is considered the crucial precondition for flow to emerge: a fit of skills and task demands. This is basically a manipulation check regarding the effectiveness of the experimental manipulation of skills-demands-compatibility.

Fit of Skills and Task Demands In most of our studies perceived fit of skills and task demands is assessed by asking participants to respond to the item "To what degree did the demands of the game (task) match your ability?" on a scale ranging from (1) "not at all" to (7) "completely."

Perception of Time To assess participants' perception of time we typically ask participants to indicate on a horizontal line (10 cm in length) with end-points labelled "very short" and "very long" their subjective estimate of the length of time they spent on the game or task. Given that previous work based on the experience sampling method revealed that higher intrinsic motivation is associated with a subjective experience of time passing more quickly (Conti 2001), time perception seems to be a valid indicator of one distinct component of the experience of intrinsic motivation.

Level of Self-Consciousness According to flow theory, a deep concentration on the activity is characteristic of flow experiences and is associated with a reduced level of reflexive self-consciousness (Csikszentmihalyi 1975). In our studies, we typically assess the degree to which participants experience a reduction in self-consciousness with a scale including items such as "During engagement in the game (task) all thoughts regarding personal issues that are currently bothering me were essentially extinguished." and "During engagement in the game (task) I have been reflecting on me and my behavior" (reverse coded).

Feeling of Control Flow theorists argue that a sense of control reflects one crucial element of the flow experience (Csikszentmihalyi 1975). However, sense of control can reflect different things (e.g., sense of *control over outcomes* versus sense of control over how the activity is proceeding [reflecting *procedural control*]). In our studies, we typically focus on the former component of control using a scale designed to assess the perceived control over outcomes (sample items read "I had the necessary skill to play the game successfully;" "I knew exactly what I had to do." and "I think I performed well in the game."). Note that this measure of perceived control over outcomes can be fruitfully used to document that the three experimental conditions (boredom, adaptive, overload) represent three *distinct* experiential states (as indicated by high, middle, and low scores on the measure of perceived control).

Involvement and Enjoyment Experiencing task engagement as rewarding in and of itself is the most crucial and characteristic feature of intrinsic motivation (Rheinberg 2008). We typically assess this experience with a scale designed to assess involvement in and enjoyment of the activity (sample items read "I was strongly involved in what was happening in the game;" "I was not involved" [reversed]; "I was thrilled;" "I'd love to play the game again;" and "I would consider buying the game for private use.") It is noteworthy that the measure of involvement and enjoyment contains items that assess the desire to engage in the activity again in the future, which reflects the willingness to engage in the activity in a free choice setting. Accordingly, we think that the scale also covers the fifth element of flow experience (*intrinsic motivation*) since willingness to engage in the relevant activity in a free choice time period is often seen as a crucial indicator of intrinsic motivation. We acknowledge the fact that applying an actual free choice measure would be a more stringent assessment of intrinsic motivation (and actually we did make use of such a measure in one study, cf. Keller et al. 2011b). Nonetheless, it seems fair to conclude that the self-report involvement and enjoyment scale at least partially captures this component of intrinsic motivation.

Mood Given that the flow experience is frequently related to positive affect and therefore interpreted as a state that is likely to foster subjective well-being, we assessed participants' mood state after task engagement in some of our experimental studies (e.g. Keller et al. 2011a, b). The mood index that we used contains four items where participants indicated how they currently feel on 9-point scales with endpoints labelled *very bad – very good, unhappy – happy, sad – cheerful, depressed – serene*.

21.2.3 Assessment of Physiological Processes

In addition to the assessment of experiential aspects based on self-report, we are applying a psychophysiological perspective in our research on the flow experience. This is based on the notion that a psychophysiological approach is meaningful for various reasons. First, a truly *comprehensive* analysis of a psychological phenomenon requires the consideration of physiological processes complementing the examination of cognitive, affective and behavioral mechanisms. Second, the assessment of physiological indicators provides researchers with options to identify the emergence and intensity of a certain state in the participant via *online measurement*, that is, right at the time when the person is undergoing a certain treatment or engaged in a critical activity. Third, it stands to reason that participants are not capable of accurately reporting processes and states because many processes and states are not (or not adequately) accessible via introspection (cf. Nisbett and Wilson 1977) and social desirability may also play a role resulting in biased self-reports. Finally, recent developments (also in research on the flow experience) in psychological research document the enormous potential to extend our understanding of psychological phenomena based on psychophysiological analyses. A prominent example is the psychological research on stress, but it is also true regarding other fields such as research on aggression, depression, trauma, or trust.

Considering the defining elements of the flow experience and the proposed trigger of flow (skills-demands-compatibility which can also be conceptualized as working at the limit of one's ability), specific physiological indicators seem particularly interesting to study. First, it seems worthwhile to assess *endocrinological parameters* that have been documented as being reliable indicators of the level of stress a person is experiencing (specifically, cortisol; cf. Kirschbaum and Hellhammer 1989, 2000). Of note, Mason (1968) reported that personal involvement is a potent stimulus known to activate the HPA axis. Given that flow experiences are associated with strong involvement it stands to reason that increased cortisol levels may be observed in individuals in a state of flow. Besides, it is well established that engagement in challenging tasks (such as public speaking, cf. Bassett et al. 1987; or airplane captains conducting multiple takeoffs and landings, cf. Kakimoto 1985) typically results in raised levels of cortisol. Accordingly, increased levels of cortisol may also emerge under the challenging conditions of a skills-demands-compatibility. We include the assessment of *salivary cortisol* in some of our studies in order to empirically address these considerations (in part of our studies we also assessed *adrenocorticotropic hormone* [ACTH] – a precursor of the cortisol response – based on blood samples).

Second, in view of the fact that it appears somewhat questionable whether individuals can accurately report on the degree to which they were self-conscious during a certain episode, it seems promising to build on previous work in the field of social neuroscience documenting distinct neural correlates of the state of reduced self-consciousness. For example, Goldberg et al. (2006) reported that *brain regions* which show a strong activation under introspection (left inferior frontal cortex) are inhibited under conditions of high task demands. Accordingly, one can expect that these brain regions are down-regulated in a state of flow reflecting reduced self-consciousness. We tested this notion in a recent *fMRI study* (Ulrich et al. 2014) applying a specific scanning technique (continuous arterial spin labeling). In our initial fMRI study, magnetic resonance imaging data were acquired on a 3.0 T Magnetom Allegra (Siemens AG, Erlangen, Germany) head-only MRI system using a single channel transmit-receive head coil. Perfusion imaging was performed using *continuous arterial spin labeling* (CASL, Wang et al. 2003; for details on the sequence used, see also Adolph et al. 2010; Groen et al. 2011).

Third, we recently started empirical work focusing on the *cardiovascular system*. The theoretical rationale underlying this work refers to a prominent model in social psychophysiology – the biopsychosocial model of challenge and threat (Blascovich and Tomaka 1996; Tomaka et al. 1993). The proponents of this model argue that distinct patterns of cardiovascular activity can be used to identify whether a person is in a state of challenge or threat. According to this account, two parameters are particularly important to detect challenge and threat on a cardiovascular level: Cardiac Output (CO, the amount of blood pumped by the heart per time unit) and Total Peripheral Resistance (TPR). Challenge is indicated by a relatively large increase (relative to baseline) of CO and a relatively large decrease of TPR. In contrast, threat is indicated by a (small) increase of CO accompanied by an increase of TPR. In our studies testing for cardiovascular correlates of the flow experience, we examine electrocardiographic signals (ECG), impedance-cardiographic signals (ICG) and blood pressure signals, which are continuously measured during task engagement. A Biopac MP150 system (Biopac Systems Inc., Goleta, CA) can be used to collect these signals. The technical settings we are working with are similar to those described in some detail by Does et al. (2012). We make use of a continuous non-invasive blood pressure monitoring system (CNAP™ Monitor 500), which is applied on the participant's left arm and hand (therefore only right-handed participants are examined). Moreover, Acknowledge software (BIOPAC Systems Inc., Goleta CA) serves not only to record data, but also to perform the scoring of the data.

It should be noted that the advantage of using CO and TPR as indicators based on the biopsychosocial model of challenge and threat in comparison to analyses focusing on heart rate (HR), heart rate variability (HRV) or blood pressure (BP) lies in the fact that these indicators can be associated with fairly specific states. Other indicators (such as HR, HRV, BP or galvanic skin response) are clearly less specific.

In order to provide an overview regarding the findings we obtained in our (primarily experimental) studies, exemplary findings will be presented and discussed in this section in a condensed form. The results mentioned and displayed in the paragraph on experiential processes represent the general pattern of findings that we observed in a series of studies applying the experimental paradigms described above. That is, although data obtained in single studies will be presented (which may appear selective), they can be considered as exemplary and essentially representative for our findings in other studies we conducted so far.

21.3 Results Regarding Experiential Processes

On the measure of *perceived fit of skills and task demands* the typical finding observed in our studies is displayed in Fig. 21.5 and shows an inverted U-shaped pattern. This reveals that the adaptive condition was indeed experienced as a situation of skills-demands compatibility (relative to boredom and overload conditions). Thus, the algorithm implemented in our experimental paradigms seems to be successful in manipulating the crucial boundary condition for flow to emerge.

As already mentioned in the description of our experimental paradigms, findings on the measure of *time perception* should be interpreted keeping in mind that overload is (at least partially) operationalized in our paradigms by way of limiting the time period participants have available to edit a response. Accordingly, relatively low estimates on the measure of time spent on the task can be expected not only

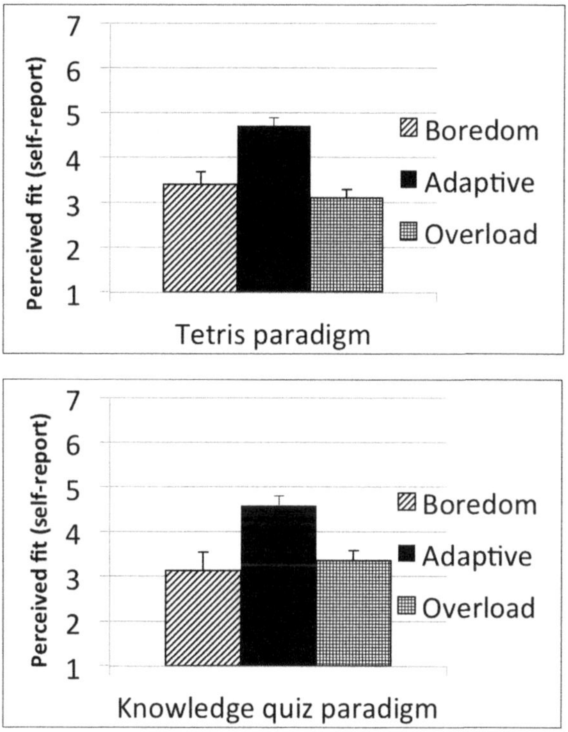

Fig. 21.5 Perceived fit of skills and task demands (self-reported scores)

under adaptive conditions but under overload conditions as well. As can be seen in Fig. 21.6, the time perception scores follow a U-shaped pattern in the Tetris paradigm, whereas relatively low time estimates emerged under adaptive and overload conditions in the knowledge quiz paradigm. This indicates that the perception of time as passing quickly is not a phenomenon that is exclusively linked to a state of flow, but can emerge under conditions of overload as well.

In some of our more recent studies using the mental arithmetic paradigm, we also included a self-report measure assessing the degree to which participants experienced a *loss of self-consciousness*. Figure 21.7 displays the pattern observed in one of these studies indicating that in line with flow theory participants reached significantly higher levels on this measure under adaptive conditions as compared to conditions of boredom and overload. Of note, in some studies we found that conditions of overload can also be associated with a relatively low level of self-consciousness. That is, similar to our findings on the measure of time perception, reduced self-consciousness (at least as assessed with a self-report instrument) is not a phenomenon that is exclusively linked to a state of flow, but can be observed under conditions of overload, too. Note that we also addressed this component of the flow experience (reduced self-consciousness) with a focus on neuronal processes (see below) – which provides further insights regarding this component of the flow experience and complements the findings based on self-report.

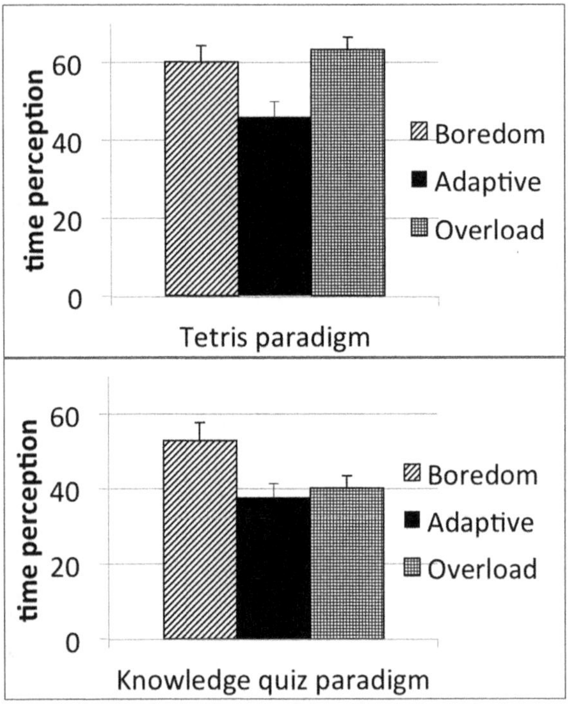

Fig. 21.6 Time perception (self-reported scores; higher scores = longer time estimates)

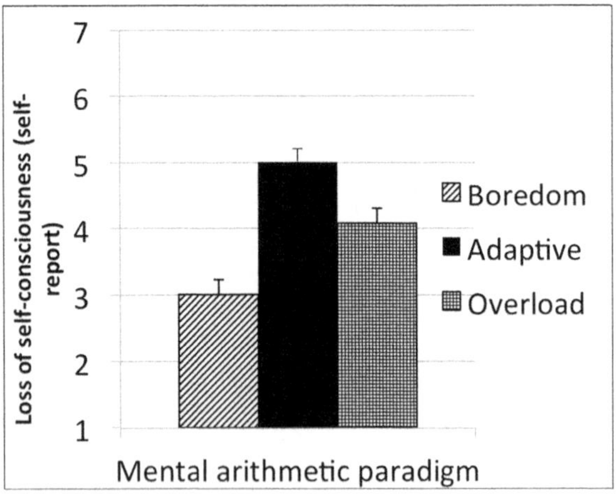

Fig. 21.7 Scores on index assessing loss of self-consciousness

A consideration of the extent to which individuals *perceived control* during task engagement can be particularly worthwhile when one is not only interested in the state of flow, but also in a differentiation of the states of boredom and overload. It is evident that the level of perceived control (over outcomes) should be modest at best under conditions of overload, whereas boredom should be associated with a high level of perceived control (specifically in our experimental settings where we operationalize the three conditions basically with reference to the difficulty of the game or task), with adaptive conditions falling in between. Figure 21.8 reveals that a linear decline in perceived control (across the conditions of boredom, adaptive and overload) is actually what can be observed.

The component of the flow experience that is probably most frequently addressed (and assessed) in flow research so far reflects *intrinsic motivation* as expressed in involvement in and enjoyment of the activity. Figure 21.9 shows two exemplary findings obtained in studies using the Tetris and the knowledge quiz paradigm. Both patterns of results show that the highest level of involvement and enjoyment emerged under adaptive conditions (which differed significantly from both boredom and overload conditions). Of note, the effect of the experimental variation is robust when the level of performance in the game or task is controlled for. That is, involvement and enjoyment is not a function of actual performance (success in the game or task as reflected in the number of questions correctly answered in the knowledge quiz or lines completely filled in the Tetris game) but determined by other more subjective factors (specifically, the perceived fit of skills and task demands).

Given that the flow experience is frequently related to positive affect and therefore interpreted as a state that is likely to foster subjective well-being, it is interesting to note that in some of our experimental studies we assessed participants' mood state after task engagement (e.g. Keller et al. 2011a, b). In these studies we found no meaningful effects on the respective mood scale (see Fig. 21.10). The failure to find significant effects on mood indicates that it seems not meaningful to interpret the flow experience merely as a state of "having fun" or "feeling good." The observed divergence in the effect that the skills-demands-compatibility manipulation exerted on the measures of experiential processes assessed in our studies suggests that experiencing a fit of skills and task demands is likely to trigger fairly specific experiential (and physiological, see below) mechanisms that differentiate this state from other (positive) experiences (such as relaxation).

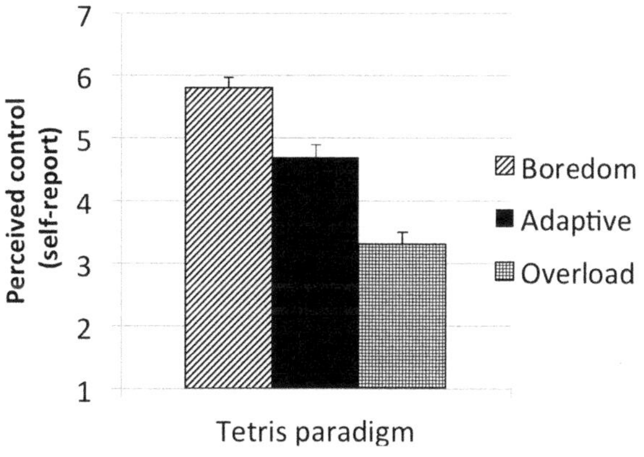

Fig. 21.8 Scores observed on index assessing perceived control

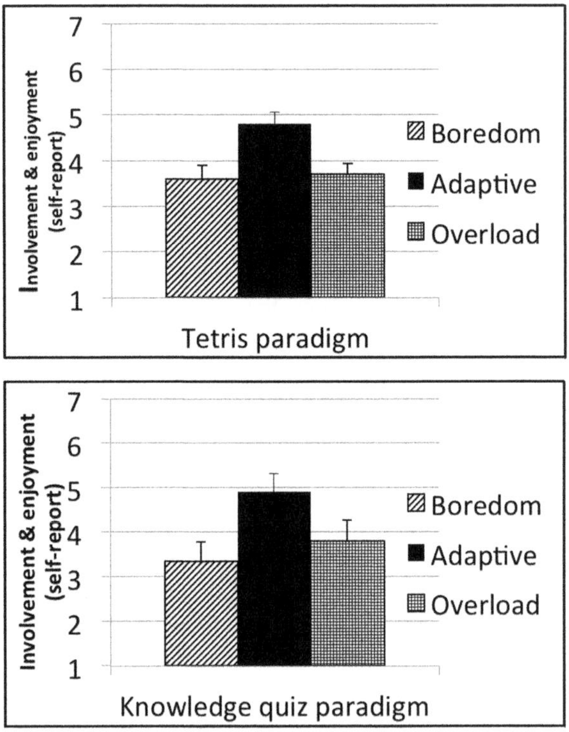

Fig. 21.9 Scores observed on index assessing involvement and enjoyment

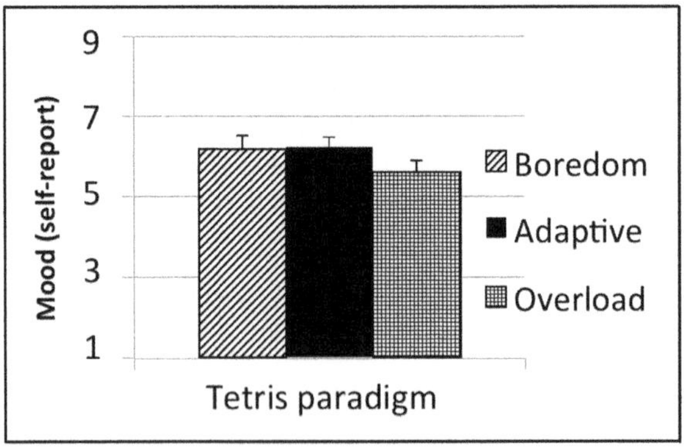

Fig. 21.10 Scores observed on mood index

21.4 Results Regarding Physiological Processes

As discussed above, there is reason to assume that increased *cortisol* levels may be observed in individuals in a state of flow. The rationale underlying this assumption refers to the fact that flow experiences are obviously characterized by a deep involvement in the relevant activity and typically emerge under conditions where

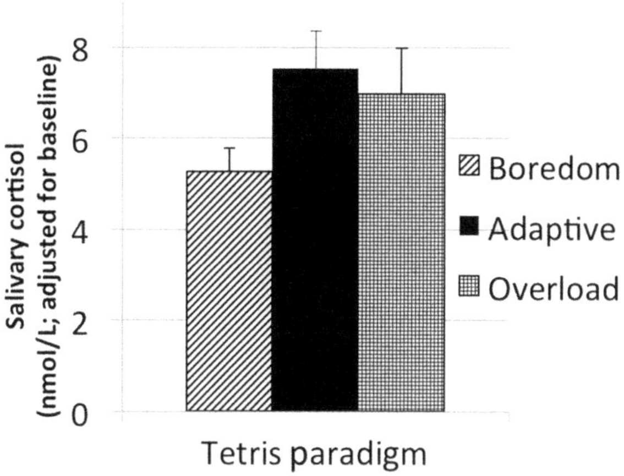

Fig. 21.11 Cortisol levels (assessed in saliva)

individuals engage in a skill-related activity under circumstances where they are confronted with challenging demands (at the limit of their ability). We tested the endocrine response in participants collecting saliva samples prior to and after task engagement (following established procedures, see Keller et al. 2011a, b) in the Tetris paradigm. As can be seen in Fig. 21.11, the obtained results are well in line with the notion that engagement in the Tetris game under adaptive conditions is associated with a stress response as reflected in substantially higher cortisol levels than those observed in participants under boredom conditions. In this case, the cortisol level under adaptive conditions was even slightly (but not significantly) higher compared to the overload condition. This may be attributable to the fact that participants may cope with overload in the Tetris paradigm by way of "giving up" for some moments. That is, when the game reaches a speed level that is hardly manageable any longer, participants simply refrain from any attempts to arrange the objects until the speed level is either down-regulated by one step (as implemented in the algorithm) or until a new (i.e., empty) playing field is presented. These strategies can serve as a stress-buffer providing at least some moments of relaxation.

Building on the findings obtained with salivary cortisol samples, we conducted a follow-up study where we collected blood samples that allowed for an assessment of *adrenocorticotropic hormone* – a precursor of the cortisol response (cf. Melmed et al. 2011). In this study, we applied the mental arithmetic paradigm (varying the order of task conditions between participants: order 1 = boredom-flow-overload; order 2 = flow-boredom-overload, order 3 = overload- flow-boredom) and observed a pattern pretty similar to that obtained in the cortisol study (see Fig. 21.12). Again, participants' endocrine response to the activity was much stronger under adaptive and overload conditions compared to boredom conditions. In the interpretation of the difference scores (ACTH assessed at baseline minus ACTH assessed after task engagement) one should take into account that ACTH levels typically show a circadian trend similar to cortisol levels (with an early morning peak, a continuous decline over daytime and a relatively steep decline in the morning hours; cf. Young

Fig. 21.12 ACTH levels (assessed in serum)

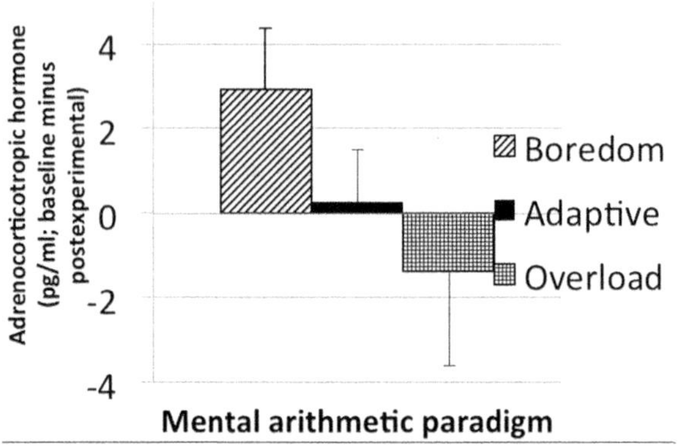

et al. 2001). The positive difference score under boredom conditions reflects the usual steep decline in the morning (given that all participants were assessed in the morning in our study, starting time for data collection at 8:45 a.m.). This decline was compensated by task engagement under adaptive conditions and overcompensated under overload conditions. Accordingly, these findings again indicate that engagement in an activity under adaptive (and overload) conditions is associated with a stress response as reflected in the corresponding ACTH response. In combination, the cortisol and ACTH findings suggest that working on a task or playing a game under adaptive conditions that result in experiential processes characteristic of the state of flow is associated with a stress response on the physiological level. It should be noted that so far we do not have much data available concerning physiological reactions occurring during longer episodes in a state of flow. Accordingly, we cannot tell whether the observed endocrine responses reflect only brief peaks that may level out after a little while. However, in case the endocrine levels remained high across longer episodes in flow, this would indicate that it may not be particularly sensible to propagate the advice to maximize time in flow since it is well established that chronically elevated levels of stress puts individuals' health at risk (Lee et al. 2002; Raber 1998; Reiche et al. 2004; Ohlin et al. 2004).

Given that we obtained initial evidence documenting reduced self-consciousness under adaptive conditions in our studies including the self-report measure assessing loss of self-consciousness, we applied a physiological approach in an *fMRI study* and assessed whether distinct brain regions in the prefrontal cortex known to be involved in processes of self-reflection are down-regulated under adaptive conditions. As our findings revealed, this seems to be the case (see Fig. 21.13); for more detailed information regarding this study, see Ulrich et al. 2014). Note that self-referential processing has been particularly linked with the medial prefrontal cortex (MPFC; Brewer et al. 2011; D'Argembeau et al. 2007; Gusnard et al. 2001; Jenkins and Mitchell 2011; Johnson et al. 2009; Northoff et al. 2006; van Buuren et al. 2010; Whitfield-Gabrieli et al. 2011; Zysset et al. 2003). A lesion study could even demonstrate that damage to the MPFC eliminated self-referential processing (Philippi et al. 2012). Given these prior results, we therefore conclude that the flow-associated

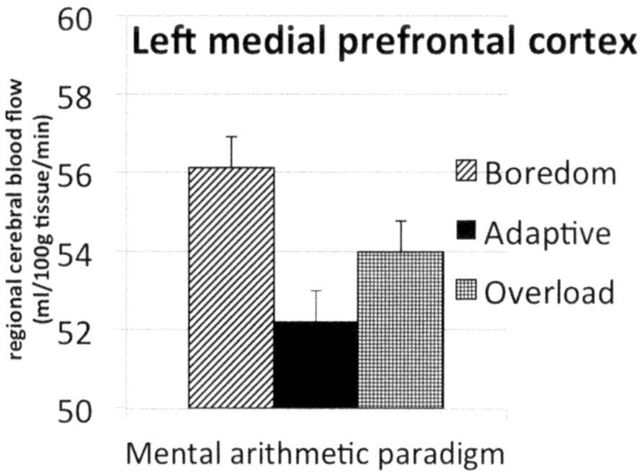

Fig. 21.13 Neural activity in the left prefrontal cortex assessed with perfusion imaging

decrease in MPFC activity as observed in our study, represents one of the main features of flow experiences, that is, a reduction in self-reflection. It should be noted that while some researchers failed to find a similar pattern of neural activity in the prefrontal cortex under conditions of flow in a functional near infrared spectroscopy study (Harmat et al. 2015), we were able to replicate the pattern in a standard fMRI block design using classical blood oxygenation level-dependent (BOLD) imaging (Ulrich et al. 2015).

We applied the biopsychosocial model of challenge and threat in a study where participants (passionate chess players) worked on our chess paradigm (under adaptive conditions) while we assessed various cardiovascular parameters (we computed CO and TPR scores for 60 s intervals at minute 10, 15, 20, 25, 60, 90 and 120 of task engagement). The findings revealed that in the early phase of task engagement participants reacted with a cardiovascular pattern reflecting a state of challenge (increased CO and decreased TPR relative to baseline) (See Fig. 21.14) However, this pattern reversed into one that reflects a state of threat (specifically indicated by the strong increase in TPR relative to baseline) after participants had spent 60 min (or more) on the task. Moreover, we observed that these challenge-threat patterns assessed at different times during the extended period of working on the chess paradigm (under adaptive conditions) correlates differentially with the involvement and enjoyment index. We observed a positive correlation during the early phases of working on the checkmate-in-two chess problems indicating that stronger involvement and enjoyment (assessed for the whole period of task engagement at the end of the session) was associated with a state of challenge (relatively high level of CO and low level of TPR), whereas the correlation reversed during the late phase of task engagement reflecting the fact that involvement and enjoyment was associated with a state of threat. This suggests that the subjective experience of flow as reported by individuals (here: involvement and enjoyment) can be associated with different physiological states as a function of how much time individuals spent on the task (under conditions that have been reliably documented to elicit a state of flow).

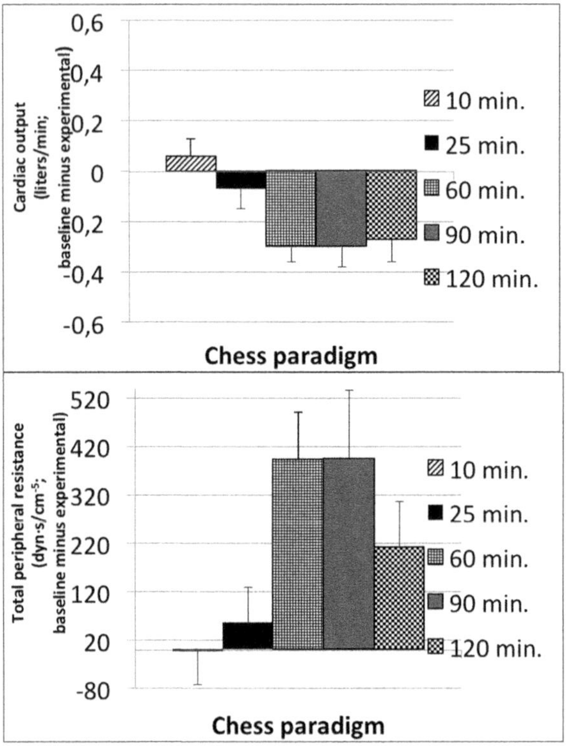

Fig. 21.14 Cardiovascular parameters (CO; TPR) assess with impedance cardiography

21.5 Discussion

Summing up the findings obtained in our flow research so far, some main conclusions seem quite evident. First, our findings reveal that the *experimental* analysis of flow is possible and provides valuable insights regarding the *causal* impact of skills-demands compatibility, which are in line with the basic notions of flow theory. Second, it is noteworthy that participants in our studies typically engage in the respective activity for only a few minutes (typically between 4 and 8 min). Accordingly, even brief episodes of working on a task (or playing a game) under (non-)adaptive conditions can trigger substantial effects. Third, the results obtained on endocrine and cardiovascular responses point to the fact that the state of flow can be associated with physiological stress responses. These findings question the "rosy picture" perspective according to which the state of flow reflects an "optimal experience" resulting in the advice to maximize time in flow in order to foster well-being and happiness. Finally, given that we were successful in developing experimental paradigms designed to manipulate the crucial boundary condition for flow to emerge, these paradigms can be applied in order to address the question which traits characterize the so-called autotelic personality (i.e., who is most prone to experience a state of flow). An answer to this basic question can be approached by way of testing personality traits as moderators of the effect the skills-demand-compatibility manipulation exerts on indicators of the flow experience (cf. Keller and Bless 2008; Keller and Blomann 2008).

21.5.1 Revisiting the Flow Experience

Reflecting on the available flow literature, it seems that the theoretical model as well as the conceptualization and measurement of flow experience may profit from some reexamination. Specifically, two aspects may profit from more systematic considerations in future flow research. First, substantial challenges in the conceptualization and measurement of the state of flow should be addressed – acknowledging the *conjunctive* nature of the flow construct. Second, the flow models proposed in the current literature are basically silent regarding variations in the *intensity* of flow.

21.5.2 The Conjunctive Nature of the Flow Construct

In diagnostic decisions, one important question refers to how scores on relevant assessment or diagnostic tests should be combined in order to make a reasonable decision which treatment a person should receive, which track a student should be assigned to or whether a job candidate should be hired. In this domain, potential decision strategies can reflect a *compensatory* or a *conjunctive* logic (cf. Cronbach and Gleser 1965). A compensatory decision rule implies that low scores on one diagnostic test (e.g., on a specific ability test) can be compensated by high scores on another diagnostic test applied in the diagnostic procedure. In contrast, a conjunctive decision rule builds on the logic that certain threshold levels must be reached on various (or each) of the applied diagnostic tests in order to classify the person into the respective category (e.g., into a group of patients suffering from a specific mental illness). The same logic can be applied to psychological phenomena or constructs such as the flow experience. In this respect it is noteworthy that the flow experience is conceptualized based on a conjunctive logic according to flow theory. That is, flow is considered a state defined by a specific *combination* of subjective experiences which co-occur: (1) a sense of control, (2) reduced level of self-consciousness, (3) altered sense of time, (4) deep involvement and enjoyment, and (5) intrinsic motivation. Accordingly, a proper assessment and operationalization of flow should take this conjunctive nature of the construct into account. However, in flow research so far (our own work included), researchers typically consider the components of the flow experience in isolation.

21.5.3 Silence Regarding Variations in the Intensity of Flow

It seems quite noteworthy that the flow models proposed in the current literature are basically silent regarding variations in the intensity of flow. This is the case, because the flow channel model (cf. Csikszentmihalyi and Rathunde 1993) as well as the quadrant or octant model (cf. Csikszentmihalyi and LeFevre 1989; Massimini and Carli 1988) refer to the boundary conditions that have to be met for a person to enter the state of flow (i.e., in essence these models conceptualize flow as a categorical variable; cf. Keller and Landhaeusser 2012). However, none of these models allows for specific predictions regarding the intensity of flow experienced by the person. Accordingly, theoretical refinements are obviously necessary in order to go beyond the basic question of whether a person will enter a state of flow (or not). It is evident that the flow experience can vary substantially in its intensity. Thus, it is high time to develop explanatory models that address this fact.

References

Adolph, O., Köster, S., Georgieff, M., Bäder, S., Föhr, K. J., Kammer, T., Herrnberger, B., & Grön, G. (2010). Xenon-induced changes in CNS sensitization to pain. *NeuroImage, 49*, 720–730.

Bassett, J. R., Marshall, P. M., & Spillane, R. (1987). The physiological measurement of acute stress (public speaking) in bank employees. *International Journal of Psychophysiology, 5*, 265–273.

Blascovich, J., & Tomaka, J. (1996). The biopsychosocial model of arousal regulation. In M. P. Zanna (Ed.), *Advances in experimental social psychology* (Vol. 28, pp. 1–51). New York: Academic.

Brewer, J. A., Worhunsky, P. D., Gray, J. R., Tang, Y. Y., Weber, J., & Kober, H. (2011). Meditation experience is associated with differences in default mode network activity and connectivity. *Proceedings of the National Academy of Sciences, 108*, 20254–20259.

Conti, R. (2001). Time flies: Investigating the connection between intrinsic motivation and the experience of time. *Journal of Personality, 69*, 1–26.

Cronbach, L. J., & Gleser, G. C. (1965). *Psychological tests and personnel decisions* (2nd ed.). Urbana: University of Illinois Press.

Csikszentmihalyi, M. (1975). *Beyond boredom and anxiety*. San Francisco: Jossey Bass.

Csikszentmihalyi, M. (1990). *Flow: The psychology of optimal experience*. New York: Harper and Row.

Csikszentmihalyi, M., & LeFevre, J. (1989). Optimal experience in work and leisure. *Journal of Personality and Social Psychology, 56*, 815–822.

Csikszentmihalyi, M., & Rathunde, K. (1993). The measurement of flow in everyday life: Towards a theory of emergent motivation. In J. E. Jacobs (Ed.), *Developmental perspectives on motivation, 1992: Nebraska symposium on motivation. Current theory and research in motivation* (Vol. 40, pp. 57–97). Lincoln: University of Nebraska Press.

D'Argembeau, A., Ruby, P., Collette, F., Degueldre, C., Balteau, E., Luxen, A., et al. (2007). Distinct regions of the medial prefrontal cortex are associated with self-referential processing and perspective taking. *Journal of Cognitive Neuroscience, 19*(6), 935–944.

Does, S., Derks, B., Ellemers, N., & Scheepers, D. (2012). At the heart of egalitarianism: How morality framing shapes cardiovascular challenge versus threat in whites. *Social Psychological and Personality Science, 3*, 747–753.

Goldberg, I. I., Harel, M., & Malach, R. (2006). When the brain loses its self: Prefrontal inactivation during sensorimotor processing. *Neuron, 50*, 329–339.
Groen, G., Sokolov, A. N., Jonas, C., Roebling, R., & Spitzer, M. (2011). Increased resting-state perfusion after repeated encoding is related to later retrieval of declarative associative memories. *PLoS ONE, 6*(5), e19985.
Gusnard, D. A., Akbudak, E., Shulman, G. L., & Raichle, M. E. (2001). Medial prefrontal cortex and self-referential mental activity: Relation to a default mode of brain function. *Proceedings of the National Academy of Sciences, 98*, 4259–4264.
Harmat, L., de Manzano, Ö., Theorell, T., Högman, L., Fischer, H., & Ullén, F. (2015). Physiological correlates of the flow experience during computer game playing. *International Journal of Psychophysiology, 97*, 1–7.
Jenkins, A. C., & Mitchell, J. P. (2011). Medial prefrontal cortex subserves diverse forms of self-reflection. *Social Neuroscience, 6*, 211–218.
Johnson, M. K., Nolen-Hoeksema, S., Mitchell, K. J., & Levin, Y. (2009). Medial cortex activity, self-reflection and depression. *Social Cognitive and Affective Neuroscience, 4*, 313–327.
Jumbo Spiele®. (2000). *Wer wird Millionär?* [Who wants to be a millionaire?]. Herscheid, Germany.
Kakimoto, Y. (1985). Effects of physiological and mental stress on crew members in relatively long flights by C-1 transport aircraft. *Reports of Aeromedical Laboratory, 26*, 131–155.
Keller, J., & Bless, H. (2008). Flow and regulatory compatibility: An experimental approach to the flow model of intrinsic motivation. *Personality & Social Psychology Bulletin, 34*, 196–209.
Keller, J., & Blomann, F. (2008). Locus of control and the flow experience: An experimental analysis. *European Journal of Personality, 607*, 589–607.
Keller, J., & Landhäußer, A. (2012). The flow model revisited. In S. Engeser (Ed.), *Advances in flow research* (pp. 51–64). Berlin: Springer.
Keller, J., Bless, H., Blomann, F., & Kleinböhl, D. (2011a). Physiological aspects of flow experiences: Skills-demand-compatibility effects on heart rate variability and salivary cortisol. *Journal of Experimental Social Psychology, 47*, 849–852.
Keller, J., Ringelhan, S., & Blomann, F. (2011b). Does skills-demands-compatibility result in intrinsic motivation? Experimental test of a basic notion proposed in the theory of flow-experiences. *Journal of Positive Psychology, 6*, 408–417.
Kirschbaum, C., & Hellhammer, D. H. (1989). Salivary cortisol in psychobiological research: An overview. *Neuropsychobiology, 22*, 150–169.
Kirschbaum, C., & Hellhammer, D. H. (2000). Salivary cortisol. In G. Fink (Ed.), *Encyclopedia of stress* (Vol. 3, pp. 379–383). San Diego: Academic.
Lee, A. L., Ogle, W. O., & Sapolsky, R. M. (2002). Stress and depression: Possible links to neuron death in the hippocampus. *Bipolar Disorder, 4*, 117–128.
Lyubomirsky, S. (2008). *The how of happiness: A scientific approach to getting the life you want.* New York: Penguin Press.
Mason, J. W. (1968). A review of psychoendocrine research on the pituitary-adrenal cortical system. *Psychosomatic Medicine, 30*, 576–607.
Massimini, F., & Carli, M. (1988). The systematic assessment of flow in daily experience. In M. Csikszentmihalyi & I. S. Csikszentmihalyi (Eds.), *Optimal experience: Psychological studies of flow in consciousness* (pp. 288–306). New York: Cambridge University Press.
Melmed, S., Kleinberg, D., & Ho, K. (2011). Pituitary physiology and diagnostic evaluation. In S. Melmed, K. Polonsky, P. Larsen, & H. Kronenberg (Eds.), *Williams textbook of endocrinology* (12th ed., pp. 175–228). Philadelphia: Elsevier Saunders.
Nisbett, R. E., & Wilson, T. D. (1977). Telling more than we can know: Verbal reports on mental processes. *Psychological Review, 84*, 231–259.
Northoff, G., Heinzel, A., de Greck, M., Bermpohl, F., Dobrowolny, H., & Panksepp, J. (2006). Self-referential processing in our brain – A meta-analysis of imaging studies on the self. *NeuroImage, 31*, 440–457.

Ohlin, B., Nilsson, P. M., Nilsson, J. A., & Berglund, G. (2004). Chronic psychosocial stress predicts long-term cardiovascular morbidity and mortality in middle-aged men. *European Heart Journal, 25*, 867–873.

Philippi, C. L., Duff, M. C., Denburg, N. L., Tranel, D., & Rudrauf, D. (2012). Medial PFC damage abolishes the self-reference effect. *Journal of Cognitive Neuroscience, 24*, 475–481.

Raber, J. (1998). Detrimental effects of chronic hypothalamic-pituitary-adrenal axis activation. From obesity to memory deficits. *Molecular Neurobiology, 18*, 1–22.

Reiche, E. M., Nunes, S. O., & Morimoto, H. K. (2004). Stress, depression, the immune system, and cancer. *Lancet Oncology, 10*, 617–625.

Rheinberg, F. (2008). Intrinsic motivation and flow. In J. Heckhausen & H. Heckhausen (Eds.), *Motivation and action* (pp. 323–348). Cambridge: Cambridge University Press.

Tomaka, J., Blascovich, J., Kelsey, R. M., & Leitten, C. L. (1993). Subjective, physiological, and behavioral effects of threat and challenge appraisal. *Journal of Personality and Social Psychology, 18*, 616–624.

Ulrich, M., Keller, J., Hönig, K., Waller, C., & Grön, G. (2014). Neural correlates of experimentally induced flow experiences. *NeuroImage, 86*, 194–202.

Ulrich, M., Keller, J., & Grön, G. (2015). Neural signatures of experimentally induced flow experiences identified in a standard fMRI block-design with BOLD imaging. *Social Cognitive and Affect Neurosciences*. doi:10.1093/scan/nsv133.

van Buuren, M., Gladwin, T. E., Zandbelt, B. B., Kahn, R. S., & Vink, M. (2010). Reduced functional coupling in the default-mode network during self-referential processing. *Human Brain Mapping, 31*, 1117–1127.

Wang, J., Aguirre, G. K., Kimberg, D. Y., Roc, A. C., Li, L., & Detre, J. A. (2003). Arterial spin labeling perfusion fMRI with very low task frequency. *Magnetic Resonance in Medicine, 49*, 796–802.

Whitfield-Gabrieli, S., Moran, J. M., Nieto-Castanon, A., Triantafyllou, C., Saxe, R., & Gabrieli, J. D. (2011). Associations and dissociations between default and self-reference networks in the human brain. *NeuroImage, 55*, 225–232.

Young, E., Carlson, N., & Brown, M. (2001). Twenty-four-hour ACTH and cortisol pulsatility in depressed women. *Neuropsychopharmacology, 25*, 267–276.

Zysset, S., Huber, O., Samson, A., Ferstl, E. C., & von Cramon, D. Y. (2003). Functional specialization within the anterior medial prefrontal cortex: A functional magnetic resonance imaging study with human subjects. *Neuroscience Letters, 335*, 183–186.

Chapter 22
Towards a Neurobiological Understanding of Reduced Self-Awareness During Flow: An Occupational Science Perspective

Gaynor Sadlo

Abstract Advances in neurobiology, including brain-scanning and physiological measurements, can now be applied to enhance our understanding of reduced self-awareness, one of flow's core symptoms. It throws light on optimal experience, since self-forgetting links to flow's positive affect, a paradox in such a highly self-aware species. This chapter synthesises empirical studies into self-awareness, and how it is down-regulated during task performance. A breakthrough was the identification of a specific neuronal network for self-awareness, discovered during brain mapping of goal-directed tasks. The network becomes active whenever tasks end, rather like a default. Evidence suggests that deep engagement in skilled (flow-like) activities dampens the network, relating somewhat to earlier concepts of hypofrontality. An occupational science perspective proposes that participation in complex activities may reduce the weight of our extreme self-awareness. The human propensity to 'occupy' ourselves through a range of activities, such as the arts, can be a major mechanism for stress-reduction. Early twentieth century observations of the restorative function of being occupied transformed into the profession of occupational therapy, arguably originally a kind of 'flow therapy'.

22.1 Introduction

From the earliest flow studies, research participants identified reduced self-awareness as a key experience (Csikszentmihalyi and Csikszentmihalyi 1988; Csikszentmihalyi 1993), and yet its mechanisms remain relatively under-researched. Evidence from qualitative investigations reveal nuances to reduced self-awareness and thus its complexity: *When I play (the violin) I lose myself, and forget my worries* (Wright et al. 2006); *When you are climbing its like your mind is just empty of everything else…you are consumed by it* (Suchoverskyte 2013); *when I don't think about*

G. Sadlo, Ph.D., PgDTCDHE DipOccThy (✉)
School of Health Sciences, University of Brighton, Eastbourne, East Sussex, UK

First Faculty of Medicine, Charles University, Prague, Czech Republic
e-mail: g.sadlo@brighton.ac.uk

L. Harmat et al. (eds.), *Flow Experience*, DOI 10.1007/978-3-319-28634-1_22

myself, I can hit the ball much better (Gallwey 2008); *you feel as if you don't exist… as if I have nothing to do with what is happening* (Csikszentmihalyi 2004); *sewing is better than valium*! (Gregory 2013). Reduced awareness can include time, other people, even bodily needs; it 'transcends the ego' (Csikszentmihalyi 2004).

Such experiences may involve varying processes, but to start we need basic understanding of the neurobiology of how task engagement can lead to self-forgetting, which is also relevant to facilitating flow, and to flow's positive effect (Csikszentmihalyi and Rathunde 1992). Suspended self-awareness is linked to the optimal human experience by which flow is famously described – joy, rapture, even ecstasy. "Being able to forget temporarily who we are seems to be very enjoyable" Csikszentmihalyi (1990: 64). Csikszentmihalyi (1993: 38) also described flow as a "rare-state of consciousness".

Before the possibilities of contemporary neuroscience and based on more than 8,000 interviews, Csikszentmihalyi (2004) hypothesised about brain function and loss of self-awareness: that the energy that normally goes into self-awareness and self-monitoring is taken instead by the processing involved in the demanding, hyper-focus of the creative thinking/high-level task. Attention seems to be switched towards, or demanded by, the activity itself, reducing the energy 'left over' to monitor such things as body awareness or awareness of time. In this view, feelings about the self disappear from consciousness, and feelings of existence are temporarily suspended, as if identity temporarily evaporates. Such matters can now be explored through brain function studies, and other physiological measurements, such as cardiac and respiratory activities (Harmat et al. 2015).

Human consciousness research is complex and interdisciplinary (Fuster 2008) while the study of self-awareness, the realm of philosophy since antiquity, is only now an emerging field in neurobiology (Lou 2015). Human beings are the most self-aware of all species (Lieberman 2013), evolved to facilitate our exceedingly complex social intelligence (Goleman 2007). The rapid expansion of neuroscience in the twenty-first century fuels advances in brain-study techniques; and now the first experimental studies specifically into the mechanisms of flow states are being published (De Manzano et al. 2010; Klasen et al. 2012; Ulrich et al. 2014, 2015; Harmat et al. 2015).

This chapter synthesises some of this research, but it is a work in progress towards the question "*How does deep engagement in (flow-type) activities reduce self-awareness*"? It relates to neuropsychology but also to occupational science, a multi-disciplinary science emerging from occupational therapy (Zemke and Clark 1996), and informing public health through such publications as *An Occupational Perspective of Health* (Wilcock and Hocking 2015). It investigates human capacities for complex activities, including personal care, leisure pursuits and productive work, and their potential for promoting or inhibiting wellbeing (Yerxa et al. 1989). The focus of occupational science and flow research are closely aligned – indeed the inaugural edition of the Journal of Occupational Science included such comparisons (Csikszentmihalyi 1993). In the early twentieth century, occupational therapy was born out of observations that when people are 'occupied' or diverted by activities such as creative arts, wellbeing was enhanced (Yerxa 1996; Clark and Larson 1993; Clark et al. 1998). *Occupy* means to fill, inhabit, take up space or time, reside in, forcibly enter or stay, keep busy and active, or hold; the Latin root *occupare* means to sieze and take over

(Oxford English Dictionary). These concepts easily connect with the deep involvement, absorption, feeling-like-being-taken-over phenomena of flow.

22.2 Method

Fuster (2008) considers that although they seem to be at odds epistomologically, it is legitimate to seek understanding of self-awareness through both the phenomenology of lived experience, and via the neural correlates of self-conscious experience, on which this paper focuses. Since the brain mechanisms of reduced self-awareness during flow indicates complex inter-relationships between several parts and functions, systematic and follow-through searches sought existing evidence using terms "self-awareness", "self-reference", "self-consciousness", "self-forgetting", "identity", "occupation", "flow", "neurobiology" and "social neuroscience" into the major search engines using varying combinations and associations. After reading the abstracts, irrelevant studies were put aside. Leads were followed up when new concepts emerged, such as the Default Mode network, trying to track the development of the particular research topic. Neuroimaging studies include (functional, and functional connectivity) magnetic resonance imaging (MRI, fMRI, fcMRI), oxygen ratios (OEF), positron emission tomography (PET) scans, functional near infrared spectroscopy (fNIRS), diffusion tensor imaging (DTI), and electroencephelography (EEG). BOLD refers to Blood Oxygenation level-dependent signals that indicate changes in activity in different brain regions (Damoiseaux and Greicius 2009).

The emerging fields of social neuroscience and social intelligence are relevant (Lieberman 2013; Goleman 2007), since we have a fundamental need to belong that requires self (conscious)-regulation (Heatherton 2011). One of the challenges facing experimental research into flow is that invasive measures can actually prevent flow (De Manzano et al. 2010), however various scans and physiological measures are beginning to reveal significant information.

The work adopts an eclectic, wide-horizon/deep-probing but critical-evaluative and chronological approach influenced by the History of Ideas methodology (Lovejoy 1933). Seldom used in health or psychological research to date, this method has shown strong potential for theory-building within occupational science, tracking the development of changing concepts over time (Wilcock and Hocking 2015). Information is sought, judged and chosen for inclusion according to its relevance to answering the missing links within research question.

22.3 Findings and Discussion

Skilled activities seem to more reliably lead to flow experiences (Harmat et al. 2015), and it is already known that uniquely human occupations such as playing music activate the higher cortical areas of the brain (Fuster 2008), responsible for our profound, planned, purposeful behaviour. Historic brain-damage observations confirmed the role of the frontal lobe in cognitive behaviour during deliberate, chosen actions (Fuster 2008), so the frontal brain areas are naturally the focus for neurobiology of flow studies. The pre-frontal areas and their association with self-awareness are now being scrutinised, within an 'explosion' of neuroscience this century. This section summarises current findings including concepts of transient hypo-frontality, the default mode network now more correctly called our self-awareness network, and (only touched on here) the human reward system.

The discovery of a default network is seen here as a breakthrough in the conceptualisation of the neurobiology of self-awareness and reduced awareness. Specific empirical studies of flow are very recent, and are leading to important findings regarding apparent opposites, such as flow being both exciting and calming. Ideas that link reduced self-awareness with positive experience are presented, leading to an occupational science hypothesis about the possible health-giving and even existential purpose of a range of absorbing activities in human life.

22.3.1 Transient Hypo-frontality

As discussed in detail in Chap. 5 by Stoll and Pithan, in this volume, the cognitive neuroscientist Arne Deitrich was one of the first to address the complex task of explaining flow states through neuroscience. His seminal papers described his transient hypo-frontality hypothesis of flow THT (Dietrich 2003, 2004, 2006; Dietrich and Audiffren 2011) which suggests that during the performance of skilled tasks, energy is temporarily directed away from the prefrontal, cortical, conscious 'explicit' brain areas towards the 'implicit' motor and sensory regions. Learning high-skill activity through multiple repetitions gradually shifts activity from the explicit, flexible, largely pre-frontal neurological systems, where we consciously initiate each movement – to the implicit performance system, including the cerebellum, when the skill gradually becomes so embodied through synaptic pathways being formed and reinforced (confirmed by Draganski et al. 2004, 2006) that soon we perform movements without conscious awareness (Dietrich 2006). Sensory-motor skilled performance is so demanding that it requires the brain's resources to be directed posteriorly, reducing activity in the frontal areas, according to this hypothesis. Higher cognitive executive functions that are not required during intense physical activities like running become less active, reducing self-consciousness (Dietrich 2006).

THT is a plausible idea that relates to qualitative flow research. Playing a Mozart concerto demands such extremely complex intellectual, sensory, motor and emotional performance that for the duration of playing, a musician cannot think about himself or his personal problems. Successful sports coaching applies this idea (Gallwey 2015), knowledge arising from professional experience rather than neuroscience. Gallwey's popular technique involves training athletes (and musicians, and workers) to consciously 'switch off' their over-critical inner voice "Self 1" and to trust the ancient powers of "Self 2" where (say) hitting a ball involves complex, highly evolved but nevertheless *unconscious* movements. Dietrich's hypothesis has made useful contributions to the field, providing a platform for other scientists (Harmat et al. 2015). The methodologies by which he built his hypothesis are not very transparent and he has no recent publications to progress these ideas, but other studies give some support.

Historically, the prefrontal cortex (PFC) became known as the human "seat of consciousness", incorporating "subjective awareness of one's self", due to its proven role in self-conscious cognitive operations like speaking (Fuster 2008: 376). Phenomenologists propose that we are self-aware whenever we are conscious (Lou 2015) but that fails to take account of how flow during task-matched skill *reduces* the sense of self-awareness. The proliferation of imaging studies reveals the "ubiquity" of heightened activity in the Medial PFC (MPFC) whenever we engage in self-referential mental activity (Heatherton 2011: 6). Dietrich's findings align in regard to that flow's reduction of self-reference indicates hypo-activity of the frontal areas. THT also seems to align to Csikszentmihalyi's (2004) psychological reasoning about flow mechanisms.

22.3.2 A Default Mode Network

During the last decade neuroscientists, not specifically looking at flow, have signified some relevant mechanisms concerning self-awareness that seem key to understanding the neurobiology of flow. The quest to identify the detailed functions of the (at least) 100 areas of the human brain led to an unexpected finding: that there is an endogenous, extensive, highly connected neuronal network that shows higher neural activity and energy consumption when a person is resting from specific cognitive or motor tasks (Raichle et al. 2001). Labelled as *the default mode network* (DMN) because 'in default', that is, at times whenever a person is NOT actively engaged in another cognitive or motor task, brain activity naturally returns to its normal self-reflection mode, where thoughts about issues of self-concern are internally generated. Spontaneous cognition, social cognition and endogenous connectivity are other relevant concepts within DMN (Di and Biswal 2014).

Building on previous fMRI and PET studies that revealed the location of brain areas involved in executive tasks such as solving mathematical problems, Raichle et al. (2001) aimed to identify the baseline activity in the human brain during its normal conscious state. Using PET when subjects were restfully awake, they found a baseline mode of brain function that is *substantially active* during rest periods, but where *activity reduces during goal-directed activities*. This default activity mode involves several areas along the mid-line – the medial prefrontal cortex (MPFC) (thinking about ourselves), and the parietal lobe (monitoring sensory stimuli) are shown to be active in the resting state. "The MPFC shows the highest baseline metabilic activity at rest, which exhibits decreases from this baseline during goal-directed activity" (Gusnard et al. 2001: 4259); and "attention-demanding tasks attenuate emotional processing". These neuroscientists acknowledge the earlier work of Ingvar (1979, 1985) who first noted that high blood flow in the cerbral cortex is associated with self-generated mental activity in the 'resting' brain, which he called *hyper*frontality. He associated this with the need to think about and plan future behaviour.

Greicius et al. (2003) discovered *functional connectivity* using fMRI in the previously hypothesised areas of the resting brain, claiming to be the first to do so. The MPFC but also dorsal and lateral areas of the PFC were found to be active, but they also revealed that parts of the brain known to be related to introspection, especially the Posteria Cingulate Cortex (PCC), show consistant activity. Self-awareness, awareness of social situations, episodic memory and semantic knowledge areas become active at rest, but reduce during focus on a task.

Thinking about one's self and one's own life is seen as higher order executive functioning, which explains why MPFC (Northoff and Bermpohl 2004) becomes very active during periods of self-awareness. Synthesising various neuroimaging studies, these scientists found strong evidence that self-referential stimuli relating to self-representation, monitoring, and evaluation are processed and integrated across various mid-line cortical structures. These match with reduced self-reference during flow experiences.

Goldberg et al. (2006) revealed through detailed fMRI techniques that there was "a complete segregation of brain areas during sensori-motor processing of a demanding perceptual task when compared with periods of introspection" (Goldberg et al. 2006: 228). They found "robust inhibition" of the areas of introspection during sensori-motor processing. Goleman (2007) highlighted a significant issue that seems related to flow's ability to reduce self-awareness, emphasising the importance of the amygdala during introspection, relating to social-evaluative threat (ST) (Brom et al. 2014). The amygdala responds to stimuli that are perceived as a risk, and heightened amygdala activity occurs during social emotions (Ruby and Decet 2004).

Another empirical study relevant to flow research is the mapping of two types of self-awareness (Farb et al. 2007). Using fMRI with meditators they discriminated the brain regions involved in two distinct forms of self-awareness: the self-across-time perceived by a sense of permanence – *me* – (narrative focus), and the self-in-the-present-moment – *I* – (experiential focus). Narrative self-reference includes higher-order concepts of self-traits, knowledge of one's past life, and future life plans, like one's life story, involved "pronounced recruitment" (p. 316) of midline cortical structures, such as the MRFC, PCC, the language areas, hippocampus, and even the cerebellum. In contrast, the in-the-now experience of self as when deliberately directing a task or focusing on present feelings or awareness of the senses, revealed *de*activation of the MPFC – and increased activation of parietal areas associated with proprioception and sensori-motor bodily experiences. These two forms of self-consciousness enable both short-term working-memory abilities, and long-term projections and remembering of personal life events. In tune with DMN findings, they noted a natural activity bias towards the narrative mode. Trained meditators can disengage the narrative to engage in momentary self-focus, which reduces anxiety disorders. This might relate to the sense of unity and calm reported during meditation (and during flow activities?).

DMN's relationship with pathological conditions fosters new insights. People with depression reveal higher activation of DMN, with over-rumination and increased negative self–thinking, compared with controls (Sheline et al. 2008). Gentili et al. (2009) used fMRF to discover that people with social phobia exhibit abnormal function of the DMN, it remaining overactive even during task conditions.

To summarise, since the new millennia, empirical evidence reveals extensive connectivity within DMN, a constellation of brain areas becoming most active during periods of heightened self-awareness. Andrews-Hanna et al. (2010) and Andrews-Hanna (2011), concluded their systematic review with evidence that we ruminate about ourselves and our social interactions via this network, whenever we are not involved in an external activity. DMN reduction during flow-like task engagement involves hypo-frontality, but several other cortical (non-frontal) areas become less active as well.

22.3.3 A Network for Self-Awareness

In September 2014, international experts synthesised current understanding of the neurobiology of self-awareness, identifying pathways for future research (Lou 2015). Collective research confirmed existence of a special mechanism that facilitates high-level social functioning through a profound capacity for self-awareness (Jonson et al. 2002). This mid-line para-limbic network is "exceedingly metabolically active in idleness and in tasks relevant to the self…. (but) decreases in activity during goal-directed action in the outside world" (Lou 2015: 121). A network that unequivocally refers to resting state parallel cortical activity in the insula, medial prefrontal cortex and the medial parietal lobe as 'hubs'. The insula's intimate connection to the amygdala and thalamus explains the strong effect of deeper mid-brain functions on the network, especially in the affective domain, including activation of the threat response. The think-tank suggested that this network should be conceptualised not so much as a *default* network DMN, but more accurately as the *network of self-awareness*, itself instrumental in developing self-awareness and its regulation.

This self-awareness network (SAN) has recently-evolved capacity to support our ever-more complex social interactions; the fronto-insular cortex is thought to be less than 100,000 years old (Greicius 2012). Interactions between the anterior and posterior hubs of the network exhibit higher-order processing such as gamma-range oscillations and regulation by dopamine (Lou 2015). We are *wired to connect* as an adaptive function (Lieberman 2013), involving the fast acting mirror and spindle cells (Uddin et al. 2007). We plan, build and wonder about our life story through time, to orchestrate our lives, aware of problems and alert to social-evaluative threats (ST) (Brom et al. 2014). It is as if efficient advantage is taken of resting times when other tasks are not being performed, to assess, rehearse, monitor and make plans to adapt our social interactions. Within flow research, the nuances of self awareness (forgetting problems, feeling at one with nature, losing one's identity) may provide further questions, inspiring specific studies. Reducing self- awareness requires down-grading large areas of brain activity, including the highest cortical domains of executive thinking, MPFC activity, and more ancient areas like the amygdla, via the ACC.

High activity in SAN can lead to anxiety states, as "our world contracts as our problems and pre-occupations loom large" (Goleman 2007: 54), while research into depression and anxiety disorders show association with an over-active network (Sheline et al. 2008). The detailed neurobiological mechanisms of the relationship between self-forgetting and flow need further specific exploration, a challenge taken up by members of the European flow-researchers' network.

22.3.4 Specific Neurobiology/Physiological Flow Studies

Recent empirical publications from the neuro/psycho/physiological flow researchers in Sweden and Germany reveal several discoveries. The studies may not be directly related to the topic of self-awareness, and yet their results may be tentatively interpreted in that relation.

De Manzano et al. (2010) used psychophysiological flow measures during piano playing by professional musicians, to discover that flow is associated with a complex interaction within the autonomic system – increased parasympathetic modulation of sympathetic activity. Skilled pianists executed high-level cognitively demanding performance that might normally be very stressful, and yet they experienced very positive emotions more associated with parasympathetic activity. This study brings first-ever more detailed biological findings to one of the paradoxes of flow experiences – that high-skill is reported as relaxing, and even transformative. In light of the findings regarding the DMN, perhaps dampening of the self-aware network reduced the self-evaluative threat for these participants. The authors also suggest that the ecstasy of flow might be part of the human reward system.

Ullen et al. (2012) studied flow-proneness in association with personality and intelligence, shedding light on the reported variability in likelihood of people experiencing flow. Would those more prone to negative emotions report fewer experiences of flow? Questionnaires integrating proneness, personality and intelligence scores found participants more likely to experience flow during leisure than work or domestic tasks. Virtually no association was found between flow proneness and intelligence, but overall positive, conscientious personalities were more likely to experience flow. Tasks that potentially elicit flow need self-awareness, tenacity and practice to develop the skills, which could be seen as marks of a more conscientious personality.

De Manzano et al. (2013) used PET scans in a neurobiological project, to find a positive correlation between flow proneness and dopamine production. Dopaminergic transmission is known as part of the human reward system, and in other species, which ties in with very early flow research where flow-type activities was seen as being affected by intrinsic motivation, positive mood, and good impulse control.

Ulrich et al. (2014) tested neural correlates of flow using fMRI during mental arithmatic, finding increased neural activity in the putamen (goal-directed behaviour and coding of outcome/effort); and in the inferior frontal gyrus (sense of control), beginning to reveal the subtleties involved in flow. Decreased MPFC (self-referential processing) and amygdala (decreased negative arousal) activity was recorded during the cognitive tasks. They specifically relate their findings to SAL, revealing support for the role of MPFC down-regulation in decreased self-referential processing, while reduced amygdala activity in this study was related to higher flow scores.

Harmat et al. (2015) extended their previous their ideas to consider how flow states can be relaxing, even during high performance. The role of the para/sympathetic systems during flow needed further physiological understanding, including seeking evidence of possible transient hypo-frontality. In an experimental study, they used physiological measures of cardiac activity and respiration, and oxygenation changes in the PFC using fNIRS, along with self-reported psychological flow questionnaires. Participants engaged in a well-known computer game that adjusts to match individual levels of just-right-challenge for optimal flow as well as low and too-difficult levels. Results partially supported the hypothesis that flow peak activity is associated with signs of a relaxed, parasympathetic state. They did not find evidence of hypo-frontality, steering the need for more research into the phenomenon of possible reduced frontal activity during flow, confounding the influence of the frontal cognitive and motor demands of a task.

The overall findings in this section reveal that during the last 5 years there has been a shift in applying neuroscience and biological studies directly to research into flow, which is providing us with deeper appreciation of the biological mechanism of flow. The tools now at our disposal are creating exciting new lines of enquiry within flow research, elaborating the psychological findings that have dominated flow research during the twentieth century.

22.4 Further Discussion: Reduced Self Awareness as Key to a Positive Mental State?

Developing understanding of the neuroscience of self-awareness is evolving from studies that map the function of all brain areas. A plausible current explanation is that lowered self-awareness reduces the threat response, possibly increasing activity within the parasympathetic (relaxation) pathways (Harmat et al. 2015), but the role of the autonomic pathways during flow is paradoxical and needs further research. Peifer's research (2012) and Keller's prolific physiological work (See Chap. 21 by Keller in this volume) has consistantly found more sympathetic involvement.

However, the specific self-forgetting studies seem to indicate that flow may bring transient relief at least from the threat of personal concerns, and thus a more enjoyable, happy state. Self-awareness can be rather a burden for us as well as a highly evolved adaptive, necessary resource, for social exclusion is a risk, and it has existentialist relevance, as we perceive our personhood as 'me' within a physical body (Tallis 2005). Increasing individualism in contemporary society with the proliferation of social media and concern about our personal image seems to accentuate self-concerns (Greenfield 2008). Reduced self-awareness thus relieves us from thinking about our life situation and even our existence. Transcendental experiences have been reported during flow, perceived as less focus on the self, with a sense of connecting with universal energy, related to our spirituality (Zolar and Marshall 2000). Brain wave research may bring promising new understanding about the oscillations that seem to be connected with spiritual experiences (Hanson 2009).

From an occupational science perspective, we can hypothesise that human beings are biologically rewarded for being ourselves, using our evolved form and function to build our occupational capacities – identified as bibedalism, highly manipulative hands, binocular vision, large brain with high cognitive potentials and extraordinary social intelligence, and sense of spirituality (Wilcock and Hocking 2015). These signify a creative species (Wilcock 2008), with neuropeptides and hormones forming part of a complex reward system. Like all species we are rewarded for survival activities that are essential to our survival, such as eating or mating, but also it seems dopamine, endorphins, opiods, and even oxytocin encourage us to engage in the highest level, flow-like activities (le Merrer et al. 2009; Kringelbach and Berridge 2010), with a 'love' for what we do and make (Ingold 2013). The brain areas implicated in reward processing seem to have similarities to SAN – PFC, PCC, striatum, inferior parietal (Nieuwenhuis et al. 2004), but further understanding is needed.

It may be that we have evolved *occupation of the mind* through flow-inducing activities as a fairly reliable way of diverting attention from self, relationships, problems and our sense of existence. Becoming distracted from our awareness of self could be a natural form of maintaining health: stress-deduction with positive effects on the immune system through reduced cortisol. Throughout history we developed many forms of this escape through dampening SAN:

- Skilled activities of all sorts (work, everyday survival, sport, music, maintaining living environment)
- Entertainment – films, theatre, concerts, galleries – all of the arts. Is this a major purpose of the arts? Imaginative life, day dreaming, digital games.
- Sex
- Learning, studying, education – seeking knowledge.
- Reading, novels (Blakely 2014)
- Hobbies, driving, shopping, crosswords.
- Gardening (Van den Berg and Custer 2011).
- Socializing with like-minded friends and family.

These present just a few ideas about self-forgetting activities. They may or may not be flow-inducing, or there may be different levels of flow, as others have speculated.

22.5 Limitations

The evidence for the mechanism for reduced self-awareness presented here is not comprehensive, and the history of ideas methodology builds an outline first – which this attempts to be – and then expands the concepts as new information arises. These various hypotheses will be supported or not over time, following further specific empirical studies. Each study forms part of a jigsaw that will gradually reveal the positive neurological effects of self-forgetting during flow. The science of attention and how human beings direct energy from one activity to another is a major issue, missing from this chapter.

22.6 Conclusion

Reduced self-awareness has been recognized as a symptom of flow for more than 40 years, and as a sign of occupation of the mind for a hundred years. Paradoxically in such a self-conscious species, it is experienced as positive, apparently contributing to optimal states. Neurobiological research is beginning to understand its properties through brain imagery and physiological research. The medial prefrontal cortex is known as a hub of self-awareness, becoming very active during introspection. Reduced prefrontal activity – or hypofrontality – can be seen as a part one of the neural mechanisms of flow, but flow activities often demand high cognitive planning and problem-solving involving other areas of the frontal cortex, which confounds such hypotheses as hypo-frontality.

The turn of the twenty-first century brought a plethora of neuroimages defining base-line brain activity, comparing areas oxygenated by different types of goal-directed tasks. An important discovery was made, relevant to understanding reduced self-awareness during flow. A consistent network becomes very active whenever the brain is 'resting' between goal-directed tasks, as if by default. Research is now seeking more detailed functional anatomy of each part of this network. Current synthesis implicates the medial prefrontal cortex, the insula, and the medial parietal 'hubs' along a medial paralimbic track, which can be conceptualized as a highly evolved system of self-awareness needed to support our complex social lives, not just a default. The insular cortex's connectivity to deeper structures supports findings from social neuroscience that self-regulation can activate the threat response. The complexity of the functions of each smaller part of the network in regard to the nuances of loss of self-awareness needs further research. Sympathetic and parasympathetic co-activation during flow is one of the most intriguing aspects for further study.

Human beings have evolved the capacity to engage in the most complex array of highly skilled tasks of any species, that seem to induce calming effects through dampening our extreme self-awareness. That our reward system apparently reinforces such behavior points towards it being an evolved trait of occupational beings. The questions raised by these findings need further research in this age of chronic stress. Biological research into flow presents a potent field in health sciences, with implications for the role of occupational therapy in physical and mental rehabilitation, and for health promotion within society. The global growth in sales of so-called stress-busting coloring-in books for adults, advertised as a tool for eliciting calm, indicates populous support for further research into the neurobiology of flow as a natural healing power.

References

Andrews-Hanna, J. R. (2011). The brain's default network and its adaptive role in internal mentation. doi:10.1177/1073858411403316. Neuroscientist 2012 18: 251 originally published online 15 June 2011.

Andrews-Hanna, J. R., Reidler, J. S., Haung, C., & Buckner, R. L. (2010). Evidence for the default network's role in spontaneous cognition. *Journal of Neurophysiology, 104*(1), 322–335.

Blakely, R. (2014, October 11). Switch off and book your way to bliss. *The Times UK.*

Brom, C., Buchtova, M., Sisler, V., Dechterenko, F., Palme, R., & Glenk, L. M. (2014). Flow, social interaction anxiety and salivary cortisol responses in serious games: A quasi-experimental study. *Computers & Education, 79*, 69–100.

Clark, F., & Larson, E. A. (1993). Developing and academic discipline: The science of occupation. In H. L. Hopkins & H. D. Smith (Eds.), *Willard and Spackman's occupational therapy* (8th ed.). Philadelphia: Lippincott.

Clark, F., Wood, W., & Larson, E. A. (1998). Occupational science: Occupational therapy's legacy for the 21st century. In M. E. Neistadt & E. B. Crepeau (Eds.), *Willard and Spackman's occupational therapy* (9th ed.). Philadelphia: Lippincott.

Csikszentmihalyi, M. (1990). *Flow: The psychology of optimal experience*. New York: Harper Perenial Modern Classics.

Csikszentmihalyi, M. (1993). Activity and happiness: Towards a science of occupation. *Journal of Occupational Science: Australia, 1*(1), 38–42.

Csikszentmihalyi, M. (2004). *TED talk.* https://www.ted.com/talks/mihaly_csikszentmihalyi_on_flow

Csikszentmihalyi, M., & Csikszentmihalyi, I. S. (Eds.). (1988). *Optimal experience: Psychological studies of flow in consciousness*. New York: Cambridge University Press.

Csikszentmihalyi, M., & Rathunde, K. (1992). The measurement of flow in everyday life: Toward a theory of emergent motivation. *Nebraska Symposium on Motivation, 40*, 57–97.

Damoiseaux, J. S., & Greicius, M. D. (2009). Greater than the sum of its parts: A review of studies combining structural connectivity and resting state functional connectivity. *Brain Stucture and Function, 213*, 525–533.

de Manzano, M., Thoerell, T., Harmat, L., & Ullen, F. (2010). The psychophysiology of flow during piano playing. *Emotion, 10*(3), 301–311.

de Manzano, O., Cervenko, S., Jucaite, A., Hellenas, O., Farde, L., & Ullen, F. (2013). Individual differences in the proneness to have flow experiences are linked to dopamine D2-receptor availability in the striatum. *NeuroImage, 67*, 1–6.

Di, X., & Biswal, B. B. (2014). Indentifying the default mode network structure using dynamic causal modelling on resting-state functional magnetic resonance imaging. *NeuroImage, 86*, 53–59.

Dietrich, A. (2003). Functional neuroanatomy of altered states of consciousness: The transient hypofrontality hypothesis. *Consciousness and Cognition, 12*, 231–256.

Dietrich, A. (2004). Neurocognitive mechanisms underlying the experience of flow. *Consciousness and Cognition, 13*, 746–761.

Dietrich, A. (2006). Transient hypofrontality as a mechanism for the psychological effects of exercise. *Psychiatry Research, 145*, 79–83.

Dietrich, A., & Audiffren, M. (2011). The reticular-activating hypofrontality (RAH) model of acute exercise. *Neuroscience & Biobehavioral Reviews, 35*, 1305–1325.

Draganski, B., Gaser, C., Busch, V., Schuierer, G., Bogdahn, U., & May, A. (2004). Neuroplasticity: Changes in grey matter induced by training. *Nature, 427*(6972), 311–312. doi:10.1038/427311a.

Draganski, B., Gaser, C., & Kempermann, G. (2006). Temporal and spatial dynamics of brain structure changes during extensive learning. *Journal of Neuroscience, 26*(23), 6314–6317. doi:10.1523/JNEUROSCI.4628-05.2006.

Farb, N. A. S., Segal, Z. V., Mayberg, H., Bean, J., McKeon, D., Fatima, Z., & Anderson, A. K. (2007). Attending to the present: Mindfulness meditation reveals distinct neural modes of self-reference. *SCAN, 2*, 313–322.

Fuster, J. M. (2008). *The prefrontal cortex*. Fourth Edition. London: Elsevier.

Gallwey, W. T. (2015). *The inner game of tennis: The ultimate guide to the mental side of peak performance*. London: Pan Books

Gentili, C., Ricciardi, E., Gobbini, M. I., Santarelli, M., Haxby, F., Peitrini, J. V., et al. (2009). Beyond Amygdala: Default mode network activity differs between patients with social phobia and healthy controls. *Brain Research Bulleton, 79*(6), 409–413.

Goldberg, I. I., Harel, M., & Malach, R. (2006). When the brain loses its self: Prefrontal inactivation during sensorimotor processing. *Neuron, 50*, 329–339. doi:10.1016/j.neuron.2006.03.015.

Goleman, D. (2007). *Social intelligence: The new science of human relationships*. New York: Arrow Books.

Greenfield, S. (2008). *I.D. -The quest for identity in the 21st century*. London: Sceptre.

Gregory, A. (2013). Unpublished dissertation. University of Brighton.

Greicius, M. D., Krasnou, B., Reiss, A. L., & Menon, V. (2003). Functional connectivity in the resting brain: A network analysis of the default mode hypothesis. PNAS, 100(1), 253–258.

Gusnard, D. A., Akdudak, E., Shulman, G. L., & Raiche, M. E. (2001). Medical prefrontal cortex and self-referential mental activity: Relation to a default mode of brain function. *PNAS, 98*(7), 4259–4264.

Hanson, R. (2009). *Buddha's brain*. Oakland: New Harpinger.

Harmat, L., de Manzano, O., Theorell, T., Hogman, L., Fischer, H., & Ullen, F. (2015). Physiological correlates of the flow experience during computer game playing. *International Journal of Psychophysiology, 97*, 1–7.

Heatherton, T. F. (2011). Neuroscience of self and self regulation. *Annual Review of Psychology, 62*, 363–390.

Ingold, T. (2013). *Making: Anthropology, archeology, art and architecture*. London: Routledge.

Ingvar, D. H. (1979). "Hyperfrontal" distribution of the cerbral grey matter flow in resting wakefulness: On the functional anatomy of the resting state. *Acta Neurologica Scandinavica, 60*, 12–25.

Ingvar, D. H. (1985). "Memory of the future": An essay on the temoral organization of conscious awareness. *Human Neurobiology, 4*(3), 127–136.

Jonson, S. C., Baxter, J. C., & Wilder, L. S. (2002). Neural correlates of self reflection. *Brain, 125*, 1814–1818.

Klasen, M., Weber, R., Kirchner, T. T., Mathiak, K. A., & Mathiak, K. (2012). Neural contributions to flow experience during video game playing. *Social Cognitive Affective Neuroscience, 7*(4), 485–495.

Kringelbach, M. L., & Berridge, K. C. (2010). The functional neuroanatomy of pleasure and happiness. *Discovery Medicine, 9*(49), 579–587.

le Merrer, Becker J., Befort B., & Kieffer B. L. (2009). Reward processing by the opioid system in the brain *Physiolog.* 2013 Social: Why our brains are wired to connect. Oxford University Press.

Lieberman, M. D. (2013). *Social: Why our brains are wired to connect*. Oxford: Oxford University Press.
Lou, H. C. (2015). Editorial: Self-awareness – An emerging field in neurology. *ACTA Paediatrica, 104*, 121–122.
Lovejoy, A. (1933). *The great chain of being: A study of the history of an idea*. Cambridge: Harvard University Press.
Northoff, G., & Bermpohl, F. (2004). Cortical midline structures and the self. *Trends in Cognitive Neurosciences, 8*, 102–107.
Peifer, C. (2012). Psycholophysiological correlates of flow experiences. In S. Engeser (Ed.), *Advances in flow research* (pp. 139–1650). New York: Springer.
Raichle, M. E., Macleod, A. M., Snyder, A. Z., Powers, W. J., Gusnard, D. A., & Shulman, G. L. (2001). A default mode of brain function. *Procedures of the National Academy of Science USA, 98*(2), 676–682.
Ruby, P., & Decet, J. (2004). How would *you* feel verses how do you think *she* would feel: A neuroimage strudy of perspective taking with social emotions. *Journal of Cognitive Neuroscience, 16*(6), 988–999.
Sheline, Y. I., Barch, D. M., Price, J. L., Rundle, M. M., Vaishnavi, S. N., Snyder, A. Z., Mintun, M. A., Wang, S., Coalson, R. S., & Raichie, M. E. (2008). The default mode network and self-referential processes in depression. *PNAS, 106*(6), 1943–1947.
Suchoversky, A. (2013). *Flow during rock-climbing*. Unpublished dissertation, University of Brighton.
Tallis, R. (2005). *I am – A philosophical inquiry into first-person being*. Edinburgh: Edinburgh University Press.
Uddin, L. Q., Iacoboni, M., Lange, C., & Keenan, P. (2007). The self and social cognition: the role of cortical midline structures and mirror neurones. *Trends in Cognitive Sciences, 11*(4), 153–157.
Ullen, F., de Manzano, O., Almeida, R., Magnussson, P. K. E., Pedeersen, N. L., Nakamura, J., et al. (2012). Proneness for psychological flow in everyday life: Association with personality and intelligence. *Personal Individual Differences, 52*, 167–172.
Ulrich, M., Keller, J., Hoenig, K., Waller, C., & Gron, G. (2014). Neural correlates of experimentally induced flow experiences. *NeuroImage, 86*, 194–202.
Ulrich, M., Keller, J., & Grön, G. (2016). Neural signatures of experimentally induced flow experiences identified in a standard fMRI block-design with BOLD imaging. *Social Cognitive and Affective Neurosciences*. 11(3): 496–507.doi:10.1093/scan/nsv133.
Van den Berg, A. E., & Custer, M. H. G. (2011). Gardening promotes neuroendocrine and affective restoration from stress. *Journal of Health Psychology, 16*(1), 3–11.
Wilcock, A. A. (2008). *An occupational perspective of health*. Thorofare: Slack.
Wilcock, A. A., & Hocking, C. (2015). *An occupational perspective of health* (3rd ed.). Thorofare: Slack Incorporated.
Wright, J., Sadlo, G., & Stew, G. (2006). Challenge-skills and mindfulness: An exploration of the conundrum of flow process. *OTJR: Occupation, Participation and Health, 26*(1), 25–32. ISSN 1539-4492.
Yerxa, E. J. (1996). Eleanor Clarke Slagle Lecture. Authentic occupational therapy. *American Journal of Occupational Therapy*, *1967XXI*(1), 1–9.
Yerxa, E., Clark, F., Jackson, J., Parham, D., Pierce, D., Stein, C., et al. (1989). An introduction to occupational science, a foundation for occupational therapy in the 21st century. *Occupational Therapy in Health Care, 6*(4), 1–17.
Zemke, R., & Clark, F. (1996). *Occupational science: The evolving discipline*. Philadelphia: F.A. Davis.
Zohar, M., & Marshall, J. (2000). *Spiritual intelligence*. London: Bloomsbury.

ERRATUM

Flow Experience

Empirical Research and Applications

László Harmat, Frans Ørsted Andersen, Fredrik Ullén, Jon Wright and Gaynor Sadlo

L. Harmat et al. (eds.), *Flow Experience*, DOI 10.1007/978-3-319-28634-1

DOI 10.1007/978-3-319-28634-1_23

The affiliation for Professor Fredrik Ullén was wrongly included as University of Aarhus, Aarhus, Denmark in the book. The correct affiliation is Department of Neuroscience, Karolinska Institutet, Stockholm, Sweden. This has been updated in this volume.

The online version of the updated original book can be found at http://dx.doi.org/10.1007/978-3-319-28634-1

L. Harmat et al. (eds.), *Flow Experience*, DOI 10.1007/978-3-319-28634-1_23

Index

L. Harmat et al. (eds.), *Flow Experience*, DOI 10.1007/978-3-319-28634-1

9783319286327